INTRODUCTION TO
Public Health

INTRODUCTION TO
Public Health

Mary Louise Fleming and Elizabeth Parker

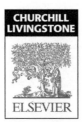

CHURCHILL
LIVINGSTONE

ELSEVIER

Sydney   Edinburgh   London   New York
Philadelphia   St Louis   Toronto

Churchill Livingstone
is an imprint of Elsevier

1006379020

Elsevier Australia. ACN 001 002 357
(a division of Reed International Books Australia Pty Ltd)
Tower 1, 475 Victoria Avenue, Chatswood, NSW 2067

ELSEVIER

© 2009 Elsevier Australia. Reprinted 2009

Every attempt has been made to trace and acknowledge copyright, but in some
cases this may not have been possible. The publisher apologises for any accidental
infringement and would welcome any information to redress the situation.

This publication has been carefully reviewed and checked to ensure that the content is
as accurate and current as possible at time of publication. We would recommend,
however, that the reader verify any procedures, treatments, drug dosages or legal
content described in this book. Neither the author, the contributors, nor the publisher
assume any liability for injury and/or damage to persons or property arising from any
error in or omission from this publication.

National Library of Australia Cataloguing-in-Publication Data

---

Introduction to public health / editors, Mary Louise Fleming, Elizabeth Parker.

ISBN: 978 0 7295 3890 9 (pbk.)

Includes index.
Bibliography.

Public health.

Fleming, Mary Louise
Parker, Elizabeth.

Dewey Number: 362.1

Publishing Editor: Sunalie Silva
Developmental Editor: Samantha McCulloch
Publishing Services Manager: Helena Klijn
Editorial Coordinator: Eleanor Cant
Edited by Matt Davies
Proofread by Tim Learner
Cover and internal design by Avril Makula
Index by Mei Yen Chua
Typeset by TnQ
Printed by Ligare

The book has been printed on paper certified
by the Programme for the Endorsement of
Forest Certification (PEFC). PEFC is
committed to sustainable forest management
through third party forest certification
of responsibly managed forests.

Contents

Introduction

Why is public health important?

An Introduction to Public Health is about the discipline of public health, the nature and scope of public health activity and the challenges that face public health in the 21st century. The book is designed as an introductory text to the principles and practice of public health. This is a complex and multifaceted area. What we have tried to do in this book is make public health easy to understand without making it simplistic. As many authors have stated, public health is essentially about the organised efforts of society to promote, protect and restore the public's health (Last 2001, Lin et al 2007, Winslow 1920). It is multidisciplinary in nature and it is influenced by genetic, physical, social, cultural, economic and political determinants of health.

How do we define public health and what are the disciplines that contribute to public health? How has the area changed over time? Are there health issues in the 21st century that change the focus and activity of public health? Yes, there are! There are many challenges facing public health now and in the future, just as there have been over the course of the history of organised public health efforts, dating from around 1850 (in the Western world).

Of what relevance is public health to the many allied health disciplines that contribute to it? How might an understanding of public health contribute to a range of health professionals who use the principles and practices of public health in their professional activities? These are the questions that this book addresses. *An Introduction to Public Health* leads the reader on a journey of discovery that concludes with not only an understanding of the nature and scope of public health but the challenges facing the field into the future.

The book is designed for a range of students undertaking health courses where such courses include a focus on advancing the health of the population. While it is imperative that people wanting to be public health professionals understand the theory and practice of public health, many other health workers contribute to effective public health practice. The book would also be relevant to a range of undergraduate students who want an introductory understanding of public health practice.

Public health is an innately political process. As we discuss in this book, there is a clear relationship between disease and the way in which society is structured. Income distribution, the allocation of resources to ensure adequate infrastructure for transport, housing and education and how much political support there is to provide adequately for these fundamental services, all impact on our health. They particularly impact on the health of certain groups within the population who do not have the financial, social and political resources to advocate for change. Why is it that we still have such disparities in health? Indigenous Australians, for example, have a life expectancy some 20 years less than the non-Indigenous population. In an egalitarian society like Australia, that prides itself on a 'fair go for all', should this be acceptable? In this book, we discuss the political, social and economic determinants of health as well as the physical and environmental issues that impact on population health.

Defining and understanding public health

Defining public health is not an easy task. This is because not everyone who works in public health agrees on a single definition. Definitions also vary from country to country. For example, the American Public Health Association (APHA) classifies public health into prevention, policy development and population health surveillance activities. It concludes:

> Public health is the practice of preventing disease and promoting good health within groups of people, from small communities to entire countries. Public health professionals rely on policy and research strategies to understand issues such as infant mortality and chronic disease in particular populations.
>
> (American Public Health Association 2008)

In the United Kingdom the Public Health Association believes that public health deals with a wide range of issues as identified below:

> [Public health]
> - is an approach that focuses on the health and wellbeing of a society and the most effective means of protecting and improving it
> - encompasses the science, art and politics of preventing illness and disease and promoting health and wellbeing addresses the root causes of illness and disease, including the interacting social, environmental, biological and psychological dimensions, as well as the provision of effective health services
> - addresses inequalities, injustices and denials of human rights, which frequently explain large variations in health locally, nationally and globally
> - works effectively through partnerships that cut across professional and organisational boundaries, and seeks to eliminate avoidable distinctions
> - relies upon evidence, judgement and skills and promotes the participation of the populations who are themselves the subject of policy and action.
>
> (UK Public Health Association 2008)

As pointed out in the introduction, public health is essentially about the organised efforts of society to promote, protect and restore the public's health (Last 2001, Lin et al 2007, Winslow 1920). It is both a science and an art in that it relies on evidence, skill and judgement, it examines the contribution of a range of factors to improving population health, it addresses inequalities and it is based on partnerships. These elements of public health will be discussed throughout the book, particularly in terms of their application to public health practice. We will be asking you to think about how you might define public health within the context of your own developing professional understanding.

To understand public health we also need to think about the contribution of both the 'art and the science' of improving the health of the population. Throughout this book, you will see many examples of how the science is used to make evidence-based decisions that lead to improvements in the health of the population.

The science of public health is about understanding the determinants of health, what works and in what circumstances. It is about using evidence as a basis for decisions about selecting interventions that work with the hard to reach and the economically and socially isolated.

The art of public health has more to do with the practice of public health and how the science is interpreted and implemented according to population needs and circumstances.

Health practitioners who work in public health also need a vision about what public health could look like in the future. As practitioners, we need to be vigilant to changing circumstances and issues. In addition, we need a set of values and ethics that underpins our practice to be brought to bear in all our public health dealings.

One final important point should be made about the differences between public health and medical care. Both have an important contribution to make to the health of the population. However, the primary focus of medical care is the individual patient and treating people who are ill, although medical practitioners do have a role in health promotion and screening directed towards the individual's care. Public health focuses on promoting health and preventing illness in the population. The problem for public health in measuring its success is that it often takes many years to see shifts in mortality and morbidity patterns as a result of a range of public health interventions introduced over many years. Take for example the case of smoking and cardiovascular disease. We know that cigarette smoking is the single largest preventable cause of death and disease in Australia. It is a major risk factor for cardiovascular disease, as well as a range of cancers and other disabling conditions. More than 19,000 Australians die each year from diseases caused by smoking (Ridolfo & Stevenson 2001). International evidence shows that well-funded, comprehensive tobacco control programs can successfully reduce tobacco use. In California, for example, mass public information and media campaigns, funded by tobacco taxes, have had a major influence on smoking behaviour (Pierce et al 1998). The problem is that these improvements are not immediately evident. It is also difficult to measure the individual contributions to change made by various different interventions.

In summary, this book covers the history and contemporary elements of public health, it includes a conversation about the determinants of health and how they shape public health practice, it discusses the important role for evidence in underpinning public health practice and it looks into the future to describe the emerging epidemics and the achievements and challenges facing public health in the 21st century.

How this book is organised

The book is organised into five sections. The five sections, and the 15 chapters within them, are outlined on the book's contents page. Each chapter is organised in the following way:
- a list of learning objectives
- an introduction
- the content of the chapter
- review questions.

The following outlines each section of the book and how each helps you to understand the complex relationships that make up contemporary public health.

Section 1 of the book introduces you to the interesting history of public health over the past 160 years since the inception of organised public health efforts. It paints a picture of the historical issues that have impacted on public health over the years. We explore definitions of public health, the principles that underpin the discipline and its multidisciplinary and multisectoral nature. We then examine the range of health professionals working in public health and why they need to comprehend the nature and scope of public health and its role in promoting, protecting and restoring the public's health. Finally, we examine the impact of public health policy and management on public health practice. You will have the opportunity to consider how public health policy decisions impact on Indigenous health, oral health and HIV/AIDS, as examples. You will come to understand the nature and function of state health departments around Australia and their relationship with the federal Department of Health and Ageing. We consider the role of not-for-profit organisations and the contribution of local government to public health.

Section 2 covers the range of factors that impact on health and, consequently, the organised efforts of public health. It lays the foundations for decisions about priorities and strategies for public health interventions. It will provide you with evidence upon which decisions are made about where to intervene, how to intervene and how to track population health changes. We give you an understanding of the fundamental principles of epidemiology, and how this discipline underpins the activities of public health. An understanding of epidemiology will enable you to make informed decisions about patterns of mortality and morbidity, and where to intervene; and, it will help you track health changes in the population and in subpopulations over time. We analyse the determinants of health – genetic, physical, social, emotional, economic and environmental. Clarity around the determinants of health will assist you in turn to understand and apply the principles of public health in your practice.

Section 3 examines the use of evidence to inform the planning and evaluation of public health activity. We begin this section by considering the ethics of public health practice. Undertaking ethical practice is essential for health professionals no matter what aspect of health you practise in. Using case study examples we provide you with a picture of how evidence can inform practice. It examines the nature of evidence being considered and it discusses the issues practitioners need to understand in order to make evidence-based decisions. The final chapter in Section 3 provides you with advice about public health planning and evaluation models and the nature and extent of their application in practice, using a range of examples in a variety of public health settings.

There are three chapters that make up **Section 4**. These chapters focus on public health interventions from disease control to health protection and health promotion. One focuses on communicable and non-communicable disease control, monitoring and surveillance. Another examines the development and relevance of environmental health to public health. Health protection traces the development and importance of environmental health and occupational health and safety to population health, and it examines the contemporary notion of ecological public health. In this section's final chapter the importance of health advancement and the promotion of health are discussed. This section should give you a good understanding of the scope of public health interventions and their application in practice.

In the final section of the book, **Section 5**, we explore the emergence of the so-called 'new epidemics' and we examine the future for public health in the 21st century. We consider the globalisation of health. Public health has become a global issue – with travel around the planet easy and accessible to many, health issues that once might have impacted on the population in a region or country are now being transported around the world. Section 5 also focuses your attention on the new epidemics such as avian influenza and severe acute respiratory syndrome (SARS), as examples. It discusses these contagious diseases as global issues that impact on population health, and the system's capacity to manage such health issues. We also deal with disaster management and emergency care in the context of natural disasters. In the final chapter of this book we think about the future of public health and the challenges facing the population, such as global warming and environmental sustainability. We also talk about the nature and scope of the public health workforce needed to meet these challenges.

Our reflection piece at the end of the book gives you a chance to consider the major challenges facing public health, where we imagine the discipline might be heading and what the consequences are for the public's health in the next 50 years.

References

American Public Health Association 2008 What is Public Health? Fact Sheet. Available: http://www.apha.org/NR/rdonlyres/C57478B8-8682-4347-8DDF-A1E24E82B919/0/what_is_PH_May1_Final.pdf 7 January 2008

Last J M 2001 A dictionary of epidemiology, 4th edn. Oxford University Press, New York

Lin V, Smith J, Fawkes S 2007 Public Health Practice in Australia: The organised effort. Allen & Unwin, Sydney

Pierce J, Gilpin E, Emery S et al 1998 Has the California tobacco control program reduced smoking? Journal of the American Medical Association 280(10):893–899

Ridolfo B, Stevenson C 2001 The quantification of drug-caused morbidity and mortality in Australia, 1998 edition. Commonwealth Department of Human Services and Health, Canberra

United Kingdom Public Health Association 2008 UKPHA Definition of Public Health. Available: http://www.ukpha.org.uk/default.asp?action=category&ID=2&order=categoryname&sort=asc&limit=0 9 Jan 2008

Winslow C E A 1920 The Untilled Field of Public Health. Science 9:23–33

About the authors

GERRY FITZGERALD

Gerry FitzGerald is Professor of Emergency Services in the School of Public Health at the Queensland University of Technology, and is responsible for developing emergency and disaster management education and research programs. He has a Bachelor of Medicine/Bachelor of Surgery degree, Bachelor of Health Administration and a Doctor of Medicine.

MARY LOUISE FLEMING

Associate Professor Mary Louise Fleming is Head of the School of Public Health at the Queensland University of Technology. She has more than 20 years' experience in teaching and research in higher education as well as public health and health promotion. Her research experience is in action research; process, impact and outcome evaluation in health promotion; and public health interventions. Mary Louise has worked as a consultant for the World Health Organization and Commonwealth and state health departments and has sat on NHMRC project grant review panels for a number of years. She has been widely published in the area of health promotion.

TRISH GOULD

Trish Gould is a research officer in the School of Public Health at the Queensland University of Technology. She has experience in public health and health promotion research, project management and coordination, writing, and editing. Trish has a MA in biological anthropology, and her interest areas include ethics, human rights, Indigenous health, and the health impacts of migration, acculturation, inequity and discrimination.

MARY-ANNE KEDDA

Mary-Anne Kedda is a senior lecturer in epidemiology in the School of Public Health at the Queensland University of Technology (QUT), and teaches in the fields of traditional epidemiology, molecular epidemiology and human genetics. Mary-Anne is also head of the Molecular Epidemiology Group in the cancer program in the Institute of Health and Biomedical Innovation at QUT, and is heavily involved with postgraduate training and research into the genetics of various hormone-related cancers.

BONNIE MACFARLANE

Bonnie Macfarlane is a lecturer in epidemiology in the School of Public Health at the Queensland University of Technology. She has experience in teaching the fundamental concepts and methods of epidemiology and the application of epidemiology to public health. She has worked on several research programs in clinical and community settings both locally and internationally. Her teaching interest areas include scientific validity and ethical research; risk communication; and how epidemiology is utilised to help plan and evaluate health services, including prevention, detection and treatment services.

ELIZABETH PARKER

Elizabeth Parker is Associate Professor and Director of Academic Programs in the School of Public Health at the Queensland University of Technology. She has teaching and research experience in public health and health promotion and an interest in Indigenous health. She worked as a senior manager in the Toronto Department of Public Health and has acted as a consultant for the Canadian Public Health Association, the Australian Government and Queensland Health.

THOMAS TENKATE

Dr Thomas Tenkate lectures in environmental health and is the postgraduate course coordinator in the School of Public Health, Queensland University of Technology. He has been an environmental health practitioner since 1990 and worked for Queensland Health for more than 10 years in a variety of environmental health investigatory, policy and research roles. His main interests are in the areas of exposure and risk assessment, food safety and communicable disease epidemiology.

XIANG-YU (JANET) HOU

Dr Xiang-Yu (Janet) Hou lectures in international health in School of Public Health, Queensland University of Technology (QUT). She has been working for QUT for almost 10 years in a variety of international health projects. Her main research interests are in social medicine, including child health.

Acknowledgements

[**MLF**] To Andrew, Lachlan and Annabel – they say 'patience is a virtue'. Thank you for demonstrating plenty of patience while wife and mother wrote and rewrote chapters of a manuscript at night and on weekends!

A special thank you to Trish Gould whose support and assistance with this manuscript has meant that Elizabeth and I could complete the job. Without Trish we would still be completing the manuscript. Thank you, Trish, for all your help and for the quality of your work.

[**EP**] A special thank you to Emma and other family and friends for your constant encouragement and forbearance during the writing and rewriting of chapters. And a special thank you to Trish Gould for her humour, endless patience and dedicated assistance.

Reviewers

ROBIN GAULD MA, PhD
Associate Professor, Department of Preventive and Social Medicine, Faculty of Medicine, University of Otago, Dunedin, New Zealand.

LESLEY HARRISON BED, MED, MA
Lecturer in health promotion, School of Human Life Sciences, Faculty of Health Science, University of Tasmania

JANET HILLER PhD, MPH, BA, Dip Soc Studs
Chair of Public Health, Deputy Head, School of Population Health and Clinical Practice Director, Adelaide Health Technology Assessment (AHTA)

LYN TALBOT RN, Grad Dip Pub & Com Health, MHlth Sc, Grad Cert Uni Teach, DrPH
Senior lecturer in public health, Department of Health and Environment, School of Public Health, La Trobe University, Melbourne

Section 1

History and definitions of public health

The first three chapters in Section 1 of this book provide you with background information about the history of public health, how the discipline is defined, its roles and responsibilities and its place within the organisational and political structures of the health system in Australia.

In Chapter 1 we discuss the history of public health. This is essentially dated from the beginnings of an organised public health effort that was focussed on containing the spread of disease, with limited knowledge about the natural history of a disease. In more recent times the complexity of the public health enterprise has become a major focus for public health activity and it is now clearly evident that there is a need for a multidisciplinary and multisectoral approach to public health endeavours. We trace the evolution of Western public health from its early beginnings to more recent times. We explore the diversity of thinking that underpinned public health activity and we trace some of the myths and superstitions that were the forerunners of more contemporary public health activities.

Chapter 2 introduces the nature and scope of public health. In this chapter, we consider various definitions of health, disease and illness and examine the changing nature of public health definitions. We explore the core functions of public health and the roles and responsibilities of public health practitioners. In the process, we discuss the way in which public health practitioners do their job and in fact who is the public health workforce and how broadly we might consider that definition. We look briefly at the role and responsibilities of various levels of government in Australia and we discuss the role of non-government organisations, associations, community organisations and advocacy groups. At the conclusion of the chapter, we briefly consider the future for public health. This issue is raised again at the end of the book.

In the final chapter in Section 1 we present you with information about public health policy and the relationship between public health and the broader health system. We discuss the breakdown of expenditure between health promotion, health protection and health surveillance and monitoring and the other components of the health system, and we ask questions about the financial and resource sustainability of our modern health care system. We also cover a number of policy initiatives in public health and consider the range of these policies and the sometimes differing requirements for action within some of the policy statements.

These three chapters provide a foundation for the book in that they define the nature and scope of health and illness and public health, its multidisciplinary and multisectoral elements and its place within the health care system.

CHAPTER 1

History and development of public health

Mary Louise Fleming

Learning objectives

After reading this chapter you should be able to:

- briefly describe the importance of public health history to contemporary public health
- understand that public health historians have a rich tradition of describing developments in population health, particularly in the past four decades
- briefly describe the ancient history of public health
- outline the key periods and activities in the modern history of Western public health
- describe and understand the important roles of political, social, environmental and economic factors as they impact on health
- consider the major factors that have influenced an understanding of contemporary public health in the past 40 years.

Introduction

This chapter and the others that follow have the study of health as their focus (as opposed to therapeutic medicine). Clearly, however, we are concerned with the way in which population health is influenced by biomedical theories and practices, and the way population health is influenced by access to therapeutic medicine. It explores the ancient history of public health to enable you to understand how civilisations often cared more about developing their cities than they did for the health of their inhabitants, and the reasons for this. We examine the modern history of Western public health dated from 1850. This date signifies the beginnings of a more organised collective effort to protect the public's health. These discussions will help you formulate your definition of public health.

You will have an entertaining journey through public health achievements and less successful outcomes by examining historical developments that have led us to a modern understanding of public health. For example, the ancient Greeks and Romans had public health measures to ensure the safety and health of their populations, for a range of social and economic reasons. Convicts arrived in Australia with many health problems and were put to work to satisfy the needs of a fledgling colony. It is important to understand the historical journey of public health and the way it is critically analysed, as it is a window into the present and the future.

The importance of the past in public health

Examining the historical evolution of public health is important because as George Rosen said:

> There can be no real comprehension of the history of public health at any period without a thorough understanding of the political, economic and social history of that period in its relation to the contemporary public health situation.
>
> (Rosen 1953 p 430)

In a similar vein, Tosh (1984) in the *Pursuit of History* commented that to know the past is to understand that things have not always been the same, and that they need not remain the same in the future.

History is also relevant because we need to be able to 'observe public health over a long period of time in order to be able to evaluate progress, or the lack of progress, in improving it' (Scally & Womack 2004 p 751). For example, Brownson and Bright (2004) discuss chronic disease control efforts in the United States in the 20th century that illustrate key concepts useful to today's public health activity. In an interesting article Ogilvie and Hamlet (2005) present a dialogue between Socrates and Panacea, the goddess of healing, in the year 2055 about the history of the Western obesity epidemic. Socrates and Panacea discuss why information to the public about this issue had little or no impact on the community; they talk about the shortcomings of environmental changes and the expectations of society around advancing economic development and access to healthy foods. At the conclusion of the article Socrates asks Panacea why the discipline that was 'fond of phrases like "primary prevention" and "going upstream" never came up with a serious challenge to obesity' (Ogilvie & Hamlet 2005 p 1547). A sobering thought for us to contemplate in the early part of the 21st century.

An understanding of how public health practitioners can influence the health of the population requires knowledge of how the discipline has evolved, and its successes and failures. The threat of infectious diseases, that as a public health community we thought had mostly been eradicated, are re-emerging as threats to the population worldwide. This is because the less we know about the aetiology, for example, of severe acute respiratory syndrome (SARS), the more quickly the disease becomes life threatening and difficult to treat effectively.

Historical awareness 'helps us to be alert to the resurgence of practice that has held sway in the past but been out of fashion in more recent times' (Scally & Womack 2004 p 752). It is important to be able to appreciate why particular approaches to public health lost favour in the past, and to determine the relevance of old approaches and their likely usefulness in thinking about new approaches. For example, the rise of coronary heart disease and cancer in the period between the two world wars led to an emphasis on adult risk factors. In more recent years lifecourse epidemiology has become more important; this is a return to a concept prevalent in the first half of the 20th century, that early life experiences influence adult mortality risk.

Historical accounts of public health up until the past 40 years were strongly influenced by public health activity in the 19th century and by the heroic works of people like Edwin Chadwick and John Snow. For example, the Englishman John Snow had the handle from the Broad Street water pump removed, which led to a rapid decline in the number of cholera cases. His work demonstrated the early use of epidemiological analysis to pinpoint more extensive outbreaks of the disease. Edwin Chadwick, as another example, and his work on improving drinking water and sanitation actually marked the end of the era of social reform in public health in favour of advances in drainage systems and other more practical solutions (Berridge 2000). When the parameters of public health are confined largely to sanitary reforms and the control of infectious diseases, it is easy to argue that although organised public health efforts did not appear until the 1850s, the foundations had been laid back through time, for example the Roman baths and aqueducts (Porter 1999). However, since the early 1960s a social history of public health has emerged where the focus is on 'economic, political, social and ideological responses to disease and the exploration of complex ways in which change both caused and was determined by the impact of epidemics' (Porter 1999 p 2).

Other more recent tensions evident in public health, such as the emergence of AIDS in the late 1980s, 'revived the historical study of stigma … and forcefully added to new debates about the social construction of everyday life (Porter 1999 p 3). Debate continues between the focus of public health on prevention and health promotion and its inability to leave its links with personal health. The tension between medical services and the community role remains unresolved today (Berridge 2000).

Understanding the factors behind this duality and placing current practice, organisational structures and political and public health philosophies within a historical framework can help us to resolve the tensions that exist within our field and increase our sense of identity and purpose. It can help us to see how we fit into the wider picture and serve to support us in our interpretation of the political and organisational structures that are part of today's environment (Scally & Womack 2004).

Historically, we can clearly see how strongly public health has been variously influenced by politics at different times. It is interesting to look back at the history of public health and to explore the political and social factors that have played a role in its evolution at various times during the past 160 years. Understanding this process provides us with more of an insight into the factors at work behind major developments, which can teach us about the many influences we need to consider, and the length of time it may take for there to be population health improvements (Perdiguero et al 2001).

The history of public health provides a useful vehicle for teaching the principles of public health. This is particularly so for health workers such as environmental health officers, nurses, general practitioners and public health workers who have a population health and prevention perspective in their work. It enriches our critical perspective of the 'social effects of initiatives undertaken in the name of public health, shows the shortcomings of public health interventions based on single factors and uses a wider time scope in the assessment of current problems' (Perdiguero et al 2001 p 667). For example, there are similar issues between the story of opium at the end of the 19th century and its cultural and legal identification, and that of tobacco and smoking at the end of the 20th century (Berridge 2000). The website for the organisation Action on Smoking and Health has the key dates in the history of anti-tobacco campaigning in the United Kingdom. If you look at this website (see www.ash.org.uk) you will see how many years passed between significant developments. It was not until the second half of the 20th century that significant progress was made on a range of fronts; however, the power of the tobacco industry still remains a major stumbling block to achieving the overall objectives of the anti-smoking campaign. The ups and downs of this story are a message to today's practitioners to consider the timescale and effort entailed in dealing with vested interests (Scally & Womack 2004).

Scally and Womack's (2004) quote is worth including in full here because it sums up why public health history is such an important aspect of our understanding of modern public health:

> An understanding of the rich and diverse history of public health cannot only support contemporary innovation but can help reduce the risk of public health practice being too narrowly focussed on specific influences on the health of individuals rather than maintaining an overview of the full range of factors at work across a population.

> (Scally & Womack 2004 p 752)

Advancing population health – medical intervention or collective action?

One of the most prominent authors writing about the factors that impacted on the changes to population health in 19th century Europe was Thomas McKeown. McKeown suggested that medical intervention, while playing a role in advancing health, was not responsible for the significant reduction in patterns of mortality and morbidity. He pointed out that medicine had not offered the nature of change that had resulted and that diseases were declining prior to the advent of effective therapy (Lewis 2003). Szreter (2002) among others has seriously challenged McKeown's thesis. Szreter (2002, 2003) indicated that McKeown was right that material living standards, such as food availability, and therefore economics, were crucial to the health of the population. However, he also argued vigorously that McKeown was wrong in failing to 'foreground the importance of politics, ideologies, states, and institutions in producing the kind of societies that distribute their material wealth, food, and living standards in a health-enhancing way for all concerned' (Szreter 2002 p 724, 2003 p 427).

McKeown's critique of the medical establishment also found support in discourse emerging from the United States, Canada and the United Kingdom that focussed on the importance of individual responsibility for health (we discuss these issues later in the chapter) (Colgrove 2002). However, Colgrove (2002) and Szreter (2002) have both suggested that McKeown had allowed his assumptions about the limited value of medical interventions and the need for social reform to predetermine his analytical categories and thus bias his interpretation of evidence.

What is clear in McKeown's argument is that nutrition and public health clearly have roles in the explanation. Along, however, with living and working conditions, urbanisation, education, aetiology of diseases, doctors and medical knowledge, mothers' attitudes, knowledge and behaviour, politics, reformers and climate (Lewis 2003).

However, McKeown's research has continued to hold a place in public health history because his research posed a fundamental question:

> Are public health ends better served by narrow interventions focussed at the level of the individual or the community, or by broad measures to redistribute the social, political, economic resources that exert such a profound influence on health status at the population level?

> (Colgrove 2002 p 728)

In answering this question, Colgrove (2002) concluded that the choice of targeted interventions versus social change should not be viewed as dichotomous or opposing choices, but as complementary to each other. The challenge for health workers is to find ways to 'integrate technical preventive and curative measures with more broad based efforts to improve all of the conditions in which people live' (Colgrove 2002 p 729).

For the sake of the public's health? The ancient history of public health

The ancient history of public health is permeated with examples of efforts to protect health. However, it was unlikely that many of those efforts were actually designed to protect the public's health but to enable other activity that would deliver a social or economic benefit to the State through having relatively healthy individuals and communities. In ancient societies collective action to advance the health of populations was reserved for promoting the comfort of elites (Porter 1999).

Actions to protect the health of the public emerge throughout history, especially those activities relating to sanitary measures to ensure safe water and food supplies. For example, the earliest records of Chinese public health practice included providing drinking wells, building ditches around houses, protecting drinking water and killing rats. Two centuries before the birth of Christ the Chinese had invented rudimentary sewers, water spray carts and toilets. There was an emphasis on providing personal hygiene and preventive practices. In addition, herbal medicines, diagnostic procedures and preventive concepts, such as feeling the pulse and acupuncture, were in use.

In Egyptian and Babylonian societies there were systems for sewage disposal and rainwater collection. Hygiene customs included personal cleanliness, frequent bathing, simple dressing and the use of 'earth closets' (the forerunner of the modern day toilet). The *Code of Hammurabi*, adopted by Babylonian society, guided the conduct of physicians and prescribed healthful practices. Temperance was recommended for all, at least three-thousand years ago.

For Greek civilisation, the emphasis was placed on the individual. Consequently, the Greeks focussed on the harmonious development of all faculties where exercise and personal cleanliness were important. Little attention was afforded to environmental protection. The *Hippocratic Oath* (attributed to Hippocrates) still guides the ethical practice of medical practitioners. Hippocrates is also credited with a treatise on environment and health. Hippocrates in the fifth century BC, and Galen in the second century AD, described what were called the four humours: phlegm (phlegmatic), blood (sanguine), black bile (melancholy) and yellow bile (choleric) (Lawson & Bauman 2001). When in harmony, these four humours are believed to be responsible for health.

By contrast, in the Roman Empire, the State, not the individual, was considered more important. This meant that the regulation of building construction, sewage disposal and the destruction of decaying goods and buildings were of fundamental concern. Town planning, street and gutter paving, establishing drainage networks and public bathing were very important aspects of Roman society because they reinforced their philosophy of the importance of the State. Both the Greeks and the Romans protected the health of the wealthy, and their military, by providing fresh food, water supply aqueducts and environmental protection laws.

Unlike the Greek and Roman eras, the Middle Ages marked a dark period in the history of public health. Throughout Europe there were major epidemics of infectious diseases. During these times, the emphasis on spiritual aspects of life increased substantially and if people were unwell, they were often thought to have done something against the will of God. Islam rose to prominence during the sixth and seventh centuries and a series of pilgrimages to Mecca saw several cholera epidemics emerge; leprosy flourished in Egypt, Asia Minor and Europe.

Between 1096 and 1248, there were six great Crusades. These events all contributed to the spread of disease as men were travelling together in large groups where disease spread easily, and with limited means to treat such outbreaks large numbers of men were lost to disease rather than to war. In the period up to 1453, a number of pandemics and epidemics emerged. Diseases that flourished during the time included cholera, bubonic plague and pulmonary anthrax. A whole variety of factors contributed to the spread of epidemics and pandemics, including poor personal hygiene, inadequate nutrition, clustering of population groups and increased contact through trade. Quarantine was the major form of intervention and prevention of further spread of disease because there was no scientific understanding of the cause and the nature of diseases, or how they were spread.

During the Renaissance, the period dated from 1453 to 1600, the emergence of individual scientific endeavour led to some understanding of the cause and the natural history of infectious disease. This increasing scientific knowledge enabled a community to put in place treatment and prevention activities that were more closely linked with an understanding of disease processes. Although these processes were not at all sophisticated, their implementation marked the beginnings of scientific medicine and the development of the medical dominance over public health. The Renaissance was also a time of increasing social density, the expansion and further development of trade between countries and general population movements, all which encouraged the development and spread of disease.

The changing history of definitions of disease

An understanding of the history of public health would not be complete without some consideration of historical definitions of health and disease. The occurrence of death and disease can only rarely be described as a matter of chance. They are influenced by a number of determinants including the social and spatial organisation of a population; the individual's genetic endowment and exposure to a range of risk factors; the physical environment; patterns of relationships and mobility; and access to health services (Perdiguero et al 2001, Scott 2004).

As the 19th century emerged, a number of disease theories formed the framework for the debate about causes of ill health. The germ (or contagion) theory held that for every disease there was a corresponding pathogen. From a modern point of view, it is difficult to understand that the phenomenon of contagion was not recognised with the first contagious disease (Fleming & Parker 2007). It was only in the 19th century that this theory gained further prominence when the theory of microorganisms could be substantiated with the aid of suitable medical apparatus such as a rudimentary microscope. By contrast, the environmental theory supported the sanitary reforms that represented the first great revolution in public health. Unfortunately, that support was based on the incorrect belief that illness was a sign of dirty air, or as it was know at the time, 'miasma'. While the theory of divine retribution suggested that a person's illness was a punishment for sinning, disease as a personal defect was another prominent theory on the cause of disease that suggested illness was attributable to an individual's social class or behaviour (Pickett & Hanlon 1990).

What becomes clear to us from the preceding discussion is that not all of the theories of disease supported the development of public health interventions. The germ theory supported the development of scientific medicine and treatment of the individual, although, with the recognition of contagious diseases, public health measures such as quarantine were introduced. The divine retribution and personal defect theories cited the cause of illness as either spiritual or the individual's class or behaviour. The personal defect theory had as its core the notion of individual responsibility for illness.

Edwin Chadwick supported the environmental theory of disease and pushed for sanitary reform; the culture of 19th-century Britain gave him the opportunity to write about the poor as the population group most often exposed to disease. They were '... less susceptible to moral influences, and the effects of education are more transient than with a healthy population; these adverse circumstances tend to produce an adult population short-lived, improvident, reckless and intemperate, and with habitual avidity to sexual gratification ...' (Pickett & Hanlon 1990 p 28).

Only the environmental theory of disease can be clearly linked with sanitary reform measures; however, even though this strategy improved the health of the population, its use was initially based on incorrect assumptions about the cause of disease. As time passed, it became clear that changing patterns of mortality and morbidity and significant decreases in the rate of death due to infectious diseases were clearly attributable, in part, to sanitary reforms. In addition, the militancy of the 19th-century working class resulted in improved wages and working conditions, and improved living standards and nutritional status, which significantly heightened people's resistance to microorganisms in air, food and drinking water. The interrelationship between the two theories of disease is evident when one considers that clean water and proper sewerage are environmental changes that work, in part, because they reduce or eliminate exposure to microbes (Fleming & Parker 2007).

In Chapter 2, we further our understanding of the concepts of health and illness in contemporary society and examine the diversity of perspectives that exist between, for example, professional and lay definitions. The ways in which professionals define health and illness are different from the ways in which other members of society conceive of them. Across time and cultures, depending on people's concerns, there have always been varied conceptions of health and illness (Waltner-Toews 2000).

The Colonial era: colonisation and health

The Colonial period extended from around 1600 to 1800. In the UK, for example, boards of health were established to examine prevalent health problems, and to protect the population from the spread of diseases caused by unsafe drinking water and tainted food supplies. Boards of health were the first employers of public health professionals. However, the ineffectiveness of the original boards of health in controlling infectious disease was partly due to the limited strategies they had at their disposal. Treatment options were minimal and often dangerous to the patient, and prevention consisted primarily of quarantine. These quarantine measures were resented by the merchants, who understandably wanted to retain the flow of goods and customers. The religious orders also resented the boards and their powers to ban public congregations during an epidemic (Lewis 2003).

Improved understanding of the causes of ill health and advances in the scientific basis of medicine further increased the possibility that people might recover from an illness when treated with procedures that were based on increasing evidence. Community sanitation legislation was introduced in England in 1837 as a mechanism to ensure at least fundamental public health activity was being pursued. Edwin Chadwick was the author of the *Report on the Sanitary Condition of the Labouring Population of Great Britain* (1842) and the initial driving force behind public health reform. In 1848 the *Public Health Act* came into being as a mechanism to remedy unsanitary conditions and to provide adequate drainage and sanitation. This Act was primarily due to the efforts of Edwin Chadwick (Porter 1999).

By 1872, a new public health Act required every statutory authority to appoint a medical officer of health. However, up until the late 1860s, more often than not, actions to improve health were likely to be for social or political ends. It was not until the early 1870s that an effective public health movement emerged in the UK.

In the colonial era, despite improved understanding of the causes of disease, actions designed to protect the public's health often came after an epidemic had established itself in a population. Isolation and quarantine were still the major mechanisms to deal with outbreaks. Public health advances in the 18th century included developing rudimentary occupational hygiene practices, considering the safety and health of workers, introducing procedures to improve infant hygiene practices and some attention to mental health issues (Lewis 2003).

Certainly, the public health movement was essential for the survival of the burgeoning cities created by 19th-century industrial capitalism (Susser 1981). Public health remained progressive, even though at times social and economic reforms were absent. The pursuit of community health at a population level was new, and the assumption of State responsibility for maintaining community health was equally so (aside from acute emergencies such as plague or other epidemics). The originality of public health was to attack disease and poverty – in the community at large – at their perceived source in the environment. Inevitably, conflict arose between the *new ethic* implicit in a definition of health that included public health and the *old ethic* implicit in the one-to-one responsibilities of physicians for individual patients (Fleming & Parker 2007, Porter 1999).

The Australian experience: colonisation and health

While Australia may have been a British colony, a somewhat different picture of public health emerged from that in 19th-century Europe and the role of public health in the aftermath of the Industrial Revolution. The first phase of public health intervention in the fledgling colony, between settlement and the early 1800s, was marked by British administration of a colony fighting for its survival (O'Connor 1991).

Lord Sydney, commenting on the establishment of the colony in New South Wales, claimed that there were two primary reasons for the settlement. These were the potential threat of escape of large numbers of prisoners from the overcrowded prisons in England and the danger of the breakout of 'infectious distempers' (Historical Records of New South Wales 1892 p 14). Other authors have commented on two further reasons for establishing a colony in New South Wales; first, the availability of materials useful to the navy in its activities in the Indian Ocean; and second, that the colony was founded to promote trade with China (Fleming & Parker 2007).

The British State was not simply reconstructed in a colonial outpost. The colonial State departed from the British model in a number of ways. In particular, differences included the force that was applied to control the convicts and the Indigenous people, and the degree of power vested in the military, a factor that permeated all aspects of the colony. A complex range of factors contributed to rises and falls in patterns of mortality and morbidity in the colonial population. These factors included the transmissibility of infections, increased population density and the creation of a permanent infectious disease 'pool'. In particular, 'new diseases' decimated segments of the Indigenous population, who were more susceptible to diseases to which their communities had not previously been exposed. Resistance levels among the colonists also fluctuated, particularly with respect to infants and children (O'Connor 1991). However, biology was not the direct determinant of the health of the colonial population, it was mediated by the colonial society's social organisation, its administration and economic development and colonial beliefs about disease causation and action needed to promote health (Fleming & Parker 2007).

How Australia matured: influences on public health development

There have been several important influences on the development of public health in Australia. Lewis (1989) articulates six major influences at the national level. These are similar to general themes identifiable in public health development overseas, but are modified by the fact that Australian society commenced its life as a convict colony. Table 1.1 outlines these major influences.

MAJOR INFLUENCE	EXPLANATION
State promotion of national efficiency and national development	Efficiency was the application of expert or scientific knowledge to economic, social and political spheres of national life. Its purpose was to advance the power and effectiveness of the nation in a world of competitive nation states and empires.
	The basis to this endeavour was the 'physical efficiency' of the population. A more positive government, guided and promoted by an elite group of experts, was advocated if the nation was to survive class conflict at home and international conflict abroad.
Bureaucratic ascendancy in Australian society	The growth of bureaucracy consequent upon the expansion of State functions. In Australia ascendancy was established in the colonial period well before the political centralisation resulting from the Second World War.
	In colonial times reliance was placed on bureaucrats for rule making and arbitrative functions.
	Since colonial times, highly successful bureaucrats have both created and administered policy in public health.
Structure of the Australian Government and the constitutional division of powers between the Australian and the state governments.	Following federation the Commonwealth was obliged, under the Constitution, to give three-quarters of its revenue back to the states, thus greatly retarding the growth of its administration.
	State jealousies and the difficulty of constitutional amendment blocked formal legal extension of Australian government functions, including health-related activities.
	However in the relatively prosperous 1920s, some growth of functions, notably in health, scientific research and overseas marketing, took place via extra-constitutional and bureaucratic means.

➡

MAJOR INFLUENCE	EXPLANATION
Existence of a well-organised and politically sophisticated medical profession.	Private practice of medicine and the professional independence from the State. The profession was ready to sanction State intervention, both in the traditional public health sphere and in health care, if the intervention was on terms it found acceptable.
Reformist Labor Party	Struggling in a capitalist economy with a government policy of collective responsibility and equitable access in health matters. Conservative parties were emphasising individual responsibility in a contributory insurance approach to health.
Advance of scientific knowledge in medicine and public health	Prominence of bacteriology shifted the focus of public health from the sanitary environment to identify infectious disease in the individual and to control by isolation and later by mass vaccination. The evolution of new disciplines in modern laboratory-based medicine, the development of powerful new diagnostic techniques and the production of new therapeutic agents gave curative medicine totally unpredicted effectiveness. New technologically intensive medicine was costly and increasingly sited in the hospital. New, more effective preventive medicine was pushing the State towards responsibility for the health of all individuals, more effective but more expensive curative medicine was creating conditions requiring greater State intervention to finance hospitals and the technological infrastructure needed for the new therapies.

TABLE 1.1: Six major influences on the development of public health in Australia (Adapted from Lewis 1989)

As noted above, most of the themes identified by Lewis within Australia were also evident at an international level. Certainly, the fundamental stages in the development of public health and the emergence of conflict between public health activity and the activities of curative medicine were evident in Australia as in other developed countries.

A general history of public health: evolution and influences

The early developments that were designed to protect the health of the public can be charted by examining a number of important phases in public health history. Table 1.2 below outlines a series of phases in the history of public health. Each of these phases is related to a particular time in history and represents the prevailing thinking of the time about the causes of diseases. This thinking was often limited and, early on in the modern history of public health, related more to preventing the spread of the disease even if it was not clear what caused the disease. What is always important for us to remember is that the history of public health has benefited over the past four decades from scholars from a range of intellectual disciplines who have broadened the study of the economic, political and social relations of health and society. A history of public health is much more about the social, economic and political influences of the time and the interplay of these influences on health, disease and population health (Porter 1999). It is no longer only a narrative about individuals and their heroic contribution to improving health.

HISTORICAL PHASE	EXAMPLES OF MAJOR HEALTH ISSUES	MEASURES TO PROTECT THE POPULATION
Miasma (1850–1880) – noxious odours caused disease	Malaria	• Environmental reforms • General cleanliness focus – *English Manual of Hygiene* as an example • Emerging rudimentary influence of medicine
Bacteriological (1880–1910)	Specific organism specific disease – plague, cholera, typhoid	• Even before isolation of specific agents, identifying certain modes of transmission of disease allowed limited public health measures to be put in place • Development of rudimentary laboratory measures • Quarantine still major form of intervention
Health resources (1910–1960)	Infectious diseases early in this period; emergence of lifestyle diseases at end of period	• Expansion of state health departments • Improvements and development of hospitals and primary source of care for ill • Expansion in nature and role of health professionals • Biomedical knowledge advances and concentration on medical focus • Voluntary health agencies established and developed • Major advances in laboratory measures
Social engineering (1960–1975)	Focus on individual health – lifestyle diseases	• Treatment focus and improvements in medical services • Advances in medical technology and increases in costs of care and treatment • Recognition of social equity aspect of health through providing medical care for all • Health education emerged to deal with individual lifestyle diseases

➡️

➡

HISTORICAL PHASE	EXAMPLES OF MAJOR HEALTH ISSUES	MEASURES TO PROTECT THE POPULATION
Old public health (1975–mid 1980s)	Lifestyle diseases; some infectious diseases	• Epidemiological studies identify determinants of health and strategies focus on factors impacting on individual health • Environmental health strategies are also considered important
New public health/health promotion (early 1980s to late 1990s)	Reduction in infectious diseases generally but emergence of diseases that have no cure – HIV/AIDS; lifestyle diseases continue; emergence of chronic diseases as a major challenge	• Health promotion • WHO *Health for All by 2000* • *Lalonde Report* – Canada • *US Surgeon General's Report* • WHO *Ottawa Charter* and elements of the charter to focus on population approach • Old versus new public health – primary health care • Continuation of tension between medical care strategies and promotion and prevention • Equitable access to promotion, treatment and prevention services • Recognition of and strategies to deal with influences of social, economic and political contributions to health and illness
Ecological public health (2000 to date)	Global warming; infectious diseases return; chronic diseases expand	• Ecological and environmental sustainability strategies • WHO *Health for All* 2010; 2020 • Strategies to encourage wise use of resources both human and material • Multidisciplinary, multisectoral strategies to deal with complexity of health issues in 21st century

TABLE 1.2: Phases in the history of public health

There are numerous ways to divide up the history of public health. Table 1.2 is one of a number of different ways of conceptualising the periods that have been seen as important phases in the modern history of public health. It should be remembered that the time periods mentioned are only a guide and that phases overlap and continue to have an influence over longer periods of time than might be suggested by this table. The table serves as an introduction to differing social, political and economic influences on health and the nature and scope of the role of individual versus collective actions to promote health in populations.

Regardless of the division, there are major themes that have emerged over time that represent significant shifts and changes in public health. These major themes have been influenced by shifting political imperatives, advancing medical knowledge, economic perspectives and social changes. Here we take four of these major shifts in the nature and scope of public health activity to present you with an overview of how change to organised efforts to promote, protect and restore the population health have occurred over the past one hundred or so years. These four major shifts include:
- environmental protection
- individualism and State involvement
- therapeutic era and medical dominance
- contemporary notions: the 'old', 'new' and 'ecological' public health.

After we introduce you to each of the major shifts in focus, there is an activity for you to undertake to help you understand each of these major shifts in focus. We ask you to think about each of these changes and the impact on public health philosophy and strategies. Some of the developments were associated with increasing knowledge, some with mechanisms that worked to protect the public even though, at the time, public health workers were not sure why they worked and some brought about a shift in professional practice and a focus on the individual rather than the population. While others recognise that population health is influenced by much greater factors than individual medical care, and that social, political and economic issues mediate the ability of individuals to make changes to their health. In more recent times, the survival of the planet as we know it has challenged public health to engage in a consideration of ecological sustainability as the ultimate goal of our civilisation.

Environment protection

The key public health activities throughout this phase ensured appropriate sanitary conditions and laws to provide clean water, adequate food supplies and the safe disposal of personal and household waste. Diseases and illness were associated with overcrowding, poor hygiene, tainted water supplies or a failure to use water for cleanliness, and contaminated food supplies. There was a divide between those with the economic and social means to ensure basic sanitation, hygiene and adequate food supplies and those with little economic or social opportunity.

ACTIVITY
- Can you think of places in Australia where even today there is inadequate access to basic environmental/sanitary structures to ensure population health?
- Without these basic measures for health, what diseases are likely to result in the population?
- What do you think are the important factors that might improve this situation?
- What are the more difficult factors that might play a role in improving the situation?
- In a country like Australia, why is it that these changes cannot be put in place and sustained?

REFLECTION

Did you identify anywhere in Australia where this problem is still a challenge for public health? Aboriginal and Torres Strait Islander populations, in some places in Australia, still live in environments that lack appropriate sanitation and housing, and where food costs are far greater than in other places in Australia. How can this problem be rectified? What role can public health practitioners play? Should the public health role be undertaken by trained Indigenous health workers? In Chapter 2, we discuss the issue of workforce development for Indigenous workers and the problems that such workers face in accessing appropriate training and remuneration for the role they play. Why do you think it is difficult to sustain the changes that are put in place in an Indigenous community? These issues will be discussed in many of the following chapters. There are no simple solutions to this complex problem.

Individualism and State involvement

This phase emerged after some of the most pressing environmental problems were brought under control, and scientific knowledge led to a far greater understanding of the natural history of diseases. In addition, the State came to see its role far more clearly as the important player in developing public health. For example, the establishment of a federal health department in Australia and the notion of a division of responsibility between state and federal systems came into play early in the 20th century. Developments of school health education programs, nursing and family planning programs and hospital services became more sophisticated and more clearly focussed on the complexity of medical care and treatment.

ACTIVITY

Look up the website for the Australian Government Department of Health and Ageing, what programs does that department sponsor that focus on population health? You can google the website and easily find the Population Health Division within the health department. Now consider the following activity.

- Write down a description of one Australian Government health program for children that is currently in place.
- Does the division discuss how the program is developed at the federal level and the role of state and territory governments? If it does what responsibility does each have?
- Think about an example in the recent press where there is an expressed tension between state/territory and Australian Government responsibility for a component of the health system? Why is this so?
- Are there examples where state/territory and federal systems are working together? Does the website give you an idea about how the relationship works? What do you think would make it easier for state/territory and federal governments to work together in public health?

REFLECTION

In an example like the one presented above there are a range of issues that you should be able to identify. If you are having difficulty considering the relationship between the Population Health Division at its activity and your state/territory health department then look at your state/territory health department website and see if there are common programs listed. How do the programs at the federal level differ in terms of structure and outcomes from state/territory initiatives? You might expect that the federal department may have more of a policy and oversight role, with the state department having more of an implementation and evaluation role. Why do you think there might be tension between the two levels of government? Can you see, or do you know of, any programs that were well integrated between state and federal governments? In Chapter 2, we discuss the division of responsibility for public health between all levels of government.

Therapeutic era

This era heralded the incredible growth in the use of drug therapies to cure a wide range of diseases, or to at least enable people to continue to live with disease that cannot be cured. Drugs such as insulin and penicillin were discovered and both these are now further refined and used, or new generations of drug therapies have replaced them through the continued advancement of biomedical science.

The therapeutic era represented a time of attention to a medical model of public health where the focus was on treating and curing health problems for the individual rather than at the population level. At the end of the 19th century, both the moral and the economic boundaries of public health were at issue, as public health agencies intruded into activities that the medical profession believed to be rightly its own. This conflict has long antecedents, but it was intensified by an historic convergence between medicine and public health (Starr 1982). We discussed this notion earlier in the chapter when we considered the changing nature of the historical analysis of public health.

The impact of scientific development further intensified the conflict between medicine and public health. This meant that public health exponents increasingly came to rely on the techniques of medicine and personal hygiene (Starr 1982). As public health authorities gradually developed a more precise conception of the sources and models of the transmission of infectious diseases, and concentrated on combating particular pathogenic organisms, attention shifted further from the environment to the individual (Fleming & Parker 2007).

An ethical justification became available for public health action in personal as well as population health. The road was open for action directed towards health that had as its central concern the personal behaviours of individuals and the contribution of a person's lifestyle to their health and wellbeing. These personal behaviours, and the ways in which the individual could modify them, became the subject of scientific judgements about the protection of the public's health.

ACTIVITY

- You've seen information on TV and in magazines about the importance of weight management and exercise, and their contribution to your health, so you decide to try to make some changes to your lifestyle. You join a fitness club and purchase some fresh fruit and vegetables. All is going well with your plan, except when you arrive at work the only coffee shop has no food to eat that fits in with your diet plan. Chips, hot dogs and greasy, stale-looking hamburgers are on offer. You're very hungry, have made good intentions and started the day well.
- You have also seen some information in the press about surgery to help you reduce weight. It has been very difficult for you to change your behaviour and your environment is not helping because of limited healthy food choices in your workplace. Perhaps surgery might make it easier for you to lose weight.
- What do you do? How do you decide on the options?

REFLECTION

This scenario illustrates one of the dilemmas of the therapeutic model that focuses on individual responsibility for health choices. While it is important that individuals accept personal responsibility for their health, this is often not easy unless structures to assist individual decisions are also in place. On a broader scale, you need the economic resources to be able to purchase food (you can't eat without money), employment is a mechanism for supporting yourself, but the level of your education and whether you have a roof over your head and appropriate transport all impact on the decisions you will make. Access to adequate food and shelter, sufficient knowledge about healthy behaviours and public health protection are considered to be widely available to the majority of the population. However, as Legge (1989 p 472) suggests, the individual focussed therapeutic approach 'overlooks', or assumes as inevitable, the economic and social inequalities that affect health chances. We also need to consider the role of surgery for the individual as a mechanism for longer term weight reduction and sustainability. Make a list of what you think are the advantages and disadvantages of surgery as a means to sustained weight reduction.

Contemporary notions: the 'old', 'new' and 'ecological' public health

We now turn our attention to a discussion of three more contemporary public health movements – the old public health, the new public health and ecological public health. The changing nature of public health roles and responsibilities, particularly over the past 160 years, has inevitably led to conflict between public health authorities and a range of other institutions and groups.

These approaches provide an insight into the changing face of the politics of health. They are contentious theoretical descriptions, and many commentators on public health have argued that all three paradigms are essential to improve and maintain the public's health (Weiss & McMichael 2004). A brief introduction to each model will set the scene for further discussion in the chapters that follow. Each of the models continues to play a role in contemporary public health as suggested by Weiss and McMichael (2004). Each has its place in a world where political, economic and social instability is still prevalent – posing many complex challenges for public health.

Old public health

The 'old public health' model is based on the discipline of epidemiology and the subject matter of the biomedical and behavioural sciences (Holman 1992). It analyses causes of disease in terms of 'factors' in the individual, and in the social and physical environment. Strategies are aimed at interrupting the 'chain of causation' for a disease, with the traditional tools being education, service provision and legislation (Legge 1989).

During the Industrial Revolution of the 19th century, the greatest triumphs of public health occurred in relation to the physical environment and occupational hazards (e.g. water, sewage, food, working conditions and housing). The environmental focus in this model still has a major role to play in addressing social inequalities and their impact on health as an example. As Grusky (2001) states, 'social inequality is the expression of lack of access to housing, health care, education, employment opportunities and status. It is the exclusion of people from full and equal participation in what we, the members of society, perceive as being valuable, important personally worthwhile and socially desirable' (Grusky 2001 p 15).

Several authors have commented on the limitations of the 'old public health' (Fleming & Parker 2007, Legge 1989, Lin et al 2007). These critiques have focussed on three issues: the knowledge–action gap; social isolation and the limits of support services; and economic inequalities in health. It has been argued that health education as one of the key strategies in the old public health makes assumptions about knowledge being a precondition of behaviour change. There are many examples, however, where people are very knowledgeable about a particular behaviour and its links with a health issue, yet they continue with the behaviour. Legge commented that the 'old public health' failed

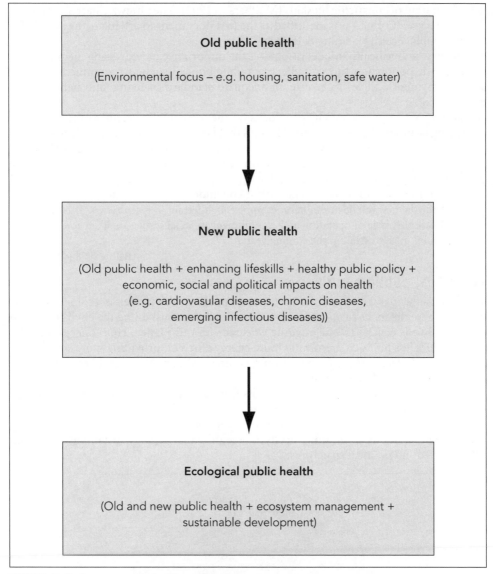

FIGURE 1.1: Contemporary public health movement

to provide a framework for 'understanding social isolation and lack of support within a broader economic and cultural framework' (1989 p 476).

Finally, many authors have commented on the limited recognition given to the contribution of economic inequalities to ill health (Baum 2008, Fleming & Parker 2007, Lin et al 2007). There is clearly a need to understand inequalities in health within a broader political context, and for addressing the underlying structural issues that lead to inequality.

New public health

The 'new public health' model represents a significant paradigm shift when compared with the 'old public health' model (Kickbusch 1989). In particular, it shifts the focus from behaviour change to healthy public policy, and it replaces the lifestyle approach with the notion of enhancing lifeskills (McPherson 1992). The Ottawa Charter for Health Promotion (WHO 1986) was identified as the first document to articulate the agenda for the new public health (Fleming & Parker 2007).

The 'new public health' model recognises the importance of addressing inequalities in health in the population through effective public policies such as economic, education and employment policies to ensure an adequate standard of living, and hence, better health for all.

Baum (2008) argues strongly for a focus on the 'new public health' as the model for advancing health in the 21st century. She says that large challenges face public health into the future in an environment where there is unstoppable yet unsustainable global growth in human population and economic activity, where international economic trends are primarily not supportive of health and where there is increasing inequity within and between countries (Baum 2008). The author concludes:

> While the new public health has met some rough terrain in recent years, its basic philosophy, style of operation and commitment to social justice are likely to stand it in good stead in the coming years.
>
> (Baum 2008 p 66)

Ecological public health

The final model in our analysis of contemporary public health models is 'ecological public health', where the focus turns to ecological sustainability. Sustaining the environment in which we live is central to our ongoing existence on this planet. This concept includes making cities less polluted, becoming more energy efficient; providing more social space and trees; and placing more emphasis on recycling, reducing waste and becoming more self-sufficient in food production.

This approach assumes that health results from a complex, dynamic, interconnected set of living systems existing in a delicate balance. It importantly considers equity, sustainability, consideration towards others and preservation. Figure 1.2 succinctly demonstrates that our community needs to recognise that ecology sustains a society and its economic and political structures.

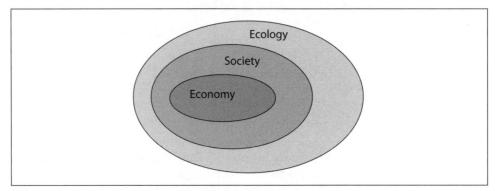

FIGURE 1.2: The relationship between ecology, society and economy

Ecological public health acknowledges that economic, environmental and social issues are interrelated and recognises the sensitive interface between the natural and built environment. As a society, we clearly need to move away from polluting and wasteful behaviours and to protect our natural, cultural, historical and human assets. We need to promote good environmental practices through collaboration and participation, and to develop products and services that are environmentally friendly. Ecological public health needs to take into account, and to be able to cost, the economic, environmental and social impacts of damaging our ecosystem and consequently our health.

These challenges will not be easy; in fact, many political, economic and social factors act as barriers to ecological sustainability. Political commitment to the notion of ecological sustainability, while growing, is certainly not comprehensive and in fact many of the emerging economies have found it hard to commit to such a concept and to associated targets to reduce carbon emissions. Australia has recently committed to the *National Strategy for Ecologically Sustainable Development*, initially endorsed by COAG in 1992. However, without a global commitment, the influence of individual nations will remain insignificant.

Applying the models

The following scenario summarises the issues we've been discussing in the final section of this chapter. The questions provide you with an opportunity to think about how a health professional might address a series of key public health issues according to his/her philosophy of public health.

Case study: Alice, a homeless woman

Alice is an 18-year-old homeless woman. She's been living on the streets for two months and does not want to go home. She has little money, is drinking a lot of alcohol with the money she has, has the flu and she has few friends. She's living in a squat with some other street people, but it's cold and inadequate. She's concerned about her flu getting worse and worried about money for food. Her money is running out. She left school at Year 11 and would like to finish school and get a job in a health-related area. She is not sure what the future holds for her but she knows that she has to try to make a break from the life she has been living. How might she do this and who might be able to help her?

ACTIVITY

- You've been appointed as a senior policy officer in a state or territory health department. In reflecting on the three major contemporary public health movements (old public health, new public health, ecological public health), list one public health action that could be suggested to assist Alice for *each* of the contemporary public health models below.

Public health model	Public health activity
Old public health	
New public health	
Ecological sustainability	

REFLECTION

How different were the actions you suggested for Alice between the old public health model and the ecological model of public health? There are a multitude of actions to assist Alice in this scenario. For example, in the 'old' public health model you may have thought that Alice needed to make personal changes to her lifestyle by finding a safe place to live and a job, and that Alice had to make this choice for herself. On the other hand, you may have felt that Alice's circumstances were created by multiple factors that she had little to no control over. How might you as a senior policy officer try to change the circumstances in which Alice finds herself?

As a future practitioner, aside from deciding on strategies for action, it is most important that you think about why you have selected a particular strategy above another and how that might improve Alice's life and possibly her health. Many would argue that strategies like providing a safe home, adequate food and a source of income would be the essential first strategies for someone in Alice's position. Others might argue that social and economic issues that make it difficult for Alice to make the necessary changes are the responsibility of governments and should be part of a range of government-managed strategies to assist Alice to find a safe environment, to provide medical care for Alice and to support her to regain her self-confidence and self-respect.

A final word

What this chapter clearly shows us is that the past is a signpost for the present and the future. The ancient history of public health, briefly presented here, demonstrates to us that even though efforts were in place at various times in history to protect the population's health, the purpose of that protection was often not for health reasons at all, but rather for social and political reasons. Throughout history, it is evident that sanitary measures and environmental protections put in place in the early years of organised efforts to protect the health of the public worked to achieve these objectives. As we have seen in this chapter, the history of public health is a rich tapestry that has been impacted on by a wide range of social, economic and political factors that have shaped society's responses to health and diseases.

Removing environmental hazards and protecting the environment marked the first public health revolution. Environmental health today is still important to public health endeavours. Providing appropriate housing, safe water supplies and adequate nutritious food are fundamental to the health of the population.

What characterised the period up until the 19th century was the general lack of scientific evidence that could be brought to bear to explain disease, its transmission and its human and social consequences. An increase in evidence about the cause of disease and its spread led to a focus on individual treatment and medical intervention. This development enabled the focus of public health to shift from the population to the individual and reinforced the dominance of the medical profession and a biomedical model of health.

Accompanying the shift to medical dominance, and an individual focus on health and illness, was the role of the State in managing health services. Increasing costs of medical treatment, drug therapies and using 'high tech' machinery to manage health conditions placed the State under extreme pressure to control health costs while providing a range of services. It also ensured that the gap between developing and developed countries and the range of public health services available would widen even further.

In the most recent past public health has moved to a 'new public health' paradigm where there is a strong focus on prevention and health promotion and using public health policy to advance the case for a focus on population health, and subsequent funds to support such a focus.

Ecological public health marks contemporary public health efforts and relies on the notion of an ecological contribution to public health that considers the environment in which we live and work, and in which our ecosystem functions, as the most important influences on population health.

In the chapter that follows, we examine contemporary public health policy and the structure and function of the organisational systems that support public health.

REVIEW QUESTIONS

1 Identify the range of approaches that contemporary historians of public health have used to understand public health history.
2 Write a paragraph or two on the work of McKeown and Szreter in describing the factors that contributed to major advances in the health of the population.
3 How did Australian public health develop and what factors contributed to the nature of these developments?
4 Identify the main themes and briefly describe the characteristics of each theme in the history of public health in Australia.
5 Describe the major themes and strategies of the 'old public health', the 'new public health' and 'ecological public health'.
6 Summarise how the history of public health can assist us in our understanding of contemporary public health.

REFERENCES

Action on Smoking and Health 2007 Key dates in the history of anti-tobacco campaigning. Available: http://www.ash.org.uk 10 Jan 2008
Baum F 2008 The new public health. 3rd edn. Oxford University Press, South Melbourne
Berridge V 2000 History of Public Health: Who needs it? Lancet 356:923–925
Brownson R C, Bright F S 2004 Chronic disease control in public health practice: Looking back and moving forward. Public Health Reports 119:230–238
Colgrove J 2002 The McKeown Thesis: A historical controversy and its enduring influence. American Journal of Public Health 92(5):725–729
Ecologically Sustainable Development Steering Committee December 1992 National Strategy for Ecologically Sustainable Development. Endorsed by the Council of Australian Governments. Available: http://www.environment.gov.au/esd/national/nsesd/strategy/index.html 12 Jan 2008
Fleming M L, Parker E 2007 Health Promotion. Principles and practice in the Australian context, 3rd edn. Allen and Unwin, Sydney
Grusky D B 2001 The Past, Present and Future of Social Inequality. Social Stratification: Class, Race, and Gender 2nd ed. Westview Press, Colorado
Historical Records of New South Wales, 1892–1901, Vol. 1, part 2, Phillip, 1783–1793, W. Britton, Government Printer, Sydney
Holman C D 1992 Something old, something new: Perspectives on five new public health movements. Health Promotion Journal of Australia 2(3):4–11
Kickbusch I 1989 Editorial, Health Promotion International 1(1):3–4
Lawson J S, Bauman A E 2001 Public Health in Australia: An Introduction, 2nd edn. McGraw-Hill, Sydney
Legge D 1989 Towards a politics of health. In: Gardner H(ed) The Politics of Health: The Australian Experience. Churchill Livingstone, Melbourne
Lewis M J (ed) 1989 Health and Disease in Australia: A history. AGPS, Canberra
Lewis M J 2003 The People's Health. Public Health in Australia, 1950 to the Present. Volume 1 and 2. Praeger, Westport
Lin V, Smith J, Fawkes S 2007 Public Health Practice in Australia: The organised effort. Allen and Unwin, Sydney
McPherson P D 1992 Health for All Australians. In: Gardner H (ed) Health Policy, Churchill Livingstone, Melbourne
O'Connor M 1991 A socio-historical study of health and medical care in New South Wales from settlement to 1850, unpublished PhD thesis, University of Queensland, Brisbane
Ogilvie D, Hamlet N 2005 Obesity: the elephant in the corner. British Medical Journal 331:1545–1548

Perdiguero E, Bernabeau J, Huertas R et al 2001 History of health, a valuable tool in public health. Journal of Epidemiology and Community Health 55:667–673

Pickett G, Hanlon J J 1990 Public Health: Administration and Practice, 9th edn. Times Mirror/Mosby College Publishing, St Louis

Porter D 1999 Health, Civilization and the State: A history of public health from ancient to modern times. Routledge, London

Rosen G 1953 Economic and Social Policy in the Development of Public Health: An Essay in Interpretation. Journal of History of Medicine and Allied Sciences 8:430

Scally G, Womack J 2004 Journal of Epidemiology and Community Health 58:751–755, doi:10.1136/jech.2003.014340

Scott W G 2004 Public policy failure in health care. Journal of American Academy of Business 5(1&2):88–94

Starr P 1982 The Social Transformation of American Medicine. Basic Books, New York

Susser M 1981 Ethical components in the definition of health. In: Caplan A L et al (eds) Concepts of Health and Disease: Interdisciplinary Perspectives. Addison-Wesley, Reading

Szreter S 2002 Rethinking McKeown: The relationship between public health and social change. American Journal of Public Health 92(5):722–725

Szreter S 2003 The population approach in historical perspective. American Journal of Public Health 93(3):421–431

Tosh J 1984 The pursuit of history. Longman, London

Waltner-Toews D 2000 The end of medicine: the beginning of health. Futures 32:655–667

Weiss R A, McMichael A J 2004 Social and environmental risk factors in the emergence of infectious diseases. Nature Medicine Supplement 10(12):s70–76

World Health Organization 1986 The Ottawa Charter for Health Promotion. First International Conference on Health Promotion, Ottawa, 21 November 1986. Available: http://www.who.int/healthpromotion/conferences/previous/ottawa/en/ 25 Jan 2008

CHAPTER 2

Defining health and public health

Mary Louise Fleming

Learning objectives

After reading this chapter you should be able to:

- define health and public health
- discuss how the concept of 'health' means different things to different individuals and be able to consider the range of factors that influence these definitions
- identify and describe the principles of public health
- recognise and describe how public health is defined and how each definition shapes the development and implementation of contemporary public health approaches
- describe the relationship between public health and other disciplines
- discuss the nature and scope of public health and the focus of the public health workers' endeavours
- understand the contribution of the World Health Organization and a number of levels of governments and organisations in Australia that contribute to public health.

Introduction

What is health? How is it defined and described? What do you mean when you describe yourself as healthy? How is public health defined? What are the fundamental principles of public health? How does public health interact with other disciplines? And how do we describe what public health workers do?

These are many of the questions that will be considered in this chapter, which is designed to help you become familiar with the principles and practices of public health. As mentioned in the previous chapter, this book is about introductory principles and concepts of public health for students. It is also relevant for health workers from a range of disciplines who want to understand and incorporate public health principles into their work.

We begin our journey by considering a fundamental issue that underpins the notion of public health, that is, the definition of health, and we consider the range and variety of definitions of health, both lay and professional.

Defining health and ill-health

Complete the simple exercise below to help you to begin thinking about how you and your friends define health.

ACTIVITY

● Ask five of your friends, classmates or family members what health means to each of them.
● What are the common themes that emerged from each of the five definitions of health?
● What was unique about the different definitions?

REFLECTION

Keep these five definitions in mind as you read, and compare them with other ways of defining health. How do you think of the term 'health'? Does it mean an absence of illness, or an ability to do all the things you want or have to do every day? Does it have more of a religious, cultural or social significance? The term health is difficult to define. How an individual defines his or her health is sometimes different compared with a professional's definition of health.

Most public health workers, or educators who work in public health, see 'health' as central to their work, and believe that the majority of people also hold health to be an important part of their lives. We clearly know that this is not the case. Much research (Baum 2002, Blaxter 1990, 2007, Fleming & Parker 2007) has been undertaken regarding the way in which people define health within the context of their daily lives.

To understand the nature and scope of public health in our society we also need to consider the variety of ways in which the term 'health' is defined. The section that follows discusses how health and illness are defined and then considers professional definitions of health.

Health and illness

Illness is primarily about how an individual experiences disease, and disease itself represents a set of signs and symptoms and medically diagnosed pathological abnormalities.

Illness can be culturally specific and may also be influenced by social, spiritual, supernatural and psychological aspects (Maher 1999). An individual lifestyle perspective has also been seen as an important dimension of health. A social view of health considers issues like the impact of social and economic factors on health, but these dimensions have often been overshadowed by the biomedical view of health.

In the 1940s, the World Health Organization (WHO) defined health as 'a state of complete physical, social and emotional wellbeing and not merely the absence of disease or infirmity' (WHO 1948). Some authors have argued that a state of health delineated by this definition is too difficult to achieve (Bircher 2005, Waltner-Toews 2000), but it certainly moved the debate about health away from an exclusive biomedical perspective.

'Health' itself is difficult to measure because it is a dynamic concept rather than something that is always the same. '... [H]ealth cannot be defined without reference to some goals ...' (Waltner-Toews 2000 p 657) and it is a 'dynamic state of wellbeing characterised by a physical, mental and social potential ...' (Bircher 2005 p 335). It is much easier to measure disease or an absence of disease than it is to measure health or wellbeing.

Lay definitions of health

Lay concepts of health and illness have been extensively researched and discussed. Blaxter (2007), quoting Kleinman, describes three ways in which health and illness have been discussed; these include professional, alternative and lay. Contemporary scholars prefer to consider lay beliefs about health and illness to be defined as 'commonsense understandings and personal experience, imbued with professional rationalization' (Blaxter 2007 p 26). In a seminal study in 1990 Blaxter, while exploring lay definitions of health and illness, found that people define health in a variety of different ways. In her research, she suggests that health is defined by people as not being ill or diseased or as being a reserve against illness. Others define health as a 'healthy life', as physical fitness or as having energy or vitality. Still others take health to mean social relationships, that is, relationships with other people or as a function of the ability to do things. For others health has meaning as psychosocial wellbeing.

Think back to your earlier activity. How do the definitions of health collected from the five people you have spoken with fit in with the different lay definitions of health and illness discussed above?

Read on and consider how others have characterised health. The following discussion introduces you to other dimensions of health that may assist you to understand how complex defining health can be, and how difficult it is to hold a single definition of health that fits with everyone's idea of the dimensions of health.

Collectively, health can be seen to represent the social, cultural and economic context of people's lives – a status, socially recognised and admired. Others believe their health is dominated by religious or supernatural forces (Durie 2004). For some, the centrality of people's relationships to the land, family and community are the central foci for health and wellbeing (Durie 2004, Thompson & Gifford 2000). For Indigenous Australians 'health' is about the totality of their environment.

'Health' to Aboriginal peoples is a matter of determining all aspects of their life, including control over their physical environment, of dignity, of community self-esteem, and of justice. It is not merely a matter of providing doctors, hospitals, medicines or the absence of disease and incapacity (National Aboriginal Health Strategy Working Party 1989 p ix).

A critical perspective

While lay definitions of health have focussed on the ways in which health is defined in the day-to-day lives of people, some authors have considered that professional definitions of health might be conceptualised as socio-political in nature. Baum (2008), for example, examines how health is defined by looking at the purposes that are achieved through particular ways of defining health. She suggests that 'health is defined by capitalist society in such a way that it becomes a "defining and controlling" mechanism. Using this definition of health means that people are defined primarily through their illness' (2008 p 10). Another way of defining health according to the author (Baum 2008) is to talk about health maintenance as an important part of being a 'good' citizen because becoming ill may mean that a person is an economic burden to society. When health is defined as individual illness, the personal dimension becomes important and the social and economic dimensions of health are not considered.

Baum (2008) explains that when health is defined more from a collective perspective there are a number of other ways it may be considered. For example, from a political perspective, health is defined by inequities in health status and influenced by environment, housing and occupational conditions. When health is measured in terms of health outcomes, defined as 'a change in the health of an individual, a group of people or population which is attributable to an intervention or series of interventions', then Baum (2002 p 12) contends that this perspective often neglects the notion that the demonstration of health outcomes is complex. She states that health outcomes are difficult to measure in the short term and that it is often better to measure health outcomes in terms of capacities rather than health status.

More recently, ecosystem health (Baum 2008, Brown et al 2005) that integrates an overall consideration of the environment and the interdependence of systems within the overall ecosystem has been espoused by ecologists who fear for the long-term sustainability of our planet.

Examining definitions of health from a critical perspective, as Baum (2002, 2008) has done, means that health as a term can be considered in a variety of different ways and can be challenged, because sometimes definitions avoid the wide-ranging social, economic and political factors that have a real and sustained impact on the health of the population. Not all theorists would necessarily agree with the analysis presented here; but this is not the point. As an educated person, you need to think about the ways in which health is defined and the limitations of a variety of definitions so that you reach your own definition on the basis of a variety of available theoretical perspectives.

We now turn our attention to consider definitions of public health. The two distinguishing features of almost all definitions of public health are (1) its focus on populations rather than on individuals and (2) efforts to promote health are organised and deliberate, and focus on collective action. Understanding how individuals may be affected by a disease or some other problem may be appropriate in certain circumstances. However, it may miss the influence on health of broader structural and socioeconomic factors.

Defining public health: an art and a science?

Public health is based on scientific principles and it uses a range of disciplines such as epidemiology, biostatistics, biology and biomedical sciences in its analysis of public health problems (Lawson & Bauman 2001, Lin et al 2007, Schneider 2006). Public health relies heavily on environmental sciences and the social and behavioural sciences. Public health is also an art in that it involves applying this scientific knowledge to a range of practical settings that require attention to issues such as the needs of the community, selecting intervention strategies and approaches that the communities need. Furthermore, public health deals with social, cultural, political and economic issues, as well as health issues.

Winslow (1920), an American public health leader in the early 20th century, defined public health as a science and an art:

> ... of preventing disease, prolonging life, and promoting physical health and efficiency through organised community efforts for the sanitation of the environment, the control of community infections, the education of the individual in principles of personal hygiene, the organization of medical and nursing services for the early diagnosis and preventive treatment of disease, and the development of the social machinery which will ensure to every individual in the community a standard of living adequate for the maintenance of health.
>
> (Winslow 1920 p 24)

In its time, this definition was very forward thinking because it identified a number of public health elements that are still considered important. For example, it refers to 'organised efforts', it considers environmental issues and infectious diseases, personal wellbeing, early diagnosis and prevention and the social dimensions of health. Little did Winslow know that many of the issues that the public health community had felt they would be able to control or eliminate have emerged again in the 21st century as major challenges.

A definition of public health that is often quoted is that of the American Institute of Medicine (1988). In that definition, public health is described as what society does to assure the conditions for people to be healthy. To do this, the definition goes on to suggest, there needs to be a countering of continuing and emerging threats to the health of the public.

What are some of these emerging threats? Environmental factors such as the effects of greenhouse gases and global warming, HIV/AIDS, avian influenza and SARS (severe acute respiratory syndrome) are significant public health issues (McMichael & Butler 2007). These 21st-century challenges require public health to return to its roots to control infectious diseases, as well as be a part of a global effort to sustain the planet and its environment for generations to come (McMichael & Butler 2007).

Public health today is recognised as being integral to promoting and sustaining the health of the population. The following definition of public health by Last (2001) supports this approach:

> … the efforts organised by society to protect, promote, and restore the people's health. It is the combination of sciences, skills and beliefs that is directed to the maintenance and improvement of the health of all the people through collective or social actions.

(Last 2001 p 145)

This definition of public health provides us with a framework from which we can gain a better understanding of the role of public health in our society. It dispels the notion that health is only concerned with curing illness and disease.

Public health is about preventing disease, illness and injury, together with promoting the quality of life of human populations. This is a very complex process and requires the committed skills and expertise of many different professional disciplines.

In Australia, similar definitions are used to describe the art and the science of public health. The Public Health Association of Australia defines public health as 'a combination of science, practical skills and beliefs that is directed to the maintenance and improvement of the health of all people. It is one of the efforts organised by society to protect, promote and restore the people's health through collective or social actions' (PHAA website). The National Public Health Partnership (NPHP), which was made up of federal, state and territory senior representatives of health ministers, agreed on a definition of public health in 1998 that states that public health is 'the organised response by society to protect and promote health and to prevent illness, injury and disability' (NPHP 2000).

What is common about most of these definitions is the notion that there is an organised desire to improve the health of the population as a whole, a sense of general public interest and a focus on the broader determinants of health (Beaglehole et al 2004). It is worthwhile stopping here to consider the meaning of the term 'determinant'. Determinants are defined in Chapter 4 as both the causes of and risk factors for health events. A wide range of determinants, including physiological, psychosocial, behavioural and risk conditions, 'can work together to influence quality of life, wellbeing, illness and disability. However, the ways in which these determinants manifest themselves in each society would depend on history, culture and politics' (Lin et al 2007 p 76).

As health workers, your knowledge and understanding of the art and science of public health will be an important element of your professional development. This knowledge and understanding will enable you to first identify the trends in the health of the population and, second, demonstrate the skills to appropriately respond to these in restoring, promoting and maintaining the health of the population.

The concepts of public health should become a little clearer to you as we further discuss its vital role in our day-to-day lives. Consider the following scenario to help you think about the contribution of public health to daily life and to enable you to begin to broaden your understanding of public health.

> ## Case study: A typical morning
>
> You get up in the morning, woken earlier than expected by the waste-disposal truck collecting outside in your street. Having completed the morning routine (shower, toilet, teeth etc.) you dress and turn on the radio for the news report. Throughout the broadcast you hear that it is Breast Cancer Awareness Week. Having realised that you are running late for the first lecture at university you quickly rush out the door and into the car. Seatbelt on and out into the usual traffic chaos. As you drive past McDonald's the sign is too enticing, and, remembering you didn't have breakfast at home, you drive through and pick up a muffin and coffee. Across the road in the local state school you notice the ambulance service has two ambulances on the oval and school students are climbing in and out of them. Finally, arriving at university you park your car as near as possible to the lecture theatre and walk the short distance to your lecture.

ACTIVITY: DAILY LIFE AND PUBLIC HEALTH

● From the scenario above, list the issues that you feel are relevant to public health.

REFLECTION

Reflect on the issues you have listed above. Did you consider any of the following issues?
● Your access to clean water, sewerage and rubbish removal and disposal?
● The radio broadcast of a media campaign, which raises your awareness of breast cancer and screening?
● Your safety on the road, which is enhanced by legislation such as that of seat-belt wearing, traffic lights and construction of road ways to maximise safety?
● Your ability to drive on roads that are maintained for safe use?
● Your purchase of food, which has been prepared with standards of hygiene that protect your health?
● The quality of the food you consumed for breakfast?
● The ambulance service visiting a school to discuss their role?
● The fact that you parked your car close to the lecture theatre and walked for a short distance to your lecture?

There are a number of activities that we take part in every day that affect our health and the public's health collectively. Public health has developed systematic ways of thinking about health issues (Schneider 2006). This systematic approach enables public health workers to tackle a health issue in a considered and deliberate fashion. However, unless public health has a collective action domain it will lack a focus on social and economic issues that are so central to supporting and maintaining changes that enhance the public's health.

If you were asked to think about how you might tackle a public health problem, you might think about it in terms of levels of prevention – primary, secondary and tertiary. Primary prevention focuses on maintaining health, for example, school health programs, seatbelts in motor vehicles, anti-smoking campaigns and physical activity and nutrition programs are primary prevention programs. Secondary prevention aims to minimise the extent of a health problem by focussing on early intervention such as prostate, bowel and breast screening. Tertiary intervention aims to minimise disability and provide rehabilitation services, such as cardiac rehabilitation.

Another way of dealing with a public health problem is to consider a chain of causation involving an agent, a host and the environment. In this case, prevention is accomplished by interrupting the chain of causation, for example, by providing immunisation, using antibiotics or purifying water.

You may, or may not, be aware that all of these actions listed above have been put into place because they have been recognised as appropriate and effective strategies that will promote health and move towards a reduction in morbidity and mortality rates throughout the population. This is one of the primary aims of public health.

For you to gain a more comprehensive understanding of public health, however, it is vital that you appreciate the underlying vision, values and core components of public health as they provide the foundations upon which strategies are developed and implemented.

Public health vision and values

Having a vision of where you think public health might be placed in the next five to 10 years is important for the discipline and for you in your practice. There are a range of factors that impact on health and public health that will have a profound effect on the nature and scope of the discipline in the next decade. Globalisation is one of those issues; other issues include the emergence of new virulent infectious diseases, an increase in chronic disease such as diabetes, the ageing population and the ever-increasing cost and the expanding technological sophistication of health care. In Chapter 13 we explore the notion of globalisation and its impact on health and in Chapter 14 we present information about the development of 'new epidemics', such as avian influenza and SARS, as examples of contemporary threats to the health of the public.

ACTIVITY
● What is your vision for public health in the next 10 years?
● Write a sentence on where you think the focus of public health will be in 10 years' time.
● What steps did you take to arrive at that decision?
● What are the implications of your decision on resources and the workforce in public health?

REFLECTION

What factors might influence what you think public health will be focussed on in 10 years' time? You might use projected data about patterns of mortality and morbidity to begin. What other sources of data or reports from places like WHO or the Australian Government might there be that you could consider? Think about the health issues you might consider to be important in 10 years' time: how do these health issues impact on the resources needed to manage them? What might the workforce look like in that time to meet the needs of the health issues and the people who might be impacted on by these health issues?

An understanding of the values that are fundamental to public health practice is vital as these values, whether they are explicit or not, will impact on the nature of public health policy and practice. The traditional values of public health are described by Lawson and Bauman (2001) as 'consistent public health principles'. The authors refer to three major principles as follows:
· using scientific evidence as a basis for action
· focussing on the health of all sections of the population
· emphasising a collective action dimension (Lawson & Bauman 2001 p 5).

In Chapter 1, we discussed the history of public health and the emergence of a scientific basis for decision making on health issues. Using scientific evidence as a basis for action is just as important today as it was two centuries ago when it was first introduced. It is the fundamental underpinning of public health practice. In Chapter 4, we continue to pursue the importance of epidemiology as a discipline that contributes significantly to decisions about public health practice. In Chapter 8 we discuss the role of evidence in guiding practice.

Addressing health issues across population subgroups is also very important to public health. It affirms the principle of equity, which is central to public health activity. Achieving the public's health in some subpopulations is a very difficult task that constantly challenges the skills and expertise of health workers. This is because people's lives are complex and people who are focussed on providing affordable housing, transport and access to food may not think about their health as a priority.

The third issue of a 'collective action' dimension tends to be contextualised differently according to the social and cultural aspects of the society in which we live. For example, in the United States there is still a very strong emphasis on individual rights and freedom; in contrast in Australia, there is a notion of the collective good. Applied to public health this means that the community accepts laws and regulations that limit the individual's freedom, if it means that the health of the population is protected.

Core functions of public health

There are a number of different ways in which the core functions or the focus of public health have been described and defined. For example, Lawson and Bauman (2001) describe four major task categories that include health promotion and disease prevention; traditional public health functions; monitoring and surveillance; and public health policy. By contrast, Turnock (2001) describes seven key principles of public health practice that involve social justice; equity of access and equity in health outcomes; links with government; an expanding and evolving agenda; a preventive focus; a balance between science and societal needs; and an appreciation of the politics of public health.

A similar perspective is taken by Beaglehole et al (2004), who talk about the five key themes of modern public health theory and practice. According to the authors, these themes include leadership of the health system; collaborative action across sectors; multidisciplinary approaches to all determinants of health; political engagement in the development of public health policy; and partnerships with the populations served. Beaglehole et al (2004) suggest that in order to strengthen public health these main themes should be acknowledged and acted on. 'A supportive framework for public health requires strong and responsive government leadership and adequate resources for personnel and infrastructure, completed by public health research, teaching and services that use the full range of public-health sciences' (Beaglehole et al 2004 p 2086). Other authors have presented a different focus. For example, Griffiths et al (2005) discuss three key domains of public health. In the three key domains of health improvement; health protection; health service delivery and quality there is an intersecting and overlapping of activity. Health improvement includes a focus on reducing inequalities and working with partners outside the health sector. Health protection encompasses preventing and controlling infectious diseases, responding to emergencies and protecting from and dealing with environmental health hazards. Health service delivery and quality focuses on service delivery, evidence-based practice, planning and prioritising and appropriate research, audit and evaluation activities (Griffiths et al 2005).

In the United States, the concept of public health, by contrast, has been interpreted in a narrow sense when compared with Europe and Australasia. For example,

Schneider (2006) has an interesting section in her book on public health in the US where she debates the issue of individual liberty and actions that support the common good. The US has a strong tradition of upholding the rights of the individual, sometimes at the expense of the collective good. Examples include the fact that in some American states it is not against the law to drive without a seatbelt. California has a serious air pollution problem and the State has proposed a number of regulations that impact on individual behaviours. Are individuals in California prepared to change their behaviour to improve the quality of the air they breathe? What would you do?

Gostin et al (2004 pp 98–103) challenge this narrow interpretation of strategies to improve the health of Americans by discussing three effective core strategies of public health. The authors provide examples of how each strategy can be implemented. They talk about strengthening 'the governmental public health infrastructure', engaging 'non-governmental actors in partnerships for public health' and transforming national health policy so that traditional dominant investments in personal health care and biomedical research are balanced against investments in the 'multiple determinants of societal health'. The authors, however, clearly recognise the challenges that this more expansive notion of public health poses in the US and the extent of political commitment to population health that is needed.

For the past 10 or more years, efforts to define core public health competencies have occurred around the world. In the US, the UK and Australia, professional bodies and government instrumentalities have attempted to define the roles and responsibilities of public health workers. In 2000 the NPHP (2000), mentioned earlier in this chapter, defined core public health functions in Australia. These functions include the following nine areas.

1 Assess, analyse and communicate population health needs and community expectations.
2 Prevent and control communicable and non-communicable diseases and injuries through risk-factor reduction, education, screening, immunisation and other interventions.
3 Promote and support healthy lifestyles and behaviour through action with individuals, families, communities and wider society.
4 Promote, develop and support healthy public policy, including legislation, regulation and fiscal measures.
5 Plan, fund, manage and evaluate health gain and capacity-building programs designed to achieve measurable improvements in health status, and to strengthen skills, competencies, systems and infrastructure.
6 Strengthen communities and build social capital through consultation, participation and empowerment.
7 Promote, develop, support and initiate actions that ensure safe and healthy environments.
8 Promote, develop and support healthy growth and development throughout all life stages.
9 Promote, develop and support actions to improve the health status of Aboriginal and Torres Strait Islander peoples and other vulnerable groups (NPHP 2000 p 2).

The *Public Health and Education Research Program* (2007), funded by the Australian Government Department of Health and Ageing, is currently working through a consultation process to define public health practice. Five areas of practice have been defined including: health monitoring and surveillance; disease prevention and control; health protection; health promotion; and health policy planning and management. The application of research methods and professional practice form the two underpinning competency groups.

You have had an opportunity in this chapter to explore the many common themes that go to the heart of what public health practice is all about. These include collaborative action across sectors, multidisciplinary approaches, establishing partnerships, reducing inequality, and political support for public health policy. Public health professionals need to work with many other professionals outside as well as inside the health sector and to approach public health issues from a multisector perspective. What we mean by multisector in the public health context is that, for example, public health needs to work with government education, housing and transport departments to ensure that these services are available to the whole population in an equitable manner. Like *Maslow's Hierarchy of Needs* (Maslow 1999), fundamental issues of clothing, shelter and food have to be met before people will turn their attention to health-related issues. Partnerships between health and non-health agencies are important because diversity is an underpinning component of public health practice.

What do public health practitioners do?

This is an interesting question that we will consider in two parts. First we will discuss who is the public health practitioner. Second, we will consider the role of the public health worker, now and in the future.

Who is the public health workforce? Is it anyone from a health discipline who is involved in some form of public health activity, or is it much narrower, such as a community primary care worker or a public health specialist? Rotem et al (1995) conducted a study of the public health workforce and for the purposes of the study the workforce was described as:

> [p]eople who are involved in protecting, promoting and/or restoring the collective health of whole or specific populations (as distinct from activities directed to the care of individuals).
>
> (Rotem et al 1995 p 437)

They found that personnel come from a wide range of professional and occupational backgrounds and that characteristically they are described as having a high degree of versatility and flexibility (Rotem et al 1995). The study suggested that the workforce is made up of mature, highly qualified, multiskilled individuals from a variety of backgrounds, who have multiple functions to perform which are not always related to their primary training or occupation.

In a NSW state-wide consultation by Madden and Salmon (1999) the authors included a third category of health worker as one with public health components included in their professional practice such as general practitioners and community health nurses who need an understanding of population health.

Public health will increasingly become the focus of a range of different health workers as the notion of an expanding scope of practice becomes articulated further. In rural and remote areas where it is difficult to attract health workers the potential inclusion of a primary health care role for nurses and paramedics will involve a focus on prevention and promotion.

Regardless of whether you extend or refine the boundaries around a definition of the public health workforce, what is important is that regardless of where you work, the workforce is principally concerned with organised efforts to protect, promote and restore the health of the population. Chapters 10, 11 and 12 look at the application of many of the principles discussed above using a variety of different public health strategies in a range of settings.

What does the public health worker do? This is the second part of our question. The role of the public health practitioner according to van der Maesen & Nijhuis (2000 p 136) involves three important elements:

1 improving social conditions that stimulate health
2 preventing social conditions that threaten health
3 neutralising existing social conditions that cause ill health.

ACTIVITY: WHAT DO YOU THINK PUBLIC HEALTH WORKERS DO?

- How would you define the public health workforce – would your definition be broad and encompassing or narrow and restrictive?
- Why is that?
- Make a list of the range and scope of activity for the public health worker.
- Select a public health worker – this might be an environmental health officer, a community health nurse, a diabetes educator or a health promotion practitioner for the National Heart Foundation. Write down what you think a typical day might be for such a worker. Make a list of the roles and responsibilities they might have.
- How does this list relate back to the competencies we discussed earlier in the chapter?

While there are core functions for public health workers, the diversity of public health practice is still enormous. The organisation that employs you, the nature of the position, the organisational philosophy, the governance structure of the organisation, whether it is for profit or not for profit, state based or non-government, all impact on the nature and scope of the public health work you might be asked to do.

For Aboriginal and Torres Strait Islander health workers, issues such as the retention of the workforce and the variety of problems that confront health workers in communities pose real challenges. Because these health workers often work in communities with particular cultural issues and values, their needs are quite specific. Add to these issues the lack of public health qualifications for many and the fact that their level of salary is usually at the lower end of the salary scale and you have a complex range of problems. Solutions to such problems, according to Lin et al (2007), include the need for a clear career path, educational pathways and industrial award coverage if the problems of retention and stability are to be solved (Lin et al 2007 p 234).

Even though the public health worker may have different roles and functions according to the setting in which he or she works, there are common aspects of practice that all workers need to be able to perform and to understand. These functions are outlined in Box 2.1.

Box 2.1: Roles and functions for the public health workforce

- Understanding the context for public health activity and its role and functions
- Clarity around political impacts on public health
- Ability to apply a range of methodological approaches to understand data
- A theoretical understanding of the disciplines that underpin public health and their contribute to strategy selection
- Understanding a range of skills around surveillance, prevention, promotion and restoration of the population's health
- Developing and analysing policy
- Planning, implementation and evaluation
- Evidence-based practice
- Advocacy, communication and negotiation skills
- Working intersectorally and with multidisciplinary groups
- Ethical practice

Reflecting on the content covered so far, you should now be feeling confident about your understanding of what public health is, and its role and value in today's society. The complexity of public health processes should also be obvious. For public health to be effective, it cannot be undertaken on an 'ad hoc' basis and must adopt a multidisciplinary approach across a range of professions. Collaborative efforts should engage a number of organisations, both government and non-government, in attempts to strive towards positive health outcomes throughout the population. It is also important to include ethics at the forefront of our practice. Chapter 7 examines the issue of ethics in public health practice in more detail.

The WHO agenda for public health

We now turn our attention to consider public health developments and events that have occurred at an international level. These, to a large extent, have influenced the public health agenda and given direction to initiatives that have been implemented in Australia with the aims of achieving the goals of public health.

WHO has played a significant role in articulating and promoting public health, particularly in promoting the concept of 'health for all', which has been embraced by countries throughout the world, underpinning their respective health policies. For WHO, the extent of public health action has become more difficult to define and has merged with other sectors that influence health opportunities and outcomes. Consequently, WHO has a six-point action plan for health that assists in shaping activity and focus. This six-point plan is outlined in Box 2.2.

Box 2.2: WHO's six-point action plan
1 Promoting development
2 Fostering health security
3 Strengthening health systems
4 Harnessing research, information and evidence
5 Enhancing partnerships
6 Improving performance
(Source: WHO 2008)

Since 1977 WHO and other substantial international players have discussed public health within four conceptual phases (Fleming & Parker 2007). These conceptual phases are not linear in time nor are they sequential in content terms. Many second-world countries still focus on primary health care initiatives as the main aspect of their public health developments and strategies.

In the late 1970s, primary health care as espoused by the WHO *Alma Ata Declaration* stressed the importance of a slogan that said 'Health for all by the year 2000'. This primary health care philosophy spoke about the principles of equity, social justice, intersectoral collaboration, community participation and empowerment. It had as its focus the important role of health promotion and disease prevention. Health promotion is a social and political process, 'it is the process of enabling people to increase control over the determinants of health and thereby improve their health. Participation is essential to sustain health promotion action' (Nutbeam 1998 p 351). (See Chapter 12 for a detailed analysis of the nature and scope of health promotion.)

In the 1980s the lifestyle phase became prominent. At this stage of public health development, Canada was at the forefront of initiatives to focus on the lifestyles of individuals but also to stress the importance of a contribution to people's health that included social issues. Issues considered important included lifestyle, environment, socioeconomic factors and health care system reform.

In the late 1980s and early 1990s, the notion of a 'new public health' emerged. In 1986, in Ottawa, Canada, WHO produced a document called the *Ottawa Charter for Health Promotion* (WHO 1986). This charter claims that there are fundamental prerequisites for health, which are 'peace, shelter, education, food, income, a stable ecosystem, sustainable resources, social justice and equity' (WHO 1986). To promote health the charter referred to five action areas as listed in Box 2.3.

Box 2.3: The Ottawa Charter for Health Promotion

1 Build healthy policies that support health
2 Create supportive environments
3 Strengthen community action
4 Develop personal skills
5 Reorient health services.

(Source: WHO 1986)

The 'new public health' included elements of the 'old public health' and new elements of public health theory and practice. In the 'new public health', the role of public health broadened as a result of recognition that health has strong social and political dimensions. Concepts of social support and social capital became important, as did recognising the need to include a focus on public health in a number of policy debates and outcomes. The term social capital refers to the social environment and its impact on health. For example, 'a community rich in stocks of social capital' has plentiful 'membership in voluntary associations of all kinds', there is strong 'interpersonal trust between citizens' and they perceive that the community provides adequate 'mutual aid' (Lochner et al 1999 p 260). Intersectoral action and a multidisciplinary approach re-emerged as important foci for public health activity, and public health practice focussed on a wide range of health workers. An example of intersectoral collaboration would be where the health sector works with other sectors and organisations such as departments of education, housing and transport and non-government organisations such as the National Heart Foundation (NHF) to facilitate heart health messages to the public. The 'new public health' also included a substantial emphasis on the sustainability of the environment.

In more recent times the global concern for ecosystem sustainability, known in public health circles as ecological public health, has emerged as the predominant theme for public health action in the 21st century. The *Jakarta Declaration* (1997) went some way towards a focus on sustainability and globalisation. However in 2005 the *Bangkok Charter on Health Promotion* identified globalisation as a central issue for health promotion endeavours. Participants at the *Sixth Global Conference on Health Promotion,* co-hosted by WHO and the Ministry of Public Health of Thailand, adopted the charter. It identifies major challenges, actions and commitments needed to address the determinants of health in a globalised world by engaging the many actors and stakeholders critical to achieving health for all. (See Chapter 12 for a more comprehensive account of the *Ottawa Charter,* the *Jakarta Declaration* and the *Bangkok Declaration* in the evolution of health promotion policy and practice).

'Health for all by the year 2000' was clearly not achieved. WHO has reforecast its endeavours in this regard with the production of 'Health for all by 2010' although some regional areas have targets dated to 2020. The emphasis in public health in this revised focus includes sustainable development, collaboration, protection, prevention, resilience, adaptation, the emergence of chronic diseases and the re-emergence of infectious diseases.

In 2000, United Nations member states agreed on eight Millennium Development Goals (MDGs) with targets to be achieved by 2015. Four of these goals relate to health outcomes: eradicating extreme poverty and hunger; improving maternal health; reducing child mortality; and dealing with HIV/AIDS, malaria and other infectious diseases (McMichael & Butler 2007). To achieve any one of these four goals in the next eight years seems almost impossible in the context of the overwhelming range of issues impacting on population health.

In March 2005, WHO created the Commission on Social Determinants of Health (CSDH). The commission operated until May 2008. The components of the CSDH include the commissioners, partner countries, evidence-gathering knowledge networks, civil society organisations and global institutions (Irwin et al 2006 p 0749). The CSDH developed five action areas as outlined in Box 2.4.

Box 2.4: Five key action areas for the CSDH

1 Improving living and learning conditions in early childhood.
2 Strengthening social programs to provide fairer employment conditions and access to labour markets, particularly for vulnerable social groups.
3 Policies and interventions to protect people in informal employment – that is, those who work without formal contracts or social protections, often in sectors outside government regulation, such as subsistence farming, household-based enterprises, and street vending.
4 Policies across sectors to improve living conditions in urban slums.
5 Programs to address key determinants of women's health, such as access to education and economic opportunities.

(Source: Irwin et al 2006, p 0750)

These developments on the international stage are now clearly focussed on health inequalities and ecological sustainability. This clearly recognises that inequalities in health are seeded in the structures of society – economically, politically and culturally, and it will take collaborative efforts across sectors to bring good health within the reach of everyone. Chapter 13 discusses the impact of globalisation on health where many of these issues are covered in more detail. Ecological sustainability is considered in Chapters 11 and 15.

The new public health and ecological sustainability are important issues for healthy public policy to address now and in the future. In addition, public health should be conscious of socioeconomic factors that impinge on people and the social systems in which they live. The *Ottawa Charter for Health Promotion* (WHO 1986) is very relevant to the new public health and beyond, as it is said to be the first document to begin to articulate this agenda.

You will hear the term 'intersectoral approach' used often in this book. It is very relevant in developing healthy public policies as it recognises the need to harness the cooperation between governments, government departments, the private sector and non-government organisations, if policies are going to be effective in achieving the maximum positive impact on the health of the population.

In concluding this section of the chapter, it is important to remember that the 'new public health' and ecological sustainability recognise all components of people's lives and they take into account the impact that these factors have on the health of populations or subgroups of populations. For example, individuals alone are not totally responsible for their health status. Although they need to adopt positive behaviours in regard to their health, factors such as the environment in which they live, their economic status, and their culture are some of the things which, although they have little or no control over, can have a significant impact on their health. Ecological public health, with its focus on sustainable environments for health, has evolved as the main focus of public health in the 21st century.

Public health in the Australian context

In Australia, managing public health activity is multilayered and is influenced by the prevailing political thinking. In this chapter, we introduce you to the systems and organisational arrangements for public health activity. In Chapter 3 we provide you with more specific information about the health care system and its relationship to public health and the range of policy initiatives supporting public health.

The division of responsibility for public health includes the Australian Government Department of Health and Ageing, state and territory health departments, local government departments, non-government organisations, professional associations and a range of advocacy groups. In addition, people such as general practitioners and health workers in community health centres also undertake health protection and health promotion roles and responsibilities.

A number of other organisations also play a role. The National Health and Medical Research Council (NHMRC) fund public health research and make policy statements on health issues; the Australian Institute of Health and Welfare (AIHW) and the Australian Bureau of Statistics (ABS) monitor and report on health data; and universities train public health, allied health, medical and nursing professionals, and undertake research and consultancy activity in public health. Divisions of general practice also play an important role in advancing population health.

Australian Government Department of Health and Ageing

The Population Health Division and the Office of Aboriginal and Torres Strait Islander Services, within the Australian Government Department of Health and Ageing, both play a role in national leadership in important public health matters, such as communicable diseases, immunisation, nutrition and obesity, physical activity, food policy, smoking, alcohol and drug abuse. The division identifies itself as playing a number of roles in creating and supporting national endeavours in public health. These activities are listed in Box 2.5.

Box 2.5: Role of the Population Health Division, Australian Government Department of Health and Ageing

- Leadership and coordination of a range of national initiatives.
- Supporting activities aimed at understanding and controlling the determinants of disease.
- Informed decision making based on effective use of health information, and on the application of research evidence in the design of programs to improve health.
- Relationship building between staff of the department and a range of stakeholders, from states and territories through to academic institutions and non-government organisations.
- Working with these stakeholders to expand its knowledge of factors affecting the health of the population and specific at-risk groups such as Aboriginal and Torres Strait Islander communities and populations located in rural and remote Australia.

The division has identified a number of broad priorities for public health that focus on identifying and responding to emerging threats and health emergencies like SARS and avian influenza and a focus on prevention particularly in areas such as nutrition, physical activity, overweight and obesity. The division has an emphasis on responding to health issues throughout the lifecourse. It also established, in 1996, the National Public Health Partnership (NPHP), creating a framework for public health leadership and to strengthen collaboration between stakeholders. The NPHP was disbanded in 2006.

The Australian Government allocates to states a 'broadbanded' purpose grant (known as the *Public Health Outcome Funding Agreement*) for key population health programs, including drugs, women's health, cervical and breast screening and childhood immunisation.

There are a number of federally supported organisations and legislation that protect and enhance the health of the population. These include the Therapeutic Goods Administration, Food Standards Australia New Zealand, Australian Radiation Protection and Nuclear Safety Agency and the Australian Safety and Compensation Council.

To build a prevention agenda in a health system that currently expends the majority of its funds on treatment is an ongoing challenge. As the costs of treatment continue to rise, and health technology becomes more sophisticated and expensive, a focus on prevention should gain greater traction in the health system. In addition, the emergence of chronic diseases, such as diabetes, means that people will be living a large part of their lives managing conditions like this. Therefore, prevention will have to become a priority if the State is going to continue to be able to fund the health system in the way that Australians have become accustomed to. The Australian Government is attempting to make prevention a fundamental pillar of the health system. This will be a difficult task, given the strength of some health interest groups that have managed to lobby effectively with a succession of governments around their own focus and needs.

Having a health workforce able to respond to the prevention agenda is also a very important component of the equation as is the building of strong collaborations across agencies, particularly in areas like transport, education and the environment.

Another very important aspect of the leadership role at the federal level is to have in place information systems that can alert us to emerging health issues. Australia has made considerable investments in information systems development and has made significant progress in the alignment and coordination of health information. However, even though there is a good information base for public health action, one of the common criticisms of the system is that the data collection is not sufficiently timely nor is it related to particular communities of interest. Also seen as a weakness are a lack of data that track health patterns over time and insufficient comparative data (Lin et al 2007 p 216). The paucity of data around these issues makes it more difficult for public health professionals to gain access to and use appropriate information for decision making. The activity below asks you to stop and think about the role of the federal government in public health and a number of important issues that face the government in the coming years such as health care costs and funding.

ACTIVITY: ADVANCING PUBLIC HEALTH – THE AUSTRALIAN PERSPECTIVE

- In the past 10 years what have been the major foci of national developments in public health in Australia?
- What factors may have influenced national developments? For example, change in political party, health crises, changing patterns of health.
- What role can non-government organisations play in public health?

- Do you think the ecological public health movement has advanced the activities of public health in the public mind?
- How do we balance health care needs with population health needs in order to be able to fund the health system in the future?

REFLECTION

The federal government, in the past 20 or so years, has played a policy and strategic role in advancing population health. This strategic role has meant an emphasis on the policy and the identification of major areas for national development, the detail of which is often translated at state/territory and local government levels. For example, the Population Health Division has set a national agenda for healthy eating and increased physical activity. At the state/territory level that national agenda has been translated into actions that more clearly meet the needs of the population. Do you think that non-government agencies such as the Cancer Fund or the NHF have been included in policy initiatives at the federal level? How might you determine if they have been given a role? How is ecological public health defined? Ask five of your friends if they understand what ecological public health is all about. In the next chapter there will be more detail about funding for public health in a health care system where the majority of current funds are expended on care and treatment. What health professional might want funding levels to remain as they are?

State and territory governments

At the state/territory level of public health activity responsibility includes managing public hospitals and community health services; leadership and planning of public health; health surveillance; local government regulation and health promotion, including working with non-government and other organisations (Baum 2008). A summary of these functions is provided in Box 2.6.

Box 2.6: State/territory government functions
- *Health protection* – such as environmental health, drugs and poisons
- *Disease prevention* – examples include surveillance, health education, immunisation, STI (sexually transmitted infection) and cancer screening
- *Health promotion* – including a focus on physical activity, nutrition, maternal and child health, tobacco, drugs and alcohol and injury prevention
- *Policy and program support* – epidemiology, evaluation, research, workforce development, policy development within and outside the sector impacting on health, and clinical service guidelines

(Adapted from Lin et al 2007)

Other roles and responsibilities include that of the chief health officer under whose authority many health activities are located and who exercises statutory responsibilities. These include environmental protection, occupational health and safety, road and traffic authority, sport and recreation and consumer affairs. Education departments in each state have a major role to play in promotion and prevention through the health curriculum, health promoting schools and a range of other activities including *Sun Smart, Healthy Tuckshops*, drug and alcohol programs such as PROMAS (*Promoting Adjustment in Schools*) and driver education. Emergency services departments in each state also play a role in promotion and prevention. For example, with the changing scope of practice, health workers such as ambulance officers play an important role in providing information and education to the general public, and in rural and remote communities as primary health care workers.

In Queensland, like many other states, a whole-of-government approach is taken where public health and many other services form part of a more integrated approach to promotion and prevention, and the multisectoral nature of public health is recognised and supported. The success of such approaches of course depends upon political will, interdepartmental collaboration and positive interaction between all tiers of government.

Local government

Local government has a critical role to play in public health, especially in the area of legislation and creating healthy communities. Local governments' roles in public health activity vary across Australia, but more often than not still include such functions as well baby clinics, immunisation, food safety, environmental protection, a strong role in cultural and recreational activities and community development and importantly local economic development.

ACTIVITY: HEALTH IN THE PUBLIC ARENA

- On a regular basis, the media will report on public health issues, initiatives, developments, etc. The newspaper is an effective communication vehicle by which the public's awareness may be raised about an issue or an event that directly, or indirectly, impacts on the public's health. What are examples of recent newspaper articles that you can find that deal with a public health issue?

PUBLIC HEALTH ISSUES IN THE DAILY PRESS

Identify and source two articles that comment or report on a current public health issue.
Write a brief review of each newspaper article. Use the following questions to frame your comments:

- Why is it a public health issue? Think about our discussion of definitions of public health.
- What population or subpopulation is involved?
- What strategies, if any, are being implemented to address the issue or concern?
- What component or components of the public health system would take responsibility, for example, the state health department or a non-government organisation?
- What are the future ramifications if the issue or concern is not addressed?

Non-government organisations (NGOs), community organisations, professional associations and public health advocacy groups

There are a broad range of organisations and associations that support public health endeavours in Australia. That support comes in a variety of different ways. For example, large well-funded NGOs such as the cancer councils, the National Heart Foundation and Diabetes Australia have a range of roles, including information and education, fundraising, advocacy, lobbying and research, in the promotion of health and the detection and treatment of specific health issues.

Other organisations, such as professional associations, play an important role in lobbying, advocacy and policy development as well as workforce education through conferences and professional development activities. These associations include the Public Health Association of Australia, the Australian Health Promotion Association, the Australasian Epidemiology Association and the Australian Institute of Environmental Health.

A third group of organisations are those focussed on advocacy and lobbying, including the Women's Health Network, the Consumer Health Forum and the National Association of Aboriginal Community-Controlled Health Organisations (Baum 2008).

Health promotion foundations are variously integrated into state health departments or have been set up to stand independently of a departmental structure. They have an important role in funding research activities and their application and, in some jurisdictions, an advocacy and lobbying role.

To the above list, Baum (2008) adds primary health care providers and universities and research institutions. Primary health care providers include general practitioners, who play a role in screening, immunisation and the health education of patients. Universities and research institutes both have an education and research function.

The future for public health?

There are a number of emerging challenges that public health faces moving into the 21st century. These challenges include the emergence of 'new' infectious diseases, the ongoing presence of HIV/AIDS (particularly in developing countries) and the impact that overweight and obesity has on a range of health issues that impact on the population's health. Add to these issues the influence of global climate change and ecological sustainability and you have a public health system stretched to capacity across a range of fronts. As McMichael and Butler (2007) succinctly state:

> The big task is to promote sustainable environmental and social conditions that bring enduring and equitable health gains.
>
> (McMichael & Butler 2007 p 15)

Through the book, we continually return to these themes and issues as we explore the nature and scope of public health.

A final word

In this chapter, we have covered a broad range of issues that are reflective of elements of public health. We have examined definitions of health, both lay and professional; we have considered the definition, vision and values of public health; and the role of a wide range of health workers who play an important role in public health.

We have considered the role of WHO in setting a global agenda for public health and the specific role of governments at three levels in Australia from federal to state and local government. We introduced you to the range of other associations, community organisations and advocacy groups who all play important roles in improving the health of the population.

In conclusion, we briefly introduced you to public health issues emerging in the 21st century and the challenges that face professionals working in the public health field if they are to deal with these emerging issues. We return to these issues in the last chapter of the book.

In the chapter that follows, we examine contemporary public health policy initiatives and planning and management of public health activity.

REVIEW QUESTIONS

1　What do you understand by the terms health, illness, disease and public health?
2　Why should public health have a vision and what values should public health workers espouse and practice?
3　Write down the core tasks of public health, and think about how these might differ in the future.

4   Who is the public health practitioner and what do you believe to be the core functions of a public health worker?
5   Make up a table of the three levels of government in Australia and in each column describe the public health roles and responsibilities.
6   What role do NGOs play in public health?
7   List and briefly comment on the issues you believe will be facing public health in the 21st century.

REFERENCES

Baum F 2002 The new public health, 2nd edn. Oxford University Press, South Melbourne

Baum F 2008 The new public health, 3rd edn. Oxford University Press, South Melbourne

Beaglehole R, Bonita R, Horton R et al 2004 Public Health in the New Era: improving health through collaborative action. Lancet 363:2084–2086

Bircher J 2005 Towards a dynamic definition of health and disease. Medicine, Health Care and Philosophy 8:335–341

Blaxter M 1990 Health and lifestyles. Tavistock/Routledge, London, New York

Blaxter M 2007 How is Health Experienced. In: Douglas J, Earle S, Handsley S et al (eds) A reader in promoting public health. Sage Publications, London

Brown V A, Grootjans J, Ritchie J et al (eds) 2005 Sustainability and Health: Supporting global ecological integrity in public health. Allen and Unwin, Crows Nest

Durie M 2004 Understanding health and illness. International Journal of Epidemiology 33: 1138–1114

Fleming M L, Parker E 2007 Health Promotion: Principles and practice in the Australian context, 3rd edn. Allen & Unwin, Sydney

Gostin L O et al 2004 Health of the people: the highest law? The Journal of Law, Medicine and Ethics 32(3):509–515

Griffiths S, Jewell T, Donnelly P 2005 Public health in practice: the three domains of public health. Public Health 119(10):907–913

Institute of Medicine, Committee for the Study of the Future of Public Health, Division of Health Care Services 1998 The future of public health. National Academy Press, Washington DC

Irwin A, Valentine N, Brown C et al 2006 The Commission on Social Determinants of Health: Tackling the Social Roots of Health Inequities. PLoS Medicine 3(6);e106:0749–0751

Last J M 2001 A dictionary of epidemiology, 4th edn. Oxford University Press, New York

Lawson J S, Bauman A E 2001 Public health Australia: an introduction. McGraw-Hill, Sydney

Lin V, Smith J, Fawkes S 2007 Public Health Practice in Australia: The organised effort. Allen & Unwin, Sydney

Lochner K, Kawachi I, Kennedy B P 1999 Social capital: A guide to its measurement. Health and Place 5:259–270

Madden L, Salmon A 1999 Public health workforce: Results of a NSW statewide consultation on the development of the national public health workforce. NSW Public Health Bulletin 10(3):19–21

McMichael A J, Butler C D 2007 Emerging health issues: the widening challenge for population health promotion. Health Promotion International 21(Suppl 1):15–24

Maher P 1999 A review of 'traditional' Aboriginal health beliefs. Australian Journal of Rural Health 7:229–236

Maslow A H 1999 Toward a psychology of being. John Wiley, New York

National Aboriginal Health Strategy Working Party 1989 A National Aboriginal Health Strategy. Department of Aboriginal Affairs, Canberra

National Public Health Partnership 2000 Public Health Practice in Australia Today: A Statement of Core Functions. NPHP, Melbourne

Nutbeam D 1998 Health promotion glossary. Health Promotion International 13(4):349–364

Proposed Competencies for the Public Health Education Research Program (PHERP) 2007 Australian Government Department of Health and Ageing, Canberra

Public Health Association of Australia Website. Available: http://www.phaa.net.au/ 7 Jan 2008

Rotem A, Walters J, Dewdney J 1995 Editorial: The public health workforce education and training study. Australian Journal of Public Health 19(5):437–438

Schneider M-J 2006 Introduction to public health. Jones & Bartlett, Sudbury

Thompson S J, Gifford S M 2000 Trying to keep a balance: the meaning of health and diabetes in an urban Aboriginal community. Social Science & Medicine 61:1457–1472

Turnock B 2001 Public Health: What It Is and How It Works, 2nd edn. Aspen Publishers, Gaithersburg

van der Maesen L J G, Nijhuis H G J 2000 Continuing the debate on the philosophy of modern public health: social quality as a point of reference. Journal of Epidemiology and Community Health 54:134–14

Waltner-Toews D 2000 The end of medicine: the beginning of health. Futures 32:655–667

Winslow C E A 1920 The Untilled Field of Public Health. Science 9:23–33

World Health Organization 1948 Constitution. WHO. Available: http://www.searo.who.int/ LinkFiles/About_SEARO_const.pdf

World Health Organization 1986 Ottawa Charter for Health Promotion. WHO: Geneva. Available: http://www.euro.who.int/aboutwho/policy/20010827_2 26 Jul 2007

World Health Organization 2005 Bangkok Charter for Health Promotion. World Health Organization (WHO), Geneva

World Health Organization 2008 The WHO Agenda. Available: http://www.who.int/about/ agenda/en/index.html 15 Jan 2008

CHAPTER 3

Contemporary public health policy and management

Elizabeth Parker

Learning objectives

After reading this chapter, you should be able to:

- identify the terms policy, public policy and health policy, the stages of policy development and the role that values play in policymaking
- recognise contemporary international developments in public health and their impact on national policymaking and the health of Australians
- describe the basic structure and financing of Australia's health system and the role of public health within it
- identify Australia's national public health priorities and be able to critique the development of the HIV/AIDS policy, Aboriginal health policy and other contemporary policies impacting on Australia's health.

Introduction

This chapter extends your understanding of the concepts of public health and its history in order to examine contemporary public health policy, both in Australia and internationally. Changing policy contexts can influence professional practice. For example, there are increasing roles for allied health professionals in preventing and managing chronic diseases (diabetes, heart disease, specific cancers). The policy framework for chronic disease initiatives and the priorities placed on these stem from national public health policy investments, so being conversant with the process of policymaking for health in Australia will provide you with a solid foundation in your public health practice. This chapter provides an introductory overview of contemporary health priorities and points you to a series of extra readings and websites to complement the beginning of this complex set of issues. It is important knowledge because all health professionals need to be familiar with the contexts in which they practise. We also introduce you to the role of values in public policymaking and give some of examples to demonstrate this connection. The World Health Organization (WHO), which acts as a global health 'thermometer' in identifying health trends, is introduced. These health trends, identified in a recent WHO report, also impact on Australia's health policy. Australia's health care system and our national public health priorities are introduced, as are specific national health policies, for example, those targeted at improving the health of Australian Aboriginal and Torres Strait Islanders.

What is policy?

Policy has various definitions. The National Cabinet in the United Kingdom defines policy as '… the process by which governments translate their political vision into programs and actions to deliver "outcomes" … desired changes in the "real world" (Cabinet Office 1999). Policy can also be defined as a broad pattern or framework of collective action in a particular field (e.g. economic policy or health policy), based on specific decisions that aim to realise the visions and goals of that field. Policy is usually about problem solving, but it can also be about preventing a problem or minimising the impact of a problem.

Palmer and Short (2000) claimed that policy can refer to a number of intentions and actions, and some of their points have been adapted below. Policy can refer to:

- a very general statement of intentions and objectives (political leaders make policy speeches during parliamentary election campaigns with 'our policy' statements prefacing many speeches prior to elections)
- the past set of actions of government in a particular area, such as economic policy, foreign policy, refugee policy or health policy
- a specific statement of future intentions, for example, 'Our policy will allow people to take up private health insurance'
- a set of standing rules intended as a guide to action or inaction such as, 'It is our policy not to interfere in those matters that are the responsibilities of the states' (Palmer & Short 2000 p 23).

The focus of policy is usually about reform, establishing priority goals and accomplishing policy objectives. Policy can thus be seen as the exercise of argument through the use of evidence, and an ability to juggle competing interests to achieve a collective purpose. Lin and Gibson claim that 'policymaking is based on discussion and persuasion and making a good argument' (2003 p 256).

Box 3.1: Stages of the policy process

1 Identifying issues and determining goals.
2 Policy analysis: designing, determining and considering policy options and their potential consequences.
3 Identifying policy instruments: These may include laws, programs, infrastructure or informative materials.
4 Consultation and coordination. Identifying and involving the key people who have an interest in the policy process and outcomes (these are often referred to as stakeholders). This should also include those who will be affected by the policy.
5 Choosing courses of action and putting these decisions through an approval process.
6 Implementing these courses of action.
7 Evaluating the results, outcomes and consequences of the policy.
8 Adjusting the policy where necessary.

(Source: Department of the Premier and Cabinet)

Stages of the policy process

In an ideal situation, the policy process consists of a number of stages, and these are outlined in Box 3.1. In reality, there are often no discernable stages and no rational sequence because the policy process is changeable and engages many players.

Determining policy goals is often not as easy as it sounds, as interested parties and different stakeholders can analyse a problem differently, and may have varied ideas regarding the most suitable action to take.

ACTIVITY

- Pick up a national or state newspaper and scan for policy initiatives proposed by a state or the federal government; then write down how your chosen policy fits with the intentions and actions proposed by Palmer and Short (2000).

REFLECTION

Did you notice if the policy was a general statement of intentions and objectives? For example, the new federal government has issued a general statement about administering public hospitals. Was the policy that you found about past actions of government or a set of standing rules to guide action or inaction? This is an important activity as it allows you to discern differences or similarities in the intentions or objectives of policies to realise specific goals.

Policy can be seen, therefore, as a framework for actions on specific issues. Policies are also shaped by implicit values and norms, yet these are often not made explicit in the policymaking process or in the implementation of policies. Here is an example. Policies about and towards Indigenous Australians have reflected a set of social, cultural and political values that have changed over time. Protectionism was the policy enacted in the first half of the 20th century when Indigenous Australians were segregated and there was no regard for their human rights. This was perpetuated by the 'White Australia' policy. However, a period of social change began in the 1960s, with a growing 'political and social consciousness among the general community and the plight of Aboriginal people constituted an urgent human rights issue' (Couzos & Murray 2003 p 5). There were mobilisation actions by Indigenous Australians, which led to the first Aboriginal community-controlled health organisation in 1971 at Redfern. So policies about improving the health of Aboriginal and Torres Strait Islander Australians reflected an evolving set of societal values. Self-determination was a key principle in establishing and maintaining Aboriginal and Torres Strait Islander community-controlled health organisations.

Policies by their very nature cannot be value free. Values underpin how governments distribute and redistribute resources, and how judgements are made in implementing policy, as the following example by Gibson (2003) illustrates.

Case study: Breast cancer screening

In the 1980s Australian policymakers grappled with whether to introduce mammography screening for breast cancer. There was empirical evidence that mammography screening was an effective tool for early cancer detection for older women. The question was asked, 'How should we decide whether or not to introduce mammography screening?' The screening principles adopted by WHO in 1968 (Wilson & Junger 1968) came into play by posing the question not only about the importance of the disease, but also about the acceptability of the screening test to the population. The values held by women about screening and its acceptability were taken into consideration, thus, the policy combines 'empirical criteria' (the evidence of the effectiveness of mammography screening) with 'value criteria' (the acceptability of the service to women).

(Source: Gibson in Lin & Gibson 2003)

Drugs and alcohol policies are often fraught with different and sometimes conflicting viewpoints. For example, should the sale of alcohol be made more widely available or restricted? And should taxes on alcohol be increased? How should people who are users of illegal drugs be dealt with? Should they be dealt with through the criminal justice system or through rehabilitation programs? And do high-performing athletes who use illegal drugs receive different attention and treatment compared with non-athletes, and why? The next case study adapted from Lin and Gibson (2003) on harm minimisation[1] for injecting drug users shows how empirical evidence together with values, and a focus on the care of individuals, were blended into a policy framework in establishing safe injecting facilities.

Case study: Needle syringe programs

In 1986, the first needle and syringe program (NSP) began in Sydney as a pilot project to address the high prevalence of needle sharing among injecting drug users, thus reducing the spread of the human immunodeficiency virus (HIV). Other states, except for Tasmania, developed similar programs. Despite the public controversies, particularly in the late 1990s, international and Australian research demonstrated that NSP programs were effective in maintaining low rates of needle-sharing-related HIV transmission. The value of harm minimisation and empirical research are linked under a policy framework of harm minimisation, through enabling individuals to self-care and reduce harm and through the coordinated efforts of public health workers, law enforcement workers and drug user groups.

In this discussion of policy, we are reminded of the claim (at that time, a somewhat audacious one) of the great 17th century German pathologist, Rudolph Virchow – that 'political action as well as rational science is necessary to initiate action to control public health problems' (Gunn et al 2005 p 11).

ACTIVITY

- In Chapter 2 you were introduced to a number of contemporary public health issues that you may have taken for granted in a typical day, and our case studies illustrate how values play a part in policymaking. Choose one of the national public health policies (from the federal government's Department of Health and Ageing website) of interest to you and analyse what, if any, values underpin the policy. One tip might be to look at the national mental health policy. See 'Useful websites' at the end of this chapter for the government link.

REFLECTION

Did the policy statement identify any explicit values within it? For example, harm minimisation, universal access to prevention and treatment services, equity? If you are doing this activity with other students and were not unanimous in your thinking, you can see how the policymaking process is complex and embraces and considers many viewpoints and values.

We now turn to an introduction on various types of public policies.

Types of public policies

Obviously, various public policies affect the way communities live, their quality of life and access to services. A number of authors have tried to categorise different types of public policies, and these insights can assist us in analysing health policies. The following categorisation provides an insightful view of how policies are perceived.

Distributive policies

These policies involve providing services or benefits to particular sections of the population. An example would be pensions to people with a disability or older people, pensioner health benefit cards for those who qualify, Youth Allowance or building a hospital in a growing suburb. They are relatively non-controversial and are implemented 'without any noticeable reduction in the benefits provided to other groups' (Palmer & Short 2000 p 24).

Regulatory policies

These are policies that place restrictions or limitations on the behaviour of individuals and groups. For example, tobacco control policies are regulatory policies that restrict the sale of tobacco to minors, restrict smoking in public places and increase taxes on the sale of tobacco products. Regulatory policies can also include the registration of teachers, nurses and other professionals who must be licensed to practise their profession (Palmer & Short 2000).

Self-regulatory policies

These policies are those often sought by organisations as a means of 'promoting their own interest' (Palmer & Short 2000 p 24). Some actions by self-regulatory boards can be seen in the establishment of the 'Australian Council on Healthcare Standards (ACHS) that accredits hospital and nursing homes' (Palmer & Short 2000 p 24).

Redistributive policies

These policies are those that attempt to redistribute income and wealth in the population. A classic example in health is the universal health insurance scheme, Medicare, which is financed by a compulsory income tax contribution. For those who are unemployed and/or for low-income earners, health insurance is subsidised by others. The principle of 'universality' is a strong principle and value in public health, and there are other examples of such redistribution, for example, free access to cervical cancer screening and mammography screening in public hospitals and clinics, mass vaccination against childhood diseases where the costs are borne by the State and vaccination is universally available to all, irrespective of the cost (Palmer & Short 2000).

These four types of public policy are not without criticism. Hayes (2007) claims that these typologies are limited in that they don't necessarily consider the influence on policy of 'political patterning' – in other words, the political dynamics that can influence policies, particularly redistributive policies. The influence of politics on policy should be understood within the policymaking process in a democracy like Australia; especially if one considers that the derivation of the word 'policy' shares its roots with *politics, policy and polity*, that is, it is related to 'people and the needs of groups of people, be they patients, providers, communities or states' (Leeder 1999 p 74). So what are the influences of these types of policies on health outcomes?

Each of these types of policy has some bearing on the health of populations, as can be seen by the examples noted. So is there one type of policy that has a specific impact on public health? Navarro et al (2006) analysed public health outcomes and policy developments in the Organisation of Economic Cooperation and Development (OECD) countries with different political systems and various kinds of health insurance policies such as Australia's Medicare. The findings suggest that 'countries with redistributive policies were positively associated with health outcomes' (Navarro et al 2006 p 1035), and that a long period of government with pro-redistributive policies is associated with low infant mortality.

ACTIVITY

● Define 'distributive', 'redistributive', 'regulatory' and 'self-regulatory' policies. Make a list of the advantages and disadvantages of these types of public policy. How do these types of public policies impact on health policy? Write down some examples. Can you think of community groups or health professions who are influential in making public health policy? How are their voices heard?

REFLECTION

Did you notice any common themes in your list of advantages and disadvantages of these types of policies for improving the health of the population? Is it possible to have a mix of types of policies to improve population health? What community groups or health professions did you identify? Are physicians and nurses influential in the distribution of resources for public health policy? Apart from health professionals, who else is influential in setting policy directions for health?

What is policy for?

The focus of policy is on reform, and in public health, is to promote and restore the health of populations. Health policies are tools that can be used to identify, plan responses to and act on prioritised health problems. According to Manciaux and Fliedner (2005), a health problem can be considered critically significant if it:

- contributes substantially to the burden of illness in a population, in terms of prevalence and/or severity
- has the potential of becoming a significant risk to community health status and general welfare
- represents a major and identifiable financial cost to the community and/or the health care system
- is amendable to improvement, thus increasing political and public pressure for corrective action.

Health policies and priorities must be periodically revised and adapted according to changing patterns of ill health and mortality data, as the two examples of breast cancer and drug use demonstrated.

Last (2005) identified five essential ingredients of the policy processes that were influential in the public health reforms of the 19th and 20th centuries. Still totally relevant to contemporary public health policy, he summarised them as:

1 awareness that the problem exists
2 understanding the causes
3 capability to control the causes
4 the belief (sense of values) that the problem is important
5 political will.

So where do these policymaking foundations and processes sit in an international context?

International developments and their impact on contemporary health policies

In Chapter 2 you were introduced to WHO's six-point plan (WHO 2008). WHO's influence on contemporary health policy is substantial and it's important to reflect on its history. Over 50 years have passed since WHO was constituted, yet its relevance to public health policies and practice is still profound as it identifies world trends for public health action.

WHO was formed in 1946 in an international climate of hope for promoting a better, more peaceful future, after the chaos of the Second World War (1939–1945). Three physicians – from China, Norway and Brazil – proposed the formulation of a single health organisation that would address the health needs of the world's people. Their joint declaration to establish such an international health organisation was approved when the constitution was adopted in 1946. There are currently 191 member countries, and its headquarters are in Geneva, Switzerland. The WHO constitution stated:

> [t]he enjoyment of the highest attainable standard of health is one of the fundamental rights of every human being without distinction of race, religion, political belief, economic or social condition.
>
> (WHO 1946 p 1)

WHO identifies several principles that underpin global and national health policies:

- The health of all peoples is fundamental to the attainment of peace and security and is dependent upon the fullest cooperation of individuals and States.
- The achievement of any State in the promotion and protection of health is of value to all.
- Unequal development in different countries in the promotion of health and control of disease, especially communicable disease, is a common danger.
- Healthy development of the child is of basic importance; the ability to live harmoniously in a changing total environment is essential to such development.
- The extension to all peoples of the benefits of medical, psychological and related knowledge is essential to the fullest attainment of health.
- Informed opinion and active cooperation on the part of the public are of the utmost importance in the improvement of the health of the people.
- Governments have a responsibility for the health of their peoples, which can be fulfilled only by the provision of adequate health and social measures (WHO 1948).

WHO's report, *Preventing Chronic Disease: A Vital Investment* (2005), is a pivotal document that examines the rise of chronic disease in the developing world. And contrary to popular belief that chronic conditions such as heart disease, diabetes, cancers and chronic obstructive pulmonary disease (COPD) occur more frequently in countries like Australia, four out of five chronic-disease deaths in the world now occur in low- and middle-income countries. In this report, WHO has assembled global data and made recommendations for future attention. This report demonstrates the role of WHO in monitoring health across the globe.

At about the same time as WHO was being established, world leaders wanted a fresh and peaceful start to a post-world-war world and, in 1945, representatives of 50 countries met in San Francisco at the *United Nations Conference on International Organization* to draw up the *United Nations Charter*. The United Nations officially came into existence on 24 October 1945. On 10 December 1948 the General Assembly of the United Nations adopted and proclaimed the *Universal Declaration of Human Rights*, a bold and compelling document. (See the website listed at the end of the chapter for the full text of the document.) The declaration was seen as a common standard of achievement for all people and all nations and, through teaching and education, would 'promote respect for these rights and freedoms'. Article 25 (1) is relevant in our discussions on health policy. It claims that:

> [e]veryone has the right to a standard of living adequate for the health and wellbeing of himself and of his family, including food, clothing, housing and medical care and necessary social services, and the right to security in the event of unemployment, sickness, disability, widowhood, old age or other lack of livelihood in circumstances beyond his control.
>
> (United Nations General Assembly 1948 p 5)

The international policy architecture, once the domain of governments and non-government organisations, such as World Vision and other faith-based organisations, is altering with the energetic entry of private philanthropists and public–private partnerships working in health. Here is an example.

Example: The UN's Global Fund

The *Global Fund* was established in 2001 through the United Nations Secretary-General as an investment attempt to ensure that the *Millennium Development Goals* were met (see Ch 2). The *Global Fund*, administered through the World Bank, is a different mechanism from previous development assistance agencies. It is a public–private partnership (PPP) 'tasked with administering and allocating funds provided by both governments and private sector donors to countries to combat HIV/AIDS, malaria and tuberculosis' (Feachem 2007). Other public–private partnerships have been established including links between the Clinton Foundation, Global Fund, World Bank and UNICEF to assist with price reductions of AIDS drugs and diagnostics for disease identification. The Bill and Melinda Gates Foundation is a global health foundation that has funded health projects in over 100 countries, including the United States. (See the websites at the end of this chapter for more details of this enterprise.)

As you can see, the dynamics and opportunities presented in the international health policy arena create potential for learning and translation into national policy developments in Australia, to assist us in creating health opportunities and services for all.

ACTIVITY

Write down the answers to the following questions:
- What is the relevance of WHO for Australia's contemporary health policies?
- What importance can you see for Article 25 (1) in policy development in Australia, particularly the role of individual 'rights'?
- Is there scope in Australia for public–private investment in public health policy?

REFLECTION

Did you respond that WHO is relevant to Australia's policies? If so, how is it relevant? Can you give examples of its influence? What examples did you come up with for public–private investments in Australia? There are many non-government organisations such as the cancer councils that contribute to health and these are usually not for profit. Did you think of any private companies that contribute to health policies? Would private health insurance be considered? Research how private health insurance contributes to improving the public's health.

In the next section we introduce you to the Australian health care system and health policy. This is only a brief introduction as there are numerous books available for you to delve further into this topic. Some suggestions are Duckett (2007), Barraclough and Gardner (2008) and Gardner and Barraclough (2002).

Health policy and the Australian health care system

Health policy and health care policy are terms that are used interchangeably. In political and media terms, health care policy can have a focus on 'illness care' with its nearly daily focus on the funding crises of hospitals, reduction of elective waiting lists and workforce shortfalls in specific professions, particularly in rural and remote Australia. Health policy is simultaneously the goal, instrument and process by which systemic health-related decisions are made, implemented and evaluated. It is influenced by many factors including public consciousness, political power and will, scientific understanding and economic and environmental concerns.

Gardner and Barraclough (2002) claimed that 'health' in Australia includes medical and pharmaceutical services, institutions (e.g. hospitals, nursing homes and ambulance services), medical aids and appliances, non-institutional services such as community services and public health, dental services and health research. With this vast canvas illustrating how 'health' is used every day, health policy debates can range across a broad spectrum of issues! And contain many vested interests.

Health expenditure is a large sector of the economy, consuming around 9.7% of the gross domestic product[2] and a significant proportion of both Commonwealth and state government outlays (Duckett 2007 p 37). So financing the health system is always going to be a challenge, in terms of rising consumer expectations, changing patterns of disease and illness in society, treatment options and the competing interests of various health professions.

In 2003–04 Australia spent $78.3 billion on health services. Figure 3.1 shows the expenditure breakdown.

Taylor et al (2007) identify three distinct features of Australia's health system. The first is the intricate web of relationships between the Australian Government (previously called the Commonwealth of Australia) and the states and territories. The federal government maintains a critical role in funding health care for all Australians and has played an increasing role in establishing a national agenda for health priorities and coordinated action.

The second feature is Medicare – Australia's universal health insurance system – introduced in 1984. Medicare has had several iterations from Medibank that was established in 1974. Under Medicare, all Australians have equal access to care in a public hospital: 'out-of hospital medical services at no, or minimal, cost to the service user due to benefits paid under Medicare and affordable pharmaceuticals through the Pharmaceutical Benefits Scheme (PBS)' (Taylor et al 2007 p 48).

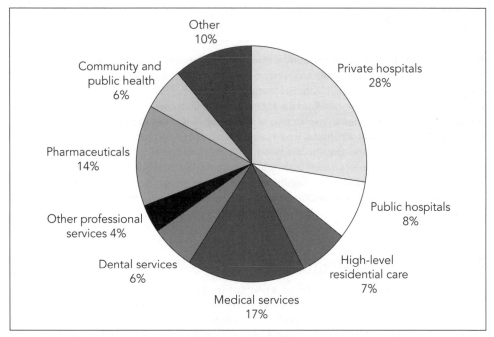

FIGURE 3.1: Distribution of recurrent health expenditure by area of the health system 2003–04

(Reproduced by permission of Oxford University Press Australia from The Australian Health Care System by Duckett © Oxford University Press)

The third feature of Australia's health care system has been the growth of the 'private sector' in health care, and 'between 1999 and 2001 there have been a number of tax incentives introduced to encourage people to take up private health insurance' (Taylor et al 2007 p 48). Taylor et al (2007) claim that this has meant individuals are paying more for their health care and are incurring more 'out of pocket' payments for services.

Another feature of Australia's health system is the role of consumers through such networks and forums as the Consumers' Health Forum of Australia, formed in the mid 1980s. The forum is important in providing feedback to the government about the community viewpoint on health issues and government health initiatives. The forum can reach approximately one million people and represents the voices of patients, consumers and health professionals in commenting on policy initiatives and being engaged in policymaking.

Duckett claims that the arguments that increasing private spending is a 'good thing' become 'somewhat muddied' 'because advocates of increased private spending are usually from wealthier groups … this disguises a redistributive intent from the poor who are more reliant on tax-funded services' (2007 p 40). So, with these distinct features of the health system, what are the roles of the various levels of government and how is health care funded? In the next section, we introduce aspects of the management of the health care system. For those of you who work in health, it is worthwhile for you to appreciate how the Australian health care system is managed.

ACTIVITY

● Are there other features of Australia's health care system that are important to consider that are not mentioned? How does public health feature in such an all-encompassing and complex health care system? Research the role of consumers in current reforms to the Australian health care system under the new government. Are there plans for an increased consumer voice in policymaking?

REFLECTION

The Australian health care system is multifaceted and complex, and it is important to reflect on the breadth of applications of the health care system and health policy on population health. Think about the issues that encompass 'health' that Gardner and Barraclough (2002) point out and examine the span of recurrent health expenditures in Figure 3.1. Is there a case to be made for increasing the community and public health investments of 6% of distribution of recurrent health expenditure? If you believe there is, what arguments would you put forward to make this case? With respect to other features of Australia's health care system, did you consider the influence of not-for-profit organisations, including church-based organisations such as Blue Care and the Salvation Army and similar organisations that deliver health services? As you can see, there are many players who contribute to the development of health policy and service delivery within the Australian health care system.

Management of health care

There are essentially three tiers of government in Australia and each has a role to play in funding and delivering health to Australians. The federal government contributes to the main policy objectives, for example establishing Medicare, and, through agreements with the states, setting the health agenda on national priorities including public health priorities. The states develop strategies for implementing the main policy objectives by the federal government, and local action, infection prevention and monitoring functions are carried out by local government.

Health financing is one of the predominant roles of the federal government, as it has the power to raise revenue through the tax system and does that also through a special Medicare levy (generally about 1.5%) of taxable income. The Medicare levy is only one component of the financing of the health system. (For a source for information on health expenditure in Australia, the Australian Institute of Health and Welfare (AIHW) presents an annual *Health Expenditure Australia* series that contains thorough information on sources of health expenditure (see the AIHW website).)

The federal government – through agreements with the states – contributes to the funding of health care in the states and territories, via a number of intergovernmental agreements and constitutional definitions (Barraclough & Gardner 2002). The Commonwealth has had an 'active role in jointly setting of priorities, goals and quality outcomes, and the States have responsibility for the delivery of services to meet agreed outcomes' (Barraclough & Gardner 2002 p 56).

Five-year *Australian Health Care Agreements* outline the funding agreements between the state/territory governments and the Commonwealth, and the directions for priority spending and conditions. Under the previous government these agreements, called specific purpose payments and general purpose grants or financial assistance grants (Taylor et al 2007), were highly contested. The new government is reviewing the Commonwealth–state arrangements including the federal government playing a larger role in managing and funding public hospitals.

Within this complex financing environment, Mooney et al (1998) in Otim et al (2004) strongly advocate for unequal per capita expenditure on Indigenous and non-Indigenous Australians in order to bring about equity, and claimed that if the federal government redeployed about 1 per cent of the health care budget, it could increase spending on Indigenous health services by about 50%. The authors claim that this would have a positive impact on health status.

The authors claim that one of the drivers for national and intergovernmental reform is the Council of Australian Governments (COAG). Established in 1992, COAG comprises the prime minister, state premiers, territory chief ministers and the president of the Australian Local Government Association (ALGA). COAG is pivotal to health reform in Australia. Indeed, when an issue reaches COAG for discussion, then it is seen to have got top priority. And in February 2006, COAG agreed on a major health reform agenda on the next five-year public hospital funding agreements that were due for signing in June 2008. See Council of Australian Governments 2006, *A New National Reform Agenda* – Communiqué, February 2006 under 'Useful websites'.

Health care costs and reform of service delivery and the health care workforce have been the focus of discussions through recent reports of the Productivity Commission where one in 17 employed Australians is working in health occupations (AIHW 2006). The Productivity Commission produced a report for COAG that focuses on the need to reform the health workforce for it to cope with the future demands for health services. The full report is contained in *Potential Benefits of the National Reform Agenda*. For an overview of the health care workforce, see Chapter 5 in Taylor et al (2007).

Despite its complexities, there are strengths in having a unified approach to health issues that affect all Australians. The Australian Government has played a pivotal role in setting a national public health policy agenda that began in the late 1980s with many subsequent initiatives to drive a 'health for all' agenda across numerous health areas. We discuss these developments in the next section.

National public health priorities

The introduction of public health policies in the 'new era of public health' began with the development of national goals and targets in the 1990s. This work built on the Better Health Commission (1986) which, for the first time in Australia, utilised policy analysis of the current health status of Australians, identified the causes underlying health problems and proposed recommendations to address these health problems. The Better Health Commission was iconic, in that it represented a 'national' approach to drawing together evidence and a national policy commitment to improving population health.

Fleming and Parker (2007) claim that, with this impetus, the Australian Health Ministers' Advisory Council (AHMAC) established a report, *Health for all Australians* (AHMAC 1988), one of the first policy attempts to focus on the health of the whole Australian community. Moreover, these developments provided an impetus for the mixture of evidence on what contributed substantially to the burden of illness in a population, in terms of prevalence and/or severity, and were coupled with a strong national government commitment to a robust and effective policymaking process that included consultations with health consumers as well as health professionals and state governments.

Twenty years on, the national public health policy agenda has evolved through a number of iterations. 'In 1990, a joint AHMAC and the National Health and Medical Research Council (NHMRC) proposed a joint working group to select initial focus areas for national agreement and action, and in 1993, a report entitled *Goals and Targets for Australia's Health in the Year 2000 and Beyond* was launched' (Fleming & Parker 2007 p 71). An optimal balance of services across a continuum from promotion to palliative services was sought, and in 1996, with the endorsement of the federal and state governments, five *National Health Priority Areas* (NHPA) were endorsed: cardiovascular health, cancer control, injury prevention and control, mental health and diabetes mellitus. In 1999, asthma was added and arthritis and musculoskeletal disorders in 2002 and dementia in 2005. Reports are provided to the Australian health ministers every two years. Fleming and Parker (2007) explain that there are specific improvements in health outcomes that are required in the priority areas. These seek to:

- monitor health outcomes and progress towards set targets
- identify the most appropriate and cost-effective points of intervention
- identify the most appropriate role for government and non-government organisations in fostering the adoption of best practice
- investigate some of the basic determinants of health, such as education, employment and socioeconomic status (National Health Priority Action Council 2002 p 8).

The national health priority areas brought together a focus on health outcomes and are identified through evidence of burden of disease and a focus on prevention and management of the health issue. The priority areas evolve through developing national policies and funding, and are important contemporary policy issues for public health. Two of the most recent national health priority areas are the *National Chronic Disease Strategy* (2006), endorsed by the Australian Health Ministers Council, and the *National Framework for Action on Dementia 2006–2010* (Australian Health Ministers' Conference 2005), to coordinate the challenges of a predicted ageing population. These are evidence of major policy strategies and national and state commitments aimed at the prevention and management of chronic conditions and dementia. For example, in the COAG agreement of February 2006, over $500 million was allocated to 'promote good health and to tackle chronic conditions through prevention and early intervention' (Taylor et al 2007 p 143), and $320 million is allocated for action on dementia. Dementia is described as a set of symptoms of a large group of illnesses that cause a progressive decline in a person's mental functioning. It is a broad term that describes a loss of memory, intellect, rationality, social skills and normal emotional reactions (Alzheimers Australia 2008).

This policy is to 'facilitate action in the areas of care and support, access and equity, information and education, research, and workforce and training as key health areas; and with the National Health and Medical Research Council, a collaborative research program was established' (Taylor et al 2007 p 140). This action on dementia reveals the integration of the evidence through research with a policy capacity and commitment to plan for programs, services through a skilled workforce able to deal with working with the aged.

In mental health, COAG has built on a number of mental health policy agreements since 1992, with the most recently endorsed national *Mental Health Action Plan 2006–2011* (COAG 2006) that targets a range of treatment and prevention initiatives.

These and other current national public health policies build on previous public health policy successes where coordinated action in developing and executing policies through consultation and coordination and, importantly, financial investments have seen changes in health outcomes. They are founded on a national health priority rhythm established through coordinated federal and state policy development and agreements. Many of these original public health policies were initiated in the 1980s and included the *National Drug Strategy*, the *National Better Health Program*, the *National Aboriginal Health Strategy*, the *National HIV/AIDS Strategy*, the *National Women's Health Program*, BreastScreen Australia and the *National Cervical Screening Program*.

ACTIVITY

● Write down what you see as the strengths of national public policy approaches to contemporary health problems. What are the limitations of a unified approach? What are the implications for public health policy development if a state or territory government has different views on implementing these policies in their state? Is there a role for consumers in national public health policy development?

REFLECTION

Did you decide there were more strengths than limitations in having a national approach to major health issues? Would it mean that without such an approach, people in different states might receive different services? What should be the role of consumers in policy development? Are there enough avenues for consumers to have a voice about public health priorities and services? If you don't believe there is, what changes would you suggest?

To explore the role of national public health policies further, we draw attention to two of these policies. The first is the *National HIV/AIDS Strategy* and the second the *National Aboriginal Health Strategy*. Australia's comprehensive national approach to responding to HIV/AIDS has long been regarded as one of the best in the world. From the endorsement of the first *National HIV/AIDS Strategy* in 1989 through to the conclusion of the third *National HIV/AIDS Strategy* in 1999, Australia has recognised the need for coordinated action in response to HIV.

The National HIV/AIDS Strategy

The *National HIV/AIDS Strategy* (Commonwealth Department of Health and Aged Care 2000) builds on an important foundation established under previous HIV/AIDS strategies – the partnership between and with affected communities, governments at all levels and medical, scientific and health care professionals.

The strategy recognised the importance of establishing and maintaining operational links with other national population health strategies and was situated within a broader communicable diseases framework. It was the links between and the integration of these responses that ensured both sustainability and maximum population health benefit.

The strategy was drafted to operate as a flexible framework for responding to the challenges it identified as well as others that emerged during its five-year term.

Policy development and implementation can seem somewhat rarefied and something that governments and sections of the health sector 'do', but what is illustrative in the policy success of most public health priorities and the HIV/AIDS policy, in particular, is the active role that those community groups affected by the virus played. Moreover, if we return to our original discussions about the role of values in public policymaking, the strategies and services had to be suitable and accessible for those affected by the virus. The unique approach adopted in Australia with the inclusion of sex workers, men affected by the AIDS virus, physicians, politicians and well-known spokespeople was a radical departure from the approach taken in the United States, and included the opening of the first needle-exchange program in Sydney. It is the breadth of the involvement of such diverse 'stakeholders' that has been attributed to its success. We alluded to the political dynamics in policymaking at the beginning of the chapter, and this case demonstrates how skilfully the key policymakers in government were able to harness various lobbyists and advocates and to put in place an agreed upon national policy. The federal Minister of Health headed the initiative. A controversial television campaign called the *Grim Reaper* that urged people to use condoms was part of the first campaign. It must be remembered that the context for policymaking was a difficult one.[3]

The National Aboriginal Health Strategy

On all measures, the health status of Aboriginal and Torres Strait Islander Australians remains very poor, with life expectancy up to 17 years less than that for the total Australian population (Australian Bureau of Statistics (ABS) & AIHW 2005). There are some differences in the demographics of the Aboriginal and Torres Strait Islander communities.

First, contrary to belief, the majority of Indigenous people live in the southern and eastern parts of Australia. While only 1% of people living in Sydney were Indigenous, these two regions alone accounted for 18% of Australia's Indigenous population (ABS 1999 p 15 in Fleming & Parker 2007). However, 29% of people in the Northern Territory were estimated to be of Indigenous origin (ABS & AIHW 2005). And the population is relatively young, with the median age being 21 years of age, while for the non-Indigenous population the corresponding figure was 36 years (ABS & AIHW 2005).

With respect to the health profile of Indigenous Australians, Murray et al (2003 p 1) argued that that was 'because some aspects are worsening points to a failure in Aboriginal health policy'. There have been numerous health policy strategies and 'accords' and funding of Aboriginal and Torres Strait Islander community-controlled health organisations in the past years, yet the social and health disadvantage of Indigenous Australia remains well documented.

The *National Aboriginal Health Strategy* was developed in 1989 and introduced a distinctive Aboriginal and Torres Strait Islander concept of health that is introduced in Chapter 1. The strategy was seen as a beginning platform for a new era on health policy development. Since then there have been a number of government publications that have emphasised the shortcomings in both health status and access to appropriate health services.

One of these preceded the development of the *National Health Strategy* and this was the influential *Royal Commission into Aboriginal Deaths in Custody* in 1988, *Enough to Make You Sick* (National Health Strategy 1992) and the National Aboriginal and Torres Strait Islander Health Council (NATSIHC) in 2003. Subsequent Aboriginal health policies were introduced that focussed on the health workforce, the competencies of such a health workforce including an initiative to develop the nutrition workforce. For example, the *National Aboriginal and Torres Strait Islander Nutrition Strategy and Action Plan* (NATSINSAP) (2000–2010) was endorsed in 2001 by the Australian health ministers as part of the national public health nutrition strategy.

The *National Strategic Framework for Aboriginal and Torres Strait Islander Health 2003–2013* (NSFATSIH) and the *Australian Government Implementation Plan 2007–2013* were established to redress the imbalance of health inequalities in Aboriginal and Torres Strait Islander communities. This new plan details the specific activities to be undertaken to realise the aims and objectives of the NSFATSIH. This plan builds on the achievements and focuses on gaps identified by these reports. (See the Office of Aboriginal and Torres Strait Islander Health website at www.aodgp.gov.au.)

The Australian Government's Department of Health and Ageing's role is 'to ensure that Aboriginal and Torres Strait Islander peoples enjoy a healthy life equal to that of the general population that is enriched by a strong living culture, dignity and justice' (Australian Government DoHA website), and to this end works with the states and territories, the National Aboriginal Community Controlled Health Organisation (NACCHO) and other community leaders and members to try to make a difference in health.

Key priorities identified in the 1989 *National Health Strategy* included building community control of Aboriginal health services, increasing Aboriginal and Torres Strait Islander participation in the health workforce, reforming the health system and increasing funding to Aboriginal and Torres Strait Islander health services. The strategy also supported increasing community education, health promotion and prevention, improving the effectiveness and adequacy of essential services such as sewerage, water supply and communication, and building effective intersect oral collaboration. It noted that Aboriginal and Torres Strait Islander communities must participate in research to ensure it is ethical and research findings must be monitored and reviewed to ensure implementation (National Aboriginal Health Strategy (NAHS) Working Party 1989). There are various strategies and different institutional arrangements for delivering health services and policies and the politics of Aboriginal and Torres Strait Islander health changes in different federal governments, reflecting again the role of values, politics and social and cultural approaches to specific policy advances. One such policy was the abolition of the Aboriginal and Torres Strait Islander Commission in 2004, and its replacement with the National Indigenous Council. Anderson (2007) argues the demise of 'self-determination' that is, the right of Indigenous Australians to participate in making decisions on issues that related to their communities' (Anderson 2007 p 138). He reminds us of the breadth of the concept of self-determination and its possibilities with new forms of structures that could be borrowed from the creation of Indigenous jurisdictions (e.g. the province of Nunavut in northern Canada) (Government of Nunuvut 2005), yet, how pivotal self-determination as a policy principle was and is in the establishment, maintenance and management of the Aboriginal and Torres Strait Islander-managed health care services. Chapter 12 profiles a successful child health program in one of the community-controlled health services.

The data on the health of Indigenous Australians remain a stark reminder of health policy gaps and complexities.

ACTIVITY

● Write down your thoughts on the following questions. Are there lessons that can be drawn from the AIDS/HIV and the Aboriginal health policy discussions? What role did social and cultural approaches to both issues have in developing improvements in health? And what was the role of a range of stakeholders in policy development?

REFLECTION

Did your lessons contain any insights that could be applied to other health issues nationally? Did engaging stakeholders play a part in ensuring a positive implementation? Were there lessons from being attuned to social and cultural approaches, and policymakers 'listening' to these?

New challenges confront Australians' health, and you will have learned how public health responds through policy and service initiatives based on compelling evidence and opportunities. Under the chronic disease umbrella, obesity has received national and international attention. Although obesity may have appeared as a 'new issue' in 2003, Lin and Robinson (2005) claim that its arrival was preceded by a National Health and Medical Research Council report in 1997, entitled *Acting on Australia's Weight: Strategic plan for the prevention of overweight and obesity*. Lin and Robinson (2005 p 3) claim that despite national cooperation on physical activity and nutrition, the public and political imagination was not captured until the issues were recast as 'obesity'. Various states have implemented a range of school-based policies, and a number of allied health professionals have joined the workforce to address chronic conditions, including obesity, yet the authors claim that the Commonwealth strategy is 'relatively weak on intersectoral policy and regulatory measures' (Lin & Robinson 2005 p 3). Again, does this speak to a policy landscape with different interests, values and therefore actions?

In New South Wales, the implementation of a number of strategies includes nutrition and physical activity programs and some negotiation with Commercial Television Australia. Lin and Robinson (2005 p 3) point out on this national policy, the Commonwealth 'apparently chose not to consider how it might exercise its relevant taxation or legislative powers' despite the evidence that public policies beyond the health system can have an impact on health. We look at the concept of healthy public policy and health promotion further in Chapter 12.

We explore briefly another public health issue that does not receive as much attention as it should, and we present a policy initiative that has been controversial and dormant for many years in Australia.

Oral health does not feature in the list of national public health priorities, yet oral health expenditure accounts for the highest expenditure of 12 chronic diseases at $3.4 billion, or 6.9% of total allocated expenditure. Most of the expenditure on chronic diseases partly reflects the use of hospitals and general practitioners, and for oral health, for out-of-hospital services, mainly dental services. The other chronic diseases by order of expenditure are coronary heart disease, osteoarthritis, depression, stroke, diabetes, asthma, kidney disease, COPD, rheumatoid arthritis, colorectal cancer, osteoporosis and lung cancer (AIHW 2005).

In the report *Australia's dental generations: the National Survey of Adult Oral Health 2004–06* (AIHW 2007), which was drawn primarily from a 2004–2006 national survey in which 14,514 Australians from 15 to 98 years of age were interviewed and 5505 of them dentally examined, those respondents of the fluoride generation (born since 1970) had about half the level of decay that their parents' generation had developed by the time they were young adults (AIHW 2007).

The prevalence of oral diseases was higher among Aboriginal and Torres Strait Islander communities and the elderly. There is a 'public dental care system with varying eligibility criteria, mostly directed at children, low-income individuals, pensioners, and defined disadvantaged groups' (Schwarz 2006 p 225).

The NHMRC completed a systematic review of fluoride and health to synthesise high-level evidence in relation to the efficacy and safety of different forms of fluoridation (NHMRC 2007). In December 2007, the Queensland Government acted to improve the oral health of Queenslanders through a public health investment to fluoridate Queensland's water supplies. The following public health case study shows a profile of poor dental health of children and the implementation of a new public health policy to improve the dental health outcomes of children through a universal public health approach of water fluoridation.

Case study: Oral health in Queensland

Queenslanders have the highest levels of tooth decay and the lowest level of access to water fluoridation in Australia. Levels of tooth decay for Queensland children are much higher than those in other states and territories, and 67% of Queensland children have experienced tooth decay by eight years of age. However, Townsville children aged five to 12 years have 45% less tooth decay than Brisbane children.

Townsville fluoridated its water in 1965 (Queensland Government water fluoridation website). The oral health program as a public health priority that provides universal access to fluoridated water supplies will be implemented to 80% of Queenslanders by 2009 and 90% by 2012 (Bligh 2007). Forty years have passed, and despite the exigencies of public health policymaking, and based on evidence internationally and from other states, the oral health status of Queenslanders should improve with this initiative.

We conclude this chapter by introducing the Australian Institute of Health and Welfare.

The role of the Australian Institute of Health and Welfare

Development of national public policies is not possible without robust data on which to make policy decisions on public health priorities. During our discussions, we have cited the Australian Institute of Health and Welfare (AIHW) and the Australian Bureau of Statistics (ABS). In Australia, the AIHW is a living powerhouse of data assemblage. It is an independent government agency established to develop, collect and disseminate reliable, timely facts on the health of Australians and their health and community services. National agreements commit all the nine governments, AIHW and the ABS to work together to develop consistent, reliable and comprehensive data on health and community services. Despite the complexity and political differences among all the players in the Australian health system, the information effort has been exceptionally successful (Madden & Reece 1999). The tools are freely available on the AIHW website at www.aihw.gov.au.

A final word

In this chapter we have introduced and discussed some definitions of policy, why policy is important and stages of policymaking. Types of policy were presented with their potential role in addressing health issues and therefore health outcomes. International health policy developments, including the roles of WHO and the United Nations and their charters were discussed, and attention was paid to the changing architecture of international policy developments with the advent of public–private partnerships and the strength of health investments by philanthropic trusts. It is impossible to discuss national health policies without some attention to the structure and financing of Australia's health system and this was touched on briefly.

Australia has a tradition of the federal government taking a lead in public health policy developments and some of the history of this tradition and its current public health priorities were introduced. Two case studies were presented – HIV/AIDS and Aboriginal Health, to compare the social, cultural and political influences on policymaking. The role of AIHW and the ABS was outlined. Finally, the issue of obesity was presented as a challenging public health priority that has captured the imagination, despite there being national cooperation on two of its key risk factors: nutrition and physical activity. A discussion on current developments on a long-term health strategy for the national health agenda was held at the *Australia 2020 Summit* in April 2008.

In summary, the health policy tools that the government employs are intended to provide the quality and wellbeing of people's lives (Bessant et al 2006 in Taylor et al 2007). These aims are positioned against a backdrop where, in an adaptation of the words of Virchow (17th century) and Walt (2004), one cannot separate policy from politics.

REVIEW QUESTIONS

1   What do you understand by the terms, policy, public policy and health policy?
2   What are the stages of policymaking?
3   What role do values and politics play in health policymaking?
4   What is the role between the government of Australia and state governments and what are the agreements that are important in funding the health system?
5   Are international organisations such as WHO relevant for Australia's health policy directions?

6   Why are there relatively fewer gains in improving Indigenous health outcomes if
    there have been policies to address the issues?
7   Why does it appear that there is more policy action on some issues and not on others?

ENDNOTES

1   'Harm minimisation links the ethical consideration of expanding the autonomy of
    the drug user with the utilitarian principle of aiming to achieve net benefit for the
    individual and the community' (Gibson 2003 p 308).
2   Gross domestic product: 'The GDP of Australia is the total market value of all goods
    and services produced within Australia in a given period of time'. Parliament of
    Australia Parliamentary Library 2005 Monthly Economic and Social Indicators.
    Available: http://www.aph.gov.au/library/pubs/mesi/FEATURES/FeatureGDP.htm
    2 Dec 2007.
3   In 2007 the Australian Broadcasting Commission (ABC) produced a documentary
    called *Rampant* that traces the Australian AIDS story.

USEFUL WEBSITES

Australian Institute of Health and Welfare: www.aihw.gov.au
Australian Institute for Policy Studies: www.aihps.org
Bill and Melinda Gates Foundation: www.gatesfoundation.org
Council of Australian Governments: www.coag.gov.au
Government of Australia Department of Health and Ageing: www.health.gov.au
Government of Australia Department of Health and Ageing, Office of Aboriginal and Torres
    Strait Islander Health: http://www.health.gov.au/internet/main/publishing.nsf/Content/Offic
    e+for+Aboriginal+and+Torres+Strait+Islander+Health-1lp
Public Health Association of Australia: www.phaa.net.au
The Clinton Foundation: www.clintonfoundation.org
The Consumers' Health Forum of Australia: www.chf.org.au
The Global Fund: www.theglobalfund.org
United Nations Children's Fund (formerly United Nations International Children's Emergency
    Fund): www.unicef.org
World Bank: www.worldbank.org

REFERENCES

Alzheimers Australia website. Available: http://www.alzheimers.org.au 16 Feb 2008
Anderson I 2007 The end of Aboriginal self-determination? Futures 39(2007):137–154
Australian Bureau of Statistics 1999 The Health and Welfare of Australia's Aboriginal and
    Torres Strait Islander Peoples. ABS, Canberra
Australian Bureau of Statistics and Australian Institute of Health and Welfare 2005 The Health
    and Welfare of Australia's Aboriginal and Torres Strait Islander Peoples. Commonwealth of
    Australia, Canberra
AHMAC Health Targets and Implementation (Health For All) Committee 1988 Health For All
    Australians. Report to the Australian Health Ministers' Advisory Council and the Australian
    Health Ministers Conference, AGPS, Canberra
Australian Health Ministers' Conference 2005 National framework for Action on Dementia
    2006–2010, NSW Dept of Health on behalf of AHMC
Australian Institute of Health and Welfare 2005 Health system expenditure on chronic diseases.
    Available: http://www.aihw.gov.au/cdarf/data_pages/health_care_costs/ 8 Feb 2008
Australian Institute for Health and Welfare 2006 Productivity Commission 2005 Australia's
    Health Workforce, research Report, Canberra. http://www.pc.gov.au/_data/assets/
    pdf_file/0003/9480/healthworkforce.pdf Feb 2008

Australian Institute of Health and Welfare 2007 Australia's dental generations: the National Survey of Adult Oral Health 2004–06. Available: http://www.arcpoh.adelaide.edu.au/

Barraclough S, Gardner H, eds 2008 Analysing health policy: a problem-oriented approach. Elsevier, Marrickville

Bessant J, Watts R, Dalton T et al 2006 Talking Policy: How Social Policy is made. In: Taylor S, Foster K, Fleming J (eds) 2008 Health Care Practice in Australia. Policy, Context and Innovations. Oxford University Press, Melbourne

Better Health Commission 1986 Looking forward to better health: Report of the Better Health Commission. Australian Government Publishing Service, Canberra

Bligh A 2007 Fluoridated to Deliver Better Oral Health for Queenslanders. Queensland Government. December 2007. Press release

Cabinet Office 1999 Modernising Government White Paper. Cm 4310. London, HMSO

Commonwealth Department of Health and Aged Care, Commonwealth of Australia 2000 National HIV/AIDS Strategy 1999–2000 to 2003–04. Commonwealth of Australia, Canberra

Council of Australian Governments (COAG) 2006 Mental Health Action Plan 2006–2011. Available: http://www.coag.gov.au/meetings/140706/docs/nap_mental_health.pdf 7 Feb 2008

Couzos S, Murray R 2003 Aboriginal primary health care. An evidence-based approach, 2nd edn. Oxford University Press, Melbourne

Department of the Premier and Cabinet 2000 Queensland Policy Handbook. Queensland Government. Available: http://www.premiers.qld.gov.au/About_the_department/publications/policies/Governing_Queensland/Policy_Handbook/cycle/stages/

Duckett S 2007 The Australian Health Care System. Oxford University Press, Melbourne

Feachem R 2007 New ways of funding development assistance. Speech given at the Lowy Institute, 16 May 2007. Available: http://www.lowyinstitute.org/Publication. asp?pid=595 3 April 2008

Fleming M L, Parker E 2007 Health Promotion: Principles and practice in the Australian context, 3rd edn. Allen & Unwin, Melbourne

Gardner H, Barraclough S 2002 Health Policy in Australia. Oxford University Press, Melbourne

General Assembly of the United Nations 1948 The Universal Declaration of Human Rights. Adopted and proclaimed by General Assembly resolution 217 A (III) of 10 December 1948. Available: http://www.un.org/Overview/rights.html 3 Dec 2007

Gibson B In: Lin V, Gibson B 2003 Evidence-based Health Policy: Problems and Possibilities. Oxford University Press, Melbourne

Government of Nunuvut. In: Anderson I 2007 The end of Aboriginal self-determination? Futures 39:137–154. Available: http://www.gov.nu.ca/english/ 16 Feb 2008

Gunn S W A, Mansourian P, Davies A et al 2005 Understanding the Global Dimensions of Health. Springer, New York

Hayes M T 2007 Policy Characteristics, Patterns of Politics, and the Minimum Wage: Toward a Typology of Redistributive Policies. Policy Studies Journal 35(3):465–480

Last J 2005 A brief history of advances toward health. In: Gunn S, Mansourian P, Davies A, Peil A, Sayers B (eds) Understanding the global dimensions of health. Springer, New York, p 3–14

Leeder S 1999 Healthy Medicine. Challenges facing Australia's health services. Allen & Unwin, Melbourne

Lin V, Gibson B 2003 Evidence-based Health Policy. Problems & Possibilities. Oxford University Press, Melbourne

Lin V, Robinson P 2005 Australian public health policy in 2003–2004. Australia and New Zealand Health Policy 2:7

Lowy Institute for International Policy 16 May 2007. Available: http://svc168.wic006v.server-web.com/Publication.asp?pid=595 7 Dec 2007

Madden R, Reece L 1999 Sharing the fruits of coordination of *health* statistics in *Australia*. Statistical Journal of the UN Economic Commission for Europe 16(1):37–47

Manciaux M, Fleidner T M 2005 World health: a mobilizing utopia? In: Gunn S W A et al (eds) Understanding the global dimensions of health. Springer, New York, pp 69–84

Mooney G H, Wiseman V L, Wiseman S J 1998 How Much Should We Be Spending on Health Services for Aboriginal and Torres Strait Islander People? Medical Journal of Australia 169(16):508–509

Murray R B, Bell K, Couzos S et al 2003 Aboriginal health and the policy process. In: Couzos S, Murray R (eds) Aboriginal primary health care: an evidence-based approach, 2nd edn. Oxford University Press, South Melbourne, p 1–37

National Aboriginal Health Strategy (NAHS) Working Party 1989 A national Aboriginal health strategy. Department of Aboriginal Affairs, Canberra

National Aboriginal and Torres Strait Islander Health Council (NATSIHC) 2003 National Strategic Framework for Aboriginal and Torres Strait Islander Health: Framework for action by Governments. Canberra: NATSIHC. Available: http://www.healthconnect.gov. au/internet/wcms/publishing.nsf/Content/health-oatsih-pubs-healthstrategy.htm/$FILE/ nsfatsihfinal.pdf 7 Dec 2007

National Health and Medical Research Council (NHMRC) 1997 Acting on Australia's Weight: Strategic plan for the prevention of overweight and obesity. Available: http://www.nhmrc. gov.au/publications/synopses/n21syn.htm 15 Feb 2008 *This publication was rescinded on 22 Sep 2006; Rescinded publications are publications that no longer represent the council's position on the matters contained therein. This means that the council no longer endorses, supports or approves these rescinded publications.*

National Health and Medical Research Council (NHMRC) 2007 Public Statement. The Efficacy and Safety of Fluoridation 2007. Adapted from: Water fluoridation information for health professionals, State of Queensland, Queensland Health 2005

National Health Priority Action Council 2006 National Chronic Disease Strategy. Australian Government Department of Health and Ageing, Canberra. Available: http://www.health.gov. au/internet/main/publishing.nsf/Content/pq-ncds 18 Feb 2008

National Health Priority Action Council 2002 Future Directions of the National Health Priority Area Initiative. Report to the Austrlaian Health Ministers' Advisory Council. Available: http://www.health.vic.gov.au/nhpa/nhpac.htm 18 Feb 2008

National Strategic Framework for Aboriginal and Torres Strait Islander Health was endorsed at the Australian Health Ministers Conference on 31 Jul 2003

Navarro V, Muntane C, Borrell C et al 2006 Politics and health outcomes. Lancet 368:1033–1037

Otim M, Anderson I, Scott I 2004 Economics and Indigenous Australian Health Policy. Centre for Study of Health and Society, University of Melbourne, Melbourne

Palmer G, Short S 2000 Health Care and Public Policy. Macmillan, Melbourne

Potential benefits of the national reform agenda 2006 Productivity Commission Research Paper: Report to the Council of Australian Governments. Productivity Commission, Canberra

Queensland Government water fluoridation website. Available: http://www.health.qld.gov.au/ fluoride/ 7 Feb 2008

Royal Commission into Aboriginal Deaths in Custody 1988 Interim Report. AGPS, Canberra

Salisbury R, Heinz J 1970 A theory of policy analysis and some preliminary applications. In: Sharkansky I (ed) Policy Analysis in Political Science. Markham, Chicago

Schwarz S 2006 Access to oral health care – an Australian perspective. Community Dentistry and Oral Epidemiology 34(3):225–231

Taylor S, Foster K, Fleming J 2007 Health Care Practice in Australia. Policy, Context and Innovations. Oxford University Press, Melbourne

Virchow R. In: Gunn S W A, Mansourian P, Davies A et al 2005 Understanding the Global Dimensions of Health. Springer, New York

Walt G 2004 Health Policy: an Introduction to Process and Power. Zed Books, London

Wilson J M G, Junger G 1968 The principles and practice of screening for disease. World Health Organization, Geneva

World Health Organization 1948 Constitution of the World Health Organization. The Constitution was adopted by the International Health Conference held in New York from 19 Jun to 22 Jul 1946, signed on 22 Jul 1946 by the representatives of 61 States, and entered into force on 7 Apr 1948. WHO, Geneva

World Health Organization Public Health Paper 34. WHO, Geneva

World Health Organization 2005 Preventing chronic diseases: a vital investment: WHO global report. Available: http://www.who.int/chp/chronic_disease_report/full_report.pdf 15 Feb 2008

World Health Organization 2008 The WHO Agenda. Available: http://www.who.int/about/agenda/en/index.html 15 Jan 2008

There are numerous books on the structure of the Australian health system and a comprehensive text is Duckett (2007). Other useful resources are the websites of the Australian Institute of Health and Welfare (www.aihw.gov.au) that publishes an annual Health Expenditure Australia series and a profile of the health of Australians in its bi-annual reports; and the Department of Health and Ageing (www.doha.gov.au), which presents the structure and priorities for attention to improve health and health care for Australians.

Section 2

Risk and determinants of health

Introduction

An examination of risk factors and the nature and range of determinants that might impact on health and illness are the issues discussed in Section 2. This section considers the important role of epidemiology in determining the factors that influence patterns of mortality and morbidity. Epidemiology is the study of factors affecting the health and illness of populations, and serves as the foundation and logic for interventions made in the interest of public health and preventive medicine. It is considered a cornerstone methodology of public health research. According to Last et al (2000), an epidemiologist investigates the occurrence of disease or other health-related conditions or events in defined populations. The control of disease in populations is often also considered to be a task for the epidemiologist.

Epidemiology has three main aims:
1 to describe disease patterns in human populations
2 to identify the causes of diseases (also known as aetiology)
3 to provide data essential for managing, evaluating and planning services for preventing, controlling and treating disease (Australasian Epidemiology Association website 2008).

Chapter 4 provides you with an introduction to epidemiology and its component parts and it gives you an idea of how useful the study of epidemiology is to public health as a fundamental discipline underpinning the subject.

Chapters 5 and 6 examine determinants of health. In recent years the social determinants of health have taken centre stage – strongly supported by the work of the World Health Organization (2005). Determinants are not just social in nature as there are a range of factors that impact on the health and wellbeing of the population, and Chapters 5 and 6 address these issues. There is a growing acknowledgement of the importance of a range of factors impacting on exposure to health hazards and risk conditions in the population. Some groups in society have a much poorer chance of achieving their full health potential as a result of their life circumstances – including political, social, economic and environmental conditions as illustrated above. These factors interact with genetic and biological factors to impact on the health and wellbeing of the population in a wide variety of ways.

Chapter 5 concentrates on the physical and environmental determinants of health. It discusses the contribution of genetic and biological factors that impact on the health of the population and subpopulations. The environment interacts with genetic and biological factors to influence health and wellbeing. Most health problems are multicausal and are influenced by a range of factors.

Social and economic factors are known to be powerful determinants of population health in modern societies. There is acknowledged scientific justification for isolating different aspects of social and economic life as the primary determinants of a population's health. Chapter 6 addresses the issue of social determinants of health and it also considers the importance of emotional determinants – issues too often neglected in political and policy deliberations about health and wellbeing.

REFERENCES

Australasian Epidemiology Association 2008 What is epidemiology? Available: http://www.aea. asn.au/home_whatisepidemiology.htm 25 Feb 2008

Last J, Spasoff R, Harris S 2000 A dictionary of epidemiology. Oxford University Press, New York

World Health Organization Secretariat of the Commission on Social Determinants of Health 2005 Action on the Social Determinants of Health: Learning from Previous Experience. A background paper prepared for the Commission on Social Determinants of Health. WHO, Geneva

CHAPTER 4

Epidemiology

Bonnie Macfarlane & Mary-Anne Kedda

Learning objectives

After reading this chapter you should be able to:

- appreciate the role of epidemiology in public health
- recognise measures of the occurrence of disease and mortality
- identify the main types of epidemiological study design
- correctly interpret reported measures of association between exposure and disease
- discuss the concepts of chance, bias and confounding.

Introduction

The aim of this chapter is to provide you with a basic understanding of epidemiology, and to introduce you to some of the epidemiological concepts and methods used by researchers and practitioners working in public health. It is hoped that you will recognise how the principles and practice of epidemiology help to provide information and insights that can be used to achieve better health outcomes for all.

Epidemiology is fundamental to preventive medicine and public health policy. Rather than examine health and illness on an individual level, as clinicians do, epidemiologists focus on communities and population health issues. The word epidemiology is derived from the Greek *epi* (on, upon), *demos* (the people) and *logos* (the study of). Epidemiology, then, is the study of that which falls upon the people. Its aims are to describe health-related states or events, and through systematic examination of the available information, attempt to determine their causes. The ultimate goal is to contribute to prevention of disease and disability and to delay mortality. The primary question of epidemiology is: Why do certain diseases affect particular population groups? Drawing upon statistics, the social and behavioural sciences, the biological sciences and medicine, epidemiologists collect and interpret information to assist in preventing new cases of disease, eradicate existing disease and prolong the lives of people who have disease.

Defining epidemiology

Epidemiology can be defined as:

> The study of the **distribution** and **determinants** of **health-related states** or events in specified **populations**, and the application of this study to **control of health problems.**

(Last 1995 p 55)

Although this may seem straightforward, it is worth taking a moment to think further about this definition. It succeeds in capturing the scope of epidemiology in a clear and concise manner. Look carefully at each of the bolded words in the definition of epidemiology given above.

Distribution refers to the pattern or frequencies of health events across not only people (who gets affected?), but also place (where does it happen?) and time (when does it happen?). **Determinants** are both the causes of and risk factors for health events, which can be living organisms (e.g. viruses and bacteria), physical entities (e.g. radiation, pollution and dangerous machinery), related to lifestyle (e.g. stress and diet), social factors (e.g. poverty) and genetic factors (e.g. specific variants in genes that are inherited at birth or even changes in genes that occur during one's life). **Health** is defined by the World Health Organization (WHO) as 'a state of complete physical, mental, and social wellbeing and not merely the absence of disease or infirmity' (WHO 1948). Health could include a specific disease state, the absence of a disease state, a quality of life rating, life expectancy or incidence of mental illness or physical injury. **Population** refers to a group of people with definable commonalities, for example, a school community or a certain ethnic group. **Control of health problems** refers to reducing the burden of a health problem in a population or community.

Objectives of epidemiology

Epidemiological studies fulfil three primary roles: description, analysis and intervention. Description allows health status to be explored between population subgroups, different geographic localities and at different times. Information that results from these descriptions can then be used to look for relationships between causal agents and diseases through analysis. Finally, the outcomes of analytic studies can be used to develop and justify the implementation of interventions, such as health promotion programs. Epidemiologic approaches can also be used to evaluate the outcomes of such interventions.

The overall objectives of epidemiology are to: investigate the cause of a disease and the associated risk factors, since knowing the cause of ill-health facilitates disease prevention and health promotion; identify syndromes and disease outbreaks using descriptions of associations of clinical phenomena in the population and to facilitate better clinical management; and describe the complete clinical picture or natural history of diseases. The outcomes of these objectives enable epidemiology to be used as a basis for strategic planning, prioritising health issues and evaluating health services.

Epidemiology works in tandem with other sciences and medicine to determine existing and potential health hazards, and also provides the basis for decisions regarding strategies to prevent such hazards from impacting heavily upon the overall health of the population.

ACTIVITY

● Think of a public health issue or activity relevant to your area of interest. Write a paragraph to explain how epidemiology could have contributed to identifying the issue or implementing an effective intervention at the population level.

REFLECTION

This activity will require you to apply your understanding of epidemiology and its objectives. What resources will you use to identify the public health issue? Try using the definition of epidemiology above to help you write the paragraph.

A brief history of epidemiology (1700s onwards)

Looking at the history of epidemiological ideas allows you to understand how scientific discoveries have fundamentally changed the ways in which humans see themselves. These days we take it for granted that many diseases can be prevented through, for example, good nutrition. However, this idea had not been proven prior to James Lind's work in preventing scurvy among British sailors by including citrus fruit in their diets in 1747 (The James Lind Library, see 'Useful websites' at the end of the chapter). Perhaps the best-known historical examples of epidemiological studies are those of John Snow and his investigations of cholera epidemics in London during the mid 1800s.

John Snow was a British physician who is considered by many epidemiologists to be the father of modern epidemiology. His story was set in 19th century London, where millions lived an impoverished life in overcrowded and unsanitary slums, susceptible to devastating outbreaks of infectious diseases such as cholera. During the early 1800s, it was thought that cholera was airborne, however Snow did not believe in the 'miasma' (bad air) theory, and was certain that the infectious agent entered the body through the mouth. In 1849 he published an essay entitled *On the Mode of Communication of Cholera* and, in August 1854, when a cholera outbreak occurred in Soho, London, Snow used epidemiological investigative skills to identify a water pump in Broad Street as the source of the disease. He had the handle of the pump removed, and cases of cholera immediately began to diminish. Although John Snow's 'germ' theory was not accepted until after his death, he was a prominent physician and certainly one of the founders of epidemiology. Should you wish to read more about the life and times of John Snow, there are a number of online resources available (see 'Useful websites' at the end of the chapter).

Measuring the occurrence of disease and death

Studying the occurrence of health conditions in human populations is the cornerstone of public health practice. Indeed, if you refer back to the definition of epidemiology, a key component is the study of the distribution of health-related states or events. Understanding the burden of disease within a population provides public health specialists with information that is vital to planning and providing health services. Measuring the health of populations can help to answer some fairly simple yet important questions. For example, how much disease is present now? How fast are new cases occurring? How long do people remain ill? How does the rate of disease or death differ over time within a population or compared with another population? Who does the disease affect? Where are they getting sick? What are the associated causes for a health condition? What strategies are effective at reducing the occurrence of a certain disease or condition?

Epidemiologists can count disease events, or go further and calculate rates and proportions for making comparisons of health status. There are several measures of disease frequency that are employed by allied health professionals such as epidemiologists. The simplest quantitative measure is a count, which merely refers to the number of people who die or become ill from any given cause. These data have limited value without information about the population size. For example, consider a study involving people who attend clinics for treating liver disease. One could say that, based on counts of those dying from liver cirrhosis, more are alcoholics than users of injected drugs. However, this tells us nothing about the risk of dying from liver cirrhosis in these two groups. For this, we would need to know how many people there are in each group.

For a count to be descriptive of a group it needs to be seen relative to the size of that group. This involves expressing a count as a proportion of a group. Imagine an outbreak of 10 influenza cases within a class of health students. This would have different significance depending on the size of the class. For example if there were 20 students, then 50% were ill; however, if there were 500 students in the class, then only 2% were ill. Clearly, these two situations would paint a different picture of disease magnitude.

A ratio describes the magnitude of one group relative to another. For example, if, of the 10 people who developed influenza, eight are men and two are women, then the sex ratio would be 8:2 male to female. Another frequently used measure is a rate, which is a measure of the frequency of occurrence of an event. A rate differs from a proportion in that it involves units of time in its calculation. There are several other measures also used in communicable disease epidemiology, such as attack rates and infection rates.

Two of the most widely used measures of disease frequency are prevalence and incidence. Prevalence refers to the number of people in a defined population who have a specific disease or condition at a certain time. Prevalence data can provide an indication of the extent of a health problem and thus assist in the planning of health services. Measuring prevalence basically involves counting cases; data on prevalence can become much more meaningful if converted into a proportion by relating it to the population from which the cases arose. Prevalence is often written or spoken in terms of a 'prevalence rate' but prevalence is actually a proportion. Prevalence does not have to refer directly to a specific point in time but can relate to a period of time. For example, we might be interested in the number of motor vehicle accidents occurring on 31 December, or we might consider the number of accidents between 1 January and 31 December. The former is referred to as 'point prevalence', while the latter is 'period prevalence'.

Prevalence can be calculated using the following equation:

$$\text{Prevalence} = \frac{\text{Number of people with the disease/condition at a specific time}}{\text{Number of people in the population at risk at a specific time}} \times 10^n$$

Example: Calculating prevalence

During a lecture on Friday afternoon, we ask all students with a headache to put up their hands, in order to calculate the prevalence of headaches in a class of 200 students. If eight students put up their hands, the prevalence of headaches is eight out of 200 students at that point in time = 4% of the class (or 40 cases per 1000 students) – this is point prevalence.

If we ask students in the same class to put up their hands if they had experienced a headache at any time during the past week, this would be period prevalence. If 15 students reported that they had experienced a headache during the past week, the period prevalence is 15 cases out of 200 students over a one-week period = 7.5% of the class per week (or 75 per 1000 students per week).

Note that period prevalence will include those with the condition at the start of the specified time period and also all the new cases (incident cases) that develop the condition over that specified time period.

Incidence refers to the number of new cases of disease, injury or death in a population during a specified time period. Unlike prevalence, it is a true rate as it always specifies a unit of time in its calculation. There are two major measures of incidence: incidence rate and cumulative incidence. Incidence rate is a more precise measure that describes the rate at which new cases occur in a population over a specified period of time. Cumulative incidence is a simpler measure of the occurrence of disease or death, and tells us the proportion of a population, from the total at risk, that develop a disease during a specified time period. As with prevalence, cumulative incidence can be expressed as a proportion, a percentage or as number of cases per population.

Incidence rate and cumulative incidence can be calculated using the following equations:

Incidence rate

$$= \frac{\text{Number of new people with the disease/condition in specified period}}{\text{Total 'person-time' at risk during specified period}} \times 10^{n}$$

Note: 'Person-time' represents the sum of each participant's time at risk.

Cumulative incidence

$$= \frac{\text{Number of new people with the disease/condition in specified period}}{\text{Number of people in the population at risk during specified period}} \times 10^{n}$$

It is important you understand the subtle differences between cumulative incidence and incidence rate. Cumulative incidence assumes that the entire population at risk at the beginning of the study period has been followed up for the whole of that specified time period. However, it is unlikely that the length of follow-up will be uniform for all participants. It is also useful to consider individuals who develop the disease of interest during the follow-up period. Epidemiologists account for these varying time periods of follow-up using incidence rates and 'person-time'. Since an incidence rate accounts for varying times of disease-free follow-up, it is considered to be a more precise measure of the occurrence of disease. If you would like to read further on the concept of person-time see *Essential Epidemiology* (Webb et al 2005 pp 37–41).

Example: Incidence of hearing loss among workers in heavy industry

Imagine you are studying the incidence of hearing loss in 8000 workers in heavy industry in Victoria, Australia. There are 750 new cases of hearing loss over a 10-year period. During those 10 years, the employees worked a total of 116,000 years of work.

What was the incidence rate of hearing loss in workers in heavy industry in Victoria over the 10-year period (in 1000 person-years)?

$$\text{Incidence rate} = \frac{\text{Number of new cases in Victoria over 10 yr}}{\text{Total person-years exposed}} \times 1000$$

$$= \frac{750}{116,000} \times 1000$$

$$= 6.47 \text{ per 1000 person years}$$

This figure can be compared with the incidence of hearing loss in people working in light industry (1.22 per 1000 person years). Hearing loss among workers in heavy industry occurs more frequently than in workers in light industry.

Continued

Example: Incidence of hearing loss among workers in heavy industry—cont'd

What is the cumulative incidence of hearing loss in these workers?

$$\text{Cumulative incidence} = \frac{\text{Number of new cases in Victoria over 10 years}}{\text{Total number of people at risk during 10 years}}$$

$$= \frac{750}{8000}$$

$$= 0.09 \text{ over 10 years}$$

You conclude that, among workers exposed to noise in heavy industry for at least 10 years, 9% developed hearing loss. This can be further interpreted as a risk statement: if workers are exposed to noise in heavy industry for at least 10 years, they have a 9% chance of developing hearing loss.

Mortality rates measure the risk of dying. Mortality patterns can be described using crude rates, age-specific rates, sex-specific rates and cause-specific rates. Crude mortality rates (CMR) are derived by the equation:

$$\text{CMR} = \frac{\text{Number of deaths in a specified time period}}{\text{Total population}} \times 10^n$$

Crude mortality rates are affected by a number of population characteristics, particularly age structure. For example in 1990, Sweden's annual death rate was 11 per 1000. This rate was higher than that of Guatemala (8 per 1000), even though life expectancy in Sweden (78 years) was greater than in Guatemala (63 years). The difference in crude mortality rates between the two countries was mainly due to differences in age structure: 18% of Sweden's population was aged over 65 years, while only 3% of Guatemala's population was over 65 years.

Crude mortality rates can be used if the frequency of death or disease is not known in subgroups, if the size of subgroups is not known and if the number of people at risk is too small to provide stable estimates. However, differences in the age structure of a population can cause misleading conclusions about health status, so age-specific rates enable more meaningful comparisons between groups. Age-specific mortality rates (ASMR) take into account the different age structures between populations, as well as the fact that the risk of mortality increases with age. ASMR are derived by the equation:

$$\text{ASMR} = \frac{\text{Number of deaths in particular age band in a specified time period}}{\text{Total population in same age band}} \times 10^n$$

There are several other measures of mortality commonly used in epidemiology, for example, the infant mortality rate (IMR) (birth to one year of age), which can be used as an indicator of the general health status of a population:

$$\text{IMR} = \frac{\text{Number of deaths in a year of children less than 1 year of age}}{\text{Number of live births in the same year}}$$

Other age-specific mortality rates include perinatal mortality (28 weeks gestation to one week of life), neonatal mortality (birth to 28 days of life) and post-neonatal mortality

(28 days to one year of age), and can be calculated by simply substituting the number of deaths with the appropriate age-specific data. This process can also be extended to calculate separate rates in other groups, for instance sex-specific rates (men and women) and cause-specific rates (different diseases).

Most introductory epidemiology textbooks discuss the measures described above; if you are interested in reading further see *Epidemiology* (Gordis 2004).

Epidemiological study design

Different types of epidemiological study design are used to answer different research questions, and each has associated advantages and disadvantages. Studies can be classified as either observational or experimental, and the distinction is an important one. Observational studies allow nature to take its course and the investigator simply observes events in different populations/groups. The investigator then seeks information about the patterns of diseases and potential risk factors or exposures. In contrast, experimental studies (also known as intervention studies) allow the investigator to actively engage in the study by deliberately manipulating an exposure to judge its effect on an outcome. Studies can also be classified as descriptive or analytical and, in some cases, a study can be both. Descriptive studies are used to describe and measure the burden of disease within a population, whereas analytical studies are carried out to evaluate the association between an exposure or characteristic and the development of a particular disease or health state.

Study designs differ with respect to the number of observations made, whether data are collected prospectively or retrospectively, the data collection procedures used, the timing of data collection, whether individuals or groups are studied and the availability of subjects/existing data. Epidemiologists use a range of study designs, as illustrated in Figure 4.1.

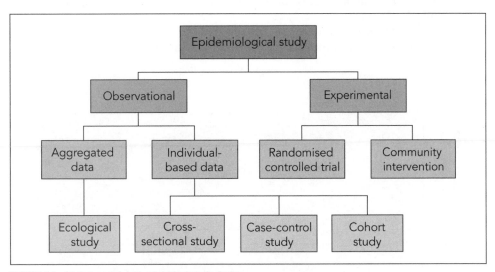

FIGURE 4.1: Main types of epidemiological study design

Observational epidemiology

For ethical reasons, many factors thought to influence disease, or protect against it, cannot be imposed upon a study population. Instead, researchers make use of naturally occurring situations, and observe and measure exposures and patterns of health in naturally occurring groups. The investigator does not intervene in any way. Among observational research designs, descriptive studies look at patterns of disease and measure the occurrence of disease and/or risk factors in a population. Analytical studies make comparisons between groups of people with and without disease, or people with and without exposures to potential risk factors for disease.

Ecological studies (sometimes called correlational studies) often constitute the first step in investigating causes of poor health. Studies examining differences in health status (e.g. death rates, disease patterns and health-risk behaviours) between groups of people (countries and regions, or within the same region at different times) are examples of ecological studies. The distinguishing factor of an ecological study is that all data on exposure and outcome are collected at the population level; there are no data on individuals (e.g. the proportion of children with asthma in 10 regions is compared with the mean level of air pollution in each region, but nothing is known about the exposure status or other characteristics of each individual child). Often ecological studies utilise data that have already been collected for other purposes, for example, census, birth and death records and periodic government health surveys. Ecological studies are most useful in helping to generate hypotheses about possible links between environmental or lifestyle exposures and disease. Trends in mortality or morbidity over time, or between populations, can reveal important information about factors that are associated with poor health. It is important to recognise, though, that any associations apparent at the group level do not necessarily hold at the individual level. Inappropriate conclusions made about individuals from ecological data constitute ecological fallacy. Finding a relationship between variables does not necessarily imply causation. We always need to be aware of other possible explanations.

An example of an ecological design is research that shows an association between international trends of dietary carbohydrate intake and oesophageal cancer (see Fig 4.2). The results suggest that an increase in oesophageal cancer rates may be associated with high carbohydrate intakes.

Note: The data points indicate the age-adjusted oesophageal adenocarcinoma rate (in millions) plotted against the total carbohydrate consumption (grams).

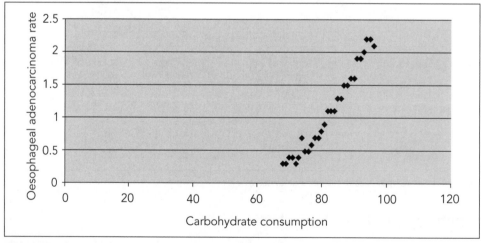

FIGURE 4.2: Oesophageal adenocarcinoma rates by carbohydrate consumption

(Source: Thompson et al 2007 Carbohydrate Consumption and Esophageal Cancer: An Ecological Assessment. American Journal of Gastroenterology 102(11):1–7. Online Early Articles, Figure 2, p 3.)

ACTIVITY

- Consider the results illustrated in Figure 4.2. Does this mean that high carbohydrate intake has a direct effect in increasing risk of oesophageal cancer? Write a short paragraph to address this question.

REFLECTION

Did you consider whether there was a biologically plausible association between dietary carbohydrate intake and oesophageal cancer? Did you think of other explanations for this association?

Cross-sectional studies

Cross-sectional (prevalence) studies are one of the most common study designs used in descriptive epidemiology. Many health surveys in which people are interviewed are cross-sectional, that is, they collect data about both exposure and outcomes at one point in time. Indeed the main feature of the design is that exposure and 'case-ness' are determined concurrently.

The study group is chosen to be a cross-section of the population, and is usually selected in a manner to be representative of the whole population. In cross-sectional studies, besides describing the characteristics of the study population, researchers often try to establish associations between the prevalence of health problems or service usage and other factors (like working conditions or economic factors that may affect service use). This design is particularly useful for studies investigating the impact of personal characteristics, such as socioeconomic status or country of birth, on health. A good example of an Australian cross-sectional study is the one conducted by the Queensland Ambulance Service (Clark et al 1999), where data were collected on every patient ($n=11,408$) who presented at Ipswich Hospital in a four-month period. Data were collected on demographic characteristics (e.g. sex, date of birth, marital status, country of origin), presentation details (e.g. arrival method, arrival date, complaint) and departure details (e.g. date of departure). This study provided a snapshot of ambulance service users at that time, and their reasons for calling an ambulance. This helped plan services and resources for the next quarter.

Case-control studies

Case-control studies are increasingly being used to investigate the causes of diseases. The principal characteristic of the case-control study design is including a group of people with the disease/outcome (cases) and a comparison group who do not have the disease (controls). Case-control studies determine the proportion of cases that were exposed, and the proportion of cases that were not exposed. The proportions of the controls that were or were not exposed are also determined. The objective of the design is to ascertain differences in the frequency of exposure between the two groups of people. We anticipate that if the exposure (e.g. rubella) is related to disease (e.g. cataracts), then the prevalence of a history of exposure will be significantly greater among cases than controls.

As case-control studies are asking about past exposures, the direction of enquiry is *retrospective*, which makes this study design susceptible to recall bias (to be covered at a later point). One of the major advantages of case-control studies is the ability to explore multiple factors within the one study, by obtaining data on a number of exposures. Representativeness of the control group is important in case-control studies to ensure that exposure prevalence in the control group is similar to that of the population from which cases arose. A case-control study conducted between January 1996 and January 1997 in Brisbane, Australia, investigated potential risk factors for campylobacter infection in infants and young children (Tenkate & Stafford 2001). In this study, ownership of pet puppies and pet chickens, as well as mayonnaise consumption, were found to be strongly associated with campylobacter infection. Can you think of reasons why these associations might have occurred? Do you think that everyone in the study would have remembered their exposure accurately? If not, what impact might that have had on the results?

Cohort studies

Cohort studies are another type of observational study design. These are also known as 'longitudinal', 'follow-up', 'prospective' or 'incidence' studies. In this type of study design, we investigate groups of people who have no apparent symptoms of the disease under study at the time they are recruited. A critical feature of a cohort study is that the study population is then observed over a period of time so that the rate of disease occurrence among people exposed to a suspected causal agent can be compared with the rate of disease occurrence among unexposed people. Participants must not have the disease at time of recruitment to ensure as much as possible that the exposure precedes the outcome/disease; however, this is difficult for diseases with a long pre-diagnosis phase. Cohort studies directly measure the risk of disease developing and provide good information about causes of disease. However, as the exposure of interest is not under the control of the researcher, there is a potential for other competing risk factors to be linked to the outcome/disease.

Cohort studies are best undertaken when the disease has a significant burden on the population. This increases the value of public health knowledge that can be gained from conducting a cohort study and also increases the likelihood that a substantial number of participants will develop the disease/outcome. Cohort studies are *prospective* in terms of direction of inquiry. A well-known Australian cohort study took place in the *Mater Mothers' Hospital–University of Queensland Study of Pregnancy* (Keeping et al 1989). The study began in 1981 as a prospective study of over 8000 pregnant women interviewed after their first clinic visit. Follow-up data collection on both mother and child occurred at six months, five years, 15 years and again when the children turned 21 in 2002. As you can imagine, there have been numerous analyses conducted using these data. One example, using data from 2500 of the mothers and their children, explored early and late lifecourse predictors of alcohol abuse and dependence in the children (Alati et al 2005). The data revealed a strong link between exposure to maternal drinking during the child's adolescence and the subsequent development of alcohol problems in that child's early adulthood. You can see that this type of study is very useful in examining the relationship between early-life exposures and later-life outcomes, but can be very challenging because it requires long-term commitments of researchers and resources.

ACTIVITY

Consider three different studies designed to investigate the effect of raspberry leaf tea on length of labour. What types of observational studies are the following designs?

- *Design 1:* A survey of women after they have delivered at the local maternity hospital, asking them about their use of raspberry leaf tea and other herbal supplements in the preceding year. Data on length of labour are collected from existing hospital medical charts upon discharge.
- *Design 2:* A study of 226 women giving birth and classified by length of labour (usual labour versus long labour), and then asked whether or not they used raspberry leaf tea during their pregnancy.
- *Design 3:* A group of 457 pregnant women, followed up from first antenatal visit to delivery, with questionnaires addressing current complementary medicine usage at each time. Women will be classified according to whether or not they used raspberry leaf tea at all, and their length of labour compared.

REFLECTION

Did you consider whether the data was collected at one point in time or if the study required participant follow-up? Did any of the studies compare cases and controls?

Experimental epidemiology

Experimental designs are principally used in clinical epidemiology where medical interventions are evaluated, but have also been used to assess population health interventions. The essence of experimental designs is comparing outcomes among exposed and non-exposed groups, but the distinguishing element is that exposure is under the control of the investigator. Experimental designs are highly controlled in an attempt to eliminate all possible sources of bias and provide the most accurate picture of causation. There are two main types of experimental studies: therapeutic trials (to treat established disease) and prophylactic trials (to prevent disease).

Randomised controlled trials

Randomised controlled trials (RCTs) are a type of experimental study in which the experimental group receives the treatment/intervention and the control group receives either no treatment/intervention or, preferably, a placebo (something that appears similar to the real treatment, but is not active) treatment/intervention.

Randomisation (also known as random assignment or random allocation) is a way of ensuring that each participant has an equal chance to receive an intervention or enter the control group. This helps to ensure that the two groups (intervention and control) are the same from the start so that any differences between groups may be attributed to the intervention. RCTs are therefore thought to give the best evidence out of all of the epidemiological study designs. An RCT has five important elements:
1 The investigator controls the exposure for each group of people to study the effect on an outcome. For example, eliminating a dietary factor (exposure) thought to cause allergy (outcome), or testing a new treatment (exposure) on a group of people to reduce morbidity (outcome).
2 The investigator has control over all elements of the research, including selecting the participants or subjects, measuring the outcome and setting the conditions within which the experiment is conducted.
3 Participants are randomly allocated to intervention or control groups.
4 Effects of the intervention (exposure) are measured by comparing the outcome in the experimental group with that in a control group.
5 The investigators and the participants should ideally be unaware of the group to which they are allocated (when both investigators and participants are unaware, this study is considered 'double-blind'; if only the participant is unaware, then it is a 'single-blind' study).

The following example describes an RCT conducted in Izmer, Turkey, assessing the efficacy of honey as a wound dressing compared with a standard topical antibacterial cream in treating patients with pressure ulcers (Gunes & Eser 2007). After five weeks of treatment, results showed that patients receiving honey dressings healed at approximately four times the rate of the patients receiving standard dressings. In this study, participants were aware of which treatment group they were in – do you think this might have influenced the results? Imagine if half the participants who received standard dressings left the study before its completion, how might this change the results?

Prophylactic/preventive trials

These studies are usually conducted in the same manner as an RCT; however, instead of recruiting participants with the disease, participants at risk of developing the disease are selected and given a potentially preventative intervention.

Community trials

Community trials may also be referred to as field trials or as community interventions. They are similar to preventive trials in that they recruit participants who are disease free but presumed to be at risk of a particular outcome or disease. Unlike preventive trials, however, community trials are conducted at a population level rather than at an individual level. Community trials are therefore used when it is not possible to offer or evaluate the intervention at the individual level. Data collection takes place 'in the field' in community trials. This study design is particularly suitable when disease rates can be influenced by interventions aimed at group behaviour. A good example of a community trial is the *10,000 Steps Rockhampton* study in Queensland that assessed the effectiveness of a whole community approach to improve levels of physical activity in the population (Brown et al 2006). In this study, instead of selecting individual participants, the researchers implemented multiple strategies across the whole Rockhampton community to improve population levels of physical activity.

ACTIVITY

Each study design in epidemiology has advantages and disadvantages associated with it. For the following studies, which study design do you think would be the most appropriate?

- *Design 1:* What is the relationship in Australia between suicide and unemployment between 1950 and 2003?
- *Design 2:* Is green tea consumption associated with prostate cancer?
- *Design 3:* Does a daily dose of vitamin C prevent the onset of the common cold among elite athletes?
- *Design 4:* Is there an association between depression and physical abuse by partners of women attending general practice?
- *Design 5:* What are the health effects of long-term exposure to heavy metals among miners in Australia?

REFLECTION

The choice of study design will primarily be dictated by the question asked and the characteristics of the outcome and exposure being studied. Other factors such as finances, ethics, time, opportunities, and prior knowledge also need to be considered. All study designs, if well conducted, will provide useful information to the researcher, although some are better than others at providing evidence for causality. For this activity, it is important for you to be able to recognise the basic types of study design and identify which are best for different types of research questions. Consider whether the gold-standard RCT is an appropriate study design before considering one of the observational designs.

Measures of association

Most epidemiological studies look for associations between different exposures and a particular health outcome. Measuring the occurrence of disease in a population (e.g. prevalence or incidence) describes the health of the population, but it does not tell us anything about the causes of disease. The frequencies of disease in each group in a study can be combined to create a statistical summary that estimates the association between an exposure and the risk of developing the disease. Two-by-two tables are a way in which data can be presented to assist in calculating measures of association. As shown in Table 4.1, a two-by-two table consists of two columns, each representing the presence or absence of disease, and two rows, each representing the presence or absence of exposure.

| | | DISEASE | | |
		YES	NO	TOTAL
Exposure	Yes	a	b	a + b
	No	c	d	c + d
Total		a + c	b + d	a + b + c + d

TABLE 4.1: Two-by-two table

Note: The cells containing a, b, c and d each represent the number of individuals with a particular combination of disease and exposure:

a = Number of people who are exposed and who have the disease
b = Number of people who are exposed and who do not have the disease
c = Number of people who are not exposed and who have the disease
d = Number of people who are not exposed and who do not have the disease

Relative risk

In RCTs and cohort studies, the objective is to determine whether there is an increased or reduced risk of a particular health outcome associated with a particular exposure or potential risk factor. In other words, whether there is an association between a specific risk factor and the disease. Both an RCT and a cohort study observe participants over a measured period of time to see if they develop a disease. This allows researchers to calculate the incidence rates in the exposed and unexposed groups, and then to compare the risk of disease in the exposed group relative to the unexposed group. This is called the relative risk. The relative risk is calculated by dividing the incidence of disease in a group of exposed people by the incidence of disease in a group of people who are not exposed to the same factor.

$$\text{Relative risk (RR)} = \frac{\text{Incidence in exposed}}{\text{Incidence in unexposed}}$$

Or alternatively, using the two-by-two table:

$$RR = \frac{a/(a+b)}{c/(c+d)}$$

Relative risks range in value from 0 to infinity. To interpret the relative risk:
- if RR = 1 there is no association (risk in exposed is equal to risk in non-exposed)
- if RR > 1 there is a positive association (risk in exposed is greater than risk in non-exposed)
- if RR < 1 there is a negative or inverse association (risk in exposed is less than risk in non-exposed).

Consider a comparison of death from coronary heart disease (outcome) between males and females (gender = exposure). One thousand women and 1000 men were recruited into a cohort study and followed over one year. Sixteen of the women and 20 of the men died from coronary heart disease within that year. The rate of death from coronary heart disease among females was 16 per 1000 person-years of observation and the rate among males was 20 per 1000 person-years of observation. A two-by-two table for this scenario would look like this:

		DEATH FROM CHD		TOTAL
		YES	NO	
Gender	M	20	980	1000
	F	16	984	1000
Total		36	1964	2000

To calculate the relative risk in this example:

$$RR = \frac{a/(a+b)}{c/(c+d)}$$

$$= \frac{20/(20+980)}{16/(16+984)}$$

$$= 1.25$$

This is interpreted as meaning that compared with females (referent group), males have a 25% increased risk of dying from coronary heart disease.

Odds ratios

Relative risk requires the ability to measure incidence however this is not always possible, for example in case-control studies. In this situation, researchers need to use another measure of association known as an odds ratio (OR). The odds ratio asks, 'What are the odds that a case was exposed relative to the odds that a control was exposed?' And, like relative risk, two-by-two tables can be helpful when calculating odds ratios (see Table 4.2).

		DISEASE	
		YES (CASES)	NO (CONTROLS)
Past exposure	Yes (exposed)	a	b
	No (not exposed)	c	d
Total		a + c	b + d

TABLE 4.2 Two-by-two table for a case-control study

To calculate an odds ratio:

$$OR = \frac{\text{Odds that a case was exposed}}{\text{Odds that a control was exposed}} = \frac{a/c}{b/d} = \frac{ad}{bc}$$

As with relative risk, odds ratios indicate something about the strength of the association between the disease and exposure. Odds ratios range in value from 0 to infinity. To interpret the odds ratio:

- if OR = 1 there is no association (and therefore the exposure is not related to the disease)

- if OR > 1 there is a positive association (and therefore the exposure is associated with an increased risk of the disease)
- if OR < 1 there is a negative or inverse association.

Example: Calculating the odds ratio for heart problems

A researcher wants to calculate the odds ratio for heart problems in men compared with women. For this question, the women would be the referent category, as the heart problems of men are being compared with women. The women are also the unexposed group. A two-by-two table for this study would look like this:

		HEART PROBLEMS		TOTAL
		YES	NO	
Gender	M	270	1280	1550
	F	90	2010	2100
Total		360	3290	3650

To calculate the odds ratio in this example, we can calculate the odds of heart problems in each group and compare them by taking the ratio of the odds:

$$\text{The odds of a heart problem in women} = \frac{90}{2010} = 0.04477$$

$$\text{The odds of a heart problem in men} = \frac{270}{1280} = 0.21094$$

$$\text{OR} = \frac{0.21094}{0.04477}$$

$$= 4.71$$

Alternatively, using the formula for odds ratios and the two-by-two table:

$$\text{OR} = \frac{ad}{bc}$$

$$= \frac{270 \times 2010}{1280 \times 90}$$

$$= \frac{542700}{115200}$$

$$= 4.71$$

This is interpreted as meaning that, compared with women, men have a 4.71-fold increased risk of heart problems.

To interpret this odds ratio we would say that, relative to women, the odds of having a heart problem were 4.71 times higher for men. In other words, men have a 4.71-fold increased risk of having heart problems compared with women.

Sources of error in epidemiological studies

Researchers cannot control the world in which they live, so there is always the potential for error and/or bias to creep into any study. Problems can arise in a variety of ways, for example a researcher may select a group of participants for a study that does not truly reflect the true population of interest; the measurement tool/s that are used may be flawed or invalid in some way and hence give imprecise measurements; or information may not be collected for all risk factors. A primary aim of good research design is to minimise problems, such as error and bias, which may alter the outcomes of a study. There are two main types of error that we need to be aware of: random error (or chance error) and systematic error (or bias). Let's start with random error; this can occur when there is random sampling variation and/or random measurement error.

Random error

If we take a sample of our population, most of the time the characteristics of the people included in our study will be similar to the population as a whole. However, it is always possible that, by chance, the sample selected is not actually representative of the population from which it was drawn. This is random sampling variation and the results that we get from collecting data from a sample of the people in the population may be slightly different from the results we would get if we had collected data from everyone in our population. Random sampling variation can affect the generalisability of a study. There is no guaranteed way of preventing random sampling error, but the likelihood of it occurring is reduced when the size of our sample increases. Sometimes you can check for random sampling error if you have information (e.g. census data) on your target population with which to compare your sample. Random measurement error refers to the random variation in measurement of key characteristics.

When you take measurements repeatedly, there is a chance that the data will vary due to a range of uncontrollable factors. For example, if you are doing research into heart disease, you may measure blood pressure; each time blood pressure is taken, the value may be the actual blood pressure, or it could be altered slightly due to fluctuations in the instrument, the procedure used or the timing of measurement. Random variability in measurement can never be entirely eliminated, however it can be minimised by the careful training of data collectors, and the use of standard protocols and routinely tested equipment. Accuracy of a particular instrument can be assessed by repeating the measurement using a 'gold standard' instrument (that is, one that has already been shown to be the most accurate option available). Random error cannot ever be completely removed, but the impact of random error on your results can be assessed through the proper use of statistical methods (this will not be covered in this text).

ACTIVITY

● An investigator wants to measure daily fat intake among adolescents and decides to ask each participant to keep a food diary that will be used to assess fat intake. Write a paragraph to describe how using a food diary might introduce error into the information that the investigator is collecting.

REFLECTION

Did you consider that, even if all the adolescents are very motivated and honest and keep an accurate record of what they have eaten over the past week, it is very difficult to convert this diary into an accurate estimate of fat intake? For example, if a participant records the evening meal as spaghetti bolognaise, we do not know how large the portion was, or if the cook used lean mince or whether they used any extra oil in the cooking. We have to make estimates about the fat content of an 'average' spaghetti bolognaise when converting the food diary into estimated fat intake. In doing so we could easily underestimate or overestimate the fat intake of the adolescent, so the potential for random measurement error in this instrument (the food diary) is high.

Systematic error

Systematic error is a much more serious problem in epidemiology than random error. Systematic error results from any trend in the collection, analysis, interpretation, publication or review of data that leads to conclusions that are systematically different from the truth. This type of bias can lead to incorrect results and consequently incorrect conclusions about the association between exposure and outcome in the study. The main types of systematic error are selection bias (sampling, participation and attrition bias), information bias and confounding.

Selection bias

Selection bias arises when there are systematic differences between people involved in a study and those not involved in a study. This could be reflected in the way the sample was selected (sampling bias) or by an individual's choice to participate after being selected by the investigators (commonly known as participation bias). It also includes the influence of continued participation in a longitudinal or cohort study (known as 'loss to follow-up' or attrition bias). In any health research project, people who are selected for a study, who volunteer to participate and who stay in the study can differ in many ways from those who are not selected, who refuse or who drop out. Some of these differences may not be important. For instance, generally men are less likely than women to participate in research, however bias only arises if gender is associated with the exposure or the outcome/s. The most important aspect of sample bias is that the participants who are selected and stay in the study may be systematically different from those who are not in the study.

Sampling bias cannot be reduced by increasing the size of a sample, nor can it be measured using statistical tests. This form of bias arises when the identification of individuals for the sample is not truly random and can affect the generalisability of the results.

The logic is quite simple. Usually samples are selected to represent a larger target population. The best way to ensure representativeness is to select individuals at random. However, it is often difficult to ensure that each person in a whole population has an equivalent chance of being selected. For example, if we want to study vitamin D deficiency among adults, how do we obtain a truly random sample? There is no fully comprehensive list of adults in the population. The best we have in Australia are the Commonwealth electoral roll, Medicare numbers and telephone number databases. Unfortunately, some people are not recorded on any of these. Also, the data vary in accuracy (people die, move addresses, change from landlines to mobile phones, do not register with Medicare and so on). When random samples are taken from these registers, we know that some individuals (e.g. people with low socioeconomic status, recent immigrants and young people) are less likely than others to be included and so are under-represented in the sample that is drawn.

Participation bias, also known as volunteer bias, occurs when there are systematic differences between the people who agree to participate in a study and those who do not. It is often the case in health research that people who volunteer for research studies have different risk factors from those who refuse. Those who decline to participate may have poorer (or perhaps better) health than participants, depending on the type of research study. This can threaten the legitimacy of conclusions. Response rates can also affect the results of a study if those who respond are systematically different to those who do not respond.

Attrition bias occurs when people who drop out of studies are systematically different from those who stay in the study ('attrition' = loss). Attrition, or loss to follow-up, is primarily a problem in long-term prospective studies, such as a cohort study or clinical trial. There are many reasons why people do not complete research studies. Sometimes people drop out because they become sicker, and researchers cannot convince them to stay involved. Some people die from causes directly related to the research, or from unrelated causes. People might drop out when they move away from the research area, or they change their attitudes towards the study. Whatever the reason, it is likely that attrition will occur in most longitudinal studies. However, attrition bias only becomes an issue if one study group has a higher attrition rate than the other/s, or if the 'drop out' is related to the outcome under study.

Information bias

Information bias (also known as measurement bias) occurs when there are either outcomes or exposures that are measured incorrectly in systematic ways, rather than random measurement error. This is known as misclassification and refers to assigning study participants to inappropriate groups or categories. The researcher may have incorrectly classified a person as being exposed to a risk factor when in fact they were not exposed to that risk factor; the data may incorrectly measure the amount of exposure classify a person as having a disease when she/he does not or not having a disease when they do.

Recall bias occurs when individuals with a disease are more likely to overestimate or underestimate their exposure than those without the disease. Recall bias is particularly an issue in retrospective studies, which ask participants for information about things that occurred some time prior to interview/survey.

Participants have also been known to intentionally (or non-intentionally) distort self-reported information, especially when responding to questions about personal behaviour. For example, someone who drinks alcohol excessively may under-report the level of consumption to provide a more 'socially acceptable' response. Similarly, when data are collected from other sources, for example, hospital records, there may be systematic errors in the availability of personal information.

Interviewer bias, also known as observer bias, occurs when the interviewer asks questions or records information in a different way for different groups (e.g. a person receiving a new drug and person receiving a placebo). Systematic error in observation, measurement, analysis and interpretation can be controlled to some extent by making the investigator/interviewer unaware of the study participant's exposure status (also known as blinding), by training the interviewer and by using structured questionnaires or interviews and tape-recording interviews.

There are other biases that can lead to inaccurate conclusions including *publication bias*, which arises when there are systematic differences between studies that are, or are not, published.

Confounding

Confounding can be an important source of error in epidemiological studies if it is not identified and dealt with appropriately. Confounding occurs when a non-causal association between a given exposure and outcome is observed as a result of a third variable. The idea is quite simple, and the experience is very common in everyday life. If you believe that exposure X causes disease Y (it seems to, and you have some data to support this), however there is really no causal association and the apparent link arises because both X and Y are related to a third factor, A.

This is called confounding and factor A is a confounder; this is shown diagrammatically in Figure 4.3. For a factor to be a confounder, it must meet the following criteria: it must be a definite risk factor for the disease (Y); it must be associated with the other exposure (X) under study; it must not be an intermediate step between exposure (X) and the disease (Y), for example, obesity → hypertension → heart disease (see figure 4.3). Hypertension could be part of the causal chain, rather than a confounder.

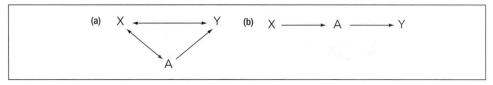

FIGURE 4.3: Diagram illustrating the relationship between (a) exposure X, disease Y and confounder A, (b) exposure X, disease Y and non-confounding factor on causal path A

ACTIVITY

- Is it possible that regular blood donation reduces the risk of heart disease? In 1998, a cohort study conducted in Finland reported that regular blood donors had an 88% reduction in risk of heart attack (Salonen et al 1998). Do you consider this to be proof that blood donation prevents heart disease?

REFLECTION

Did you consider whether there might be other factors that could explain the apparent association? For example, were the donors more health conscious and therefore less likely to have heart disease than non-donors?

Why is confounding important to an epidemiologist?

Confounding bias can undermine the efforts of research. Confounding can lead to an over- or under-estimation of association between exposure and disease, and can in fact completely mask an association or even reverse the direction of an association.

It is essential to anticipate potential sources of confounding when considering your study design. Let us consider an example in which a group of researchers want to investigate whether length of stay in hospital following cardiac surgery is associated with the type of unit to which the patient is admitted (coronary care unit versus intensive care unit). After collecting the necessary data, the researchers find a significant difference in length of stay between the two units, with intensive care patients spending, on average, two days longer in hospital (a clinically important difference!). In theory, we could stop there but, before we recommend that all hospitals introduce specialist coronary care units, what if there is another explanation for the pattern we are seeing? What if the apparent relationship between length of stay and type of unit to which each patient was admitted was confounded by a competing explanation. Is the real reason for the pattern seen? For example, it is possible that patients admitted to the coronary care unit are more likely to be those who have a planned admission, whereas patients admitted to the intensive care unit may be more likely to be emergency admissions. Emergency admissions may be in a more serious condition upon admission, with more coronary damage than elective admissions, therefore admission type (elective or emergency) could be related to length of stay, as emergency admissions could take longer to recover from surgery. So, type of admission may confound the association between admission unit and length of stay, as illustrated in Figure 4.4.

Finally, every study will be affected by some degree of error and, while strategies can be implemented to reduce chance fluctuation and bias, in practice it is impossible to eliminate all sources of error. Therefore, it is important to always consider and remain aware of the effects that error may have on the results of any epidemiological study.

ACTIVITY

- Do you ever consider alternative explanations when you hear media reports of new scientific discoveries? Think about some times when you might have done this.

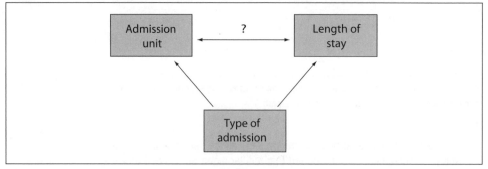

FIGURE 4.4: Diagram of relationship between admission unit and length of stay confounded by type of admission

REFLECTION

Next time you watch the news or pick up a newspaper and read a report about some new discovery, stop to think whether the researchers have considered potential confounders in their study.

Summing it all up

Epidemiology examines health from a population level rather than an individual level. A paramedic or clinician might describe myocardial infarction in individual terms of chest pain, pulse and blood pressure, while an epidemiologist would describe myocardial infarction in terms of susceptible age groups, populations and risk factors. Both types of information are important and have different uses. Current developments in epidemiology focus on the contribution of intra-individual factors (e.g. inherited genetic susceptibility) and higher level factors (e.g. social policy and climate change). However, there are, of course, many other activities that have promoted the wellbeing of the population. Clinical medicine is excellent for examining health issues within the confines of known aspects of the human body, but it is not equipped to infer cause in the absence of well-controlled experiments.

One major focus of epidemiological research has been on associations between lifestyle factors and disease. There is a continuing need to examine these associations in order to reduce disability and death. Some prominent examples of public health activities that have successfully reduced morbidity and mortality in Australia include childhood immunisation programs, needle and syringe exchange programs, anti-smoking campaigns, occupational health and safety policies, mosquito control campaigns, promoting dietary guidelines, banning toxic pesticides and mandatory use of seatbelts in cars and helmets while cycling.

Olsen et al (2001) wrote:

> In its historical evolution epidemiology's successes have largely derived from its working as the investigative component of public health, studying the distribution and determinants of health and diseases in populations. This essence should continue to be preserved in the foreseeable future by incorporating into epidemiological research the new opportunities currently arising in particular fields of genetics, environmental sciences, medicine, and health care.
>
> (Olsen et al 2001 p 15)

In order to prevent disease effectively, epidemiologists have a responsibility to not only use appropriate methods, but also to translate their findings into something of benefit to both the local and the global community.

A final word

This chapter has provided an introduction to some basic epidemiological concepts. As practicing epidemiologists, we need to build on these concepts and also consider more complex methods of assessing evidence, taking into account various measures of association and causal inference. If you are interested in exploring epidemiology further, there are numerous textbooks and online resources available, as well as formal university courses.

REVIEW QUESTIONS

1 In your own words, give a definition of epidemiology.
2 Describe how epidemiology differs from clinical medicine.
3 Describe two measures of disease frequency.
4 Discuss the differences between prevalence and incidence.
5 Explain the difference between observational and experimental study designs, giving examples of each.
6 What do relative risk and odds ratio measure?
7 What is the technical term used by epidemiologists when a third factor influences the relationship between an exposure and a disease?
8 Describe two types of systematic bias that should always be considered by epidemiologists.
9 How might you use epidemiology in your future profession?

Useful websites

Centre for Disease Control & Prevention: www.cdc.gov/excite/library/glossary
Epidemiology Supercourse: www.pitt.edu/~super1
John Snow – a historical giant in epidemiology:
http://www.ph.ucla.edu/epi/snow.html
The James Lind Library: www.jameslindlibrary.org

REFERENCES

Alati R, Najman J M, Kinner S et al 2005 Early Predictors of Adult Drinking: A Birth Cohort Study. American Journal of Epidemiology 162(11):1098–1107
Brown W J, Mummery K, Eakin E et al 2006 10,000 Steps Rockhampton: Evaluation of a Whole Community Approach to Improving Population Levels of Physical Activity. Journal of Physical Activity and Health 3(1):1–14
Clark M J, Purdie J, FitzGerald G J et al 1999 Predictors of Demand for Emergency Prehospital Care: an Australian Study. Prehospital and Disaster Medicine 14(3):167–173
Gordis L 2004 Epidemiology, 3rd edn. Elsevier Saunders, Philadelphia
Gunes UY, Eser I 2007 Effectiveness of a Honey Dressing for Healing Pressure Ulcers. Journal of Wound, Ostomy and Continence Nursing 34(2):184–190
Keeping J D, Najman J M, Morrison J et al 1989 A Prospective Longitudinal Study of Social, Psychological and Obstetric Factors in Pregnancy: Response Rates and Demographic Characteristics of the 8556 Respondents. British Journal of Obstetrics and Gynaecology 96(3):289–297
Last J M 1995 A Dictionary of Epidemiology. 4th edn. Oxford University Press, Oxford
Olsen J R, Saracci R, Trichopoulos D 2001 Teaching Epidemiology: A Guide for Teachers in Epidemiology, Public Health and Clinical Medicine. Oxford University Press, Oxford
Salonen J T, Tuomainen T P, Salonen R et al 1998 Donation of Blood Is Associated with Reduced Risk of Myocardial Infarction: The Kuopio Ischaemic Heart Disease Risk Factor Study. American Journal of Epidemiology 148(5):445–451

Tenkate T D, Stafford R J 2001 Risk Factors for Campylobacter Infection in Infants and Young Children: A Matched Case-Control Study. Epidemiology and Infection 127:399–404

Thompson C L, Khiani V, Chak A et al 2007 Carbohydrate Consumption and Esophageal Cancer: An Ecological Assessment. American Journal of Gastroenterology 102(11):1–7

Webb P, Bain C, Pirozzo S 2005 Essential Epidemiology: An Introduction for Students and Health Professionals, 1st edn. Cambridge University Press, Cambridge

World Health Organization 1948 Preamble to the Constitution of the World Health Organization as adopted by the International Health Conference, New York, 19–22 June, 1946; signed on 22 Jul 1946 by the representatives of 61 States and entered into force on 7 Apr1948

The authors would like to acknowledge those who assisted with the development of components of this chapter: Dr Diana Battistutta, Professor Michael Dunne, Kate Halton and Professor Beth Newman of the School of Public Health, QUT; and Michelle Cook, formerly of the School of Public Health, QUT.

CHAPTER 5

Physical and environmental determinants

Mary Louise Fleming & Thomas Tenkate

Learning objectives

After reading this chapter you should be able to:

- describe the meaning of the term 'determinants'
- identify and discuss the range of physical and environmental determinants that impact on health
- suggest why it is important to the practice of public health that you understand how determinants contribute to health
- understand the complexity of health and illness and the multifaceted role of health determinants
- relate determinants of health to public health activity and realise the need for multisectoral action and multiple approaches when working to improve health.

Introduction

This chapter describes physical and environmental determinants of the health of Australians, providing a background to the development of successful public health activity. Health determinants are the biomedical, genetic, behavioural, socioeconomic and environmental factors that impact on health and wellbeing. These determinants can be influenced by interventions and by resources and systems (AIHW 2006). Many factors combine to affect the health of individuals and communities. People's circumstances and the environment determine whether the population is healthy or not. Factors such as where people live, the state of their environment, genetics, their education level and income, and their relationships with friends and family are all likely to impact on their health. The determinants of population health reflect the context of people's lives; however, people are very unlikely to be able to control many of these determinants (WHO 2007a).

This chapter and Chapter 6 illustrate how various determinants can relate to and influence other determinants, as well as health and wellbeing. We believe it is particularly important to provide an understanding of determinants and their relationship to health and illness in order to provide a structure in which a broader conceptualisation of health can be placed. Determinants of health do not exist in isolation from one another. More frequently they work together in a complex system. What is clear to anyone who works in public health is that many factors impact on the health and wellbeing of people. For example, in the next chapter we discuss factors such as living and working conditions, social support, ethnicity and class, income, housing, work stress and the impact of education on the length and quality of people's lives.

In 1974 the influential *Lalonde Report* (Lalonde 1974) described key factors that impact on health status. These factors included lifestyle, environment, human biology and health services. Taking a population-health approach builds on the *Lalonde Report*, and recognises that a range of factors, such as living and working conditions and the distribution of wealth in society, interact to determine the health status of a population.

Tackling health determinants has great potential to reduce the burden of disease and promote the health of the general population. In summary, we understand very clearly now that health is determined by the complex interactions between individual characteristics, social and economic factors and physical environments; the entire range of factors that impact on health must be addressed if we are to make significant gains in population health, and focussing interventions on the health of the population or significant subpopulations can achieve important health gains.

In 2007 the Australian Government included in the list of *National Health Priority Areas* the following health issues: cancer control, injury prevention and control, cardiovascular health, diabetes mellitus, mental health, asthma, arthritis and musculoskeletal conditions. The *National Health Priority Areas* set the agenda for the Commonwealth, states and territories, local governments and not-for-profit organisations to place attention on those areas considered to be the major foci for action. Many of these health issues are discussed in this chapter and the following chapter.

Defining determinants of health

The health of individuals and populations is influenced and determined by many factors acting in various combinations. The dominant view is that health is 'multicausal' – healthiness, disease, disability and, ultimately, death are seen as the result of the interaction of human biology, lifestyle and environmental (e.g. social) factors, modified by health interventions and other measures (Marmot & Wilkinson 2006). As the Surgeon General commented in the report *Healthy People 2010*:

> Our understanding of these determinants and how they relate to one another,
> coupled with our understanding of how individual and community health
> affects the health of the nation, is perhaps the most important key to achieving
> our *Healthy People 2010* goals of increasing the quality and years of life and of
> eliminating the nation's health disparities.
>
> (Office of Disease Prevention 2007 p 23)

Health determinants can be described as those factors that raise or lower the level of health in a population or individual (Keleher & Murphy 2004). Determinants help explain and predict trends in health and explain why some groups have better or worse health than others. They are the key to preventing disease, illness and injury (AIHW 2006).

Determinants may have positive or negative effects. Factors such as tobacco smoking or low socioeconomic status increase the risk of ill health and are commonly termed 'risk factors'. Positive influences such as a high intake of fruit and vegetables are known as 'protective factors'. Unlike behaviour, some determinants such as age, sex and genetics cannot be altered. Some of these factors are the subject of this chapter. The following chapter discusses social and economic factors that determine health.

For almost all factors that impact on health the associated effect is not 'all or nothing'. For risk factors, rather than there being one point at which risk begins, there is an increasing effect as the exposure increases. For example, a person may be physically active but not in a way that increases their heart rate on a regular basis each week, and therefore, in association with inappropriate food consumption, that person has an increased risk of ill health. Although the increasing risk often starts at relatively low levels, the usual practice is to monitor a risk factor by reporting the proportion at the riskier end of the spectrum (AIHW 2006).

Determinants can vary in the extent to which they represent 'relative risk' and 'absolute risk' of developing disease. The concept of 'relative risk' has been defined and discussed in more detail in Chapter 4. If, for example, a food product provided to a small group of people was contaminated with salmonella, there would be a high relative risk of food poisoning among the group. However, as the product was only provided to the small group, there would be a relatively low absolute risk of poisoning from the food product in the population as a whole.

In addition to influencing the occurrence of new cases of disease or injury, determinants can affect the continuation and prognosis of chronic diseases and their complications (AIHW 2006). The use of health care interventions can also be regarded as a determinant in that context. Determinants can also influence how individuals function, in terms of their activities and participation in society. Aspects of the physical environment can either facilitate functioning or act as a barrier to it, as can the availability of assistance from other people or functional supports such as aids and appliances (WHO 2007b).

A complex web of determinants

Determinants are in complex interplay and range from the 'upstream' background influences (e.g. culture and wealth), with many health and non-health effects that can be difficult to quantify, to immediate or direct influences with highly specific effects on particular aspects of health. They are often described as part of broad causal 'pathways' or 'chains' that affect health (Keleher & Wilkinson 2004).

The Public Health Agency of Canada (2007) defines 11 determinants of health (see Table 5.1). Examining these issues briefly in tabular form gives you an idea of the range of factors that impact on health. Figure 5.1 collapses these many determinants into a manageable and simple framework for your consideration. Some of these determinants are discussed further in this chapter and the remaining determinants are considered in the following chapter.

Figure 5.1 presents a simple framework of determinants and their pathways. The pathways are not linear and can also occur in reverse. For example, an individual's health can influence their physical activity levels, employment status and wealth. General background factors and environmental factors can determine the nature of socioeconomic characteristics and both can influence people's health behaviour, their psychological state and factors relating to their safety. These in turn can influence biomedical factors, such as blood pressure and body weight, which may have health effects through various further pathways. At all stages along the path these various factors interact with an individual's genetic composition. This framework then shows us a simple way of organising and examining the various pathways that may occur in a range of different contexts.

DETERMINANTS OF HEALTH	DESCRIPTION
Income and social status	Much research suggests poor people are less healthy than rich people. Income distribution is a key element.
Social support networks	Support from family, friends and community is linked to health.
Employment and working conditions	Unemployment and poor health are related. More control over working conditions improves health.
Education	Low literacy levels are linked to poor health.
Physical environments	Clean air and water, healthy workplaces, safe houses, communities and roads all contribute to health.
Genetics	Inherited characteristics play a role in determining how long we live, how healthy we will be and the likelihood of contracting certain illnesses.
Personal health practices and coping skills	Physical activity, good nutrition, smoking and drinking and coping skills impact on health.
Healthy child development	Good health in childhood has a positive influence on later life.
Health services	Access to services that prevent diseases benefits health.
Gender	Different kinds of diseases and conditions affect women and men differently.
Culture	Customs and beliefs affect health.

TABLE 5.1: Determinants of health

(Source: Public Health Agency of Canada 2007)

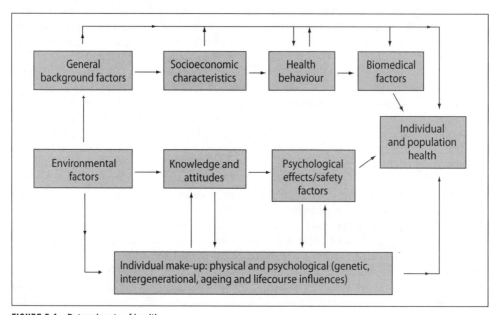

FIGURE 5.1: Determinants of health

(Adapted from AIHW 2004, figure 3.1)

An important use of determinants is to enable us to focus on where best to intervene. Turrell et al (2006) identify three broad levels of factors affecting health and how interventions might be structured based on these levels as follows:

- downstream factors include treatment systems, disease management and investment in clinical research
- midstream factors include lifestyle, behavioural and individual prevention programs
- upstream factors involve government policies and investment in population health research as examples (Keleher & Murphy 2004).

One of the important uses for this type of approach is to ensure that we direct our resources upstream to focus on issues that impact on health equity. This issue will be considered in more detail in the next chapter.

Genetics and screening

Genetic determinants are important factors impacting on individual health and they will continue to be important as nearly every disease has constitutive and/or acquired genetic components. Identifying disease susceptibility genes as well as identifying acquired somatic mutations underlying a specific disease, such as cancer, can provide vital information for a more thorough understanding of many common illnesses. This information can then be used to determine how diseases are diagnosed and how new treatments or particular drug therapies can be identified (European Commission 2007).

'Genes are the units of heredity which control the structure and function of the body by determining the structure of peptide chains that form the building blocks of enzymes and other proteins' (Harper et al 1994 p 119). A gene's role is to ensure that the amino acids are always in the same order. Genes are located at specific points in the deoxyribonucleic acid (DNA) in the cell nucleus and the DNA is arranged into 23 pairs of chromosomes. Of these, 22 are called autosomes while the other pair are the sex chromosomes. One of each pair of chromosomes is derived from each parent. There are several categories of genetic disease depending upon the location and the extent of the genetic abnormality. The categories include single-gene disorders, chromosomal disorders, disorders involving several genes and environmental influences, disorders of cytoplasmic DNA and mutations of somatic cells.

In the case of single-gene disorders, they may be autosomal dominant, for example, Huntington's disease and otosclerosis; autosomal recessive, for example, cystic fibrosis; or x-linked dominant or recessive, resulting in disorders such as muscular dystrophy and haemophilia.

Chromosomal abnormalities often cause fetal death and congenital disease. For example, about half of spontaneous abortions are linked to chromosomal abnormalities. Down syndrome is an example of a chromosomal abnormality.

The complex interplay of genetic and environmental factors is associated with the relationship between several genes at different loci on the chromosome, each with an additive effect and a variable environmental component. Characteristics determined in this multifactorial manner may be continuous or discontinuous. For a continuous multifactorial trait, such as blood pressure, there is a high continuous gradient from high blood pressure to normal blood pressure. An example of a discontinuous multifactorial variable is cleft lip and palate.

There is strong evidence of a genetic component to many conditions causing chronic illness and premature death. We must also keep in mind that the majority of diseases are multifactorial in aetiology and result from the interaction of multiple genetic and environmental factors.

Examples of the integration of genetics into public health functions in the 21st century include such activities as investigating clusters of cancer in communities, developing policies for using genetic testing to prevent iron overload in the US, population analysis of the impact of asthma interventions based on individual susceptibility, evaluating prevention effectiveness of a national campaign for early detection of colon cancer and a national assurance program to monitor the utilisation, effectiveness and impact of genetic testing. The implications for public health include treatment for affected high-risk individuals, prevention for at-risk individuals, health promotion activities among the general population and with regard to the environment, crop modification, pharmaceuticals and the cloning of animals, as examples.

However, genetic screening raises ethical, social and legal concerns around the privacy and confidentiality of genetic information, fairness in the use of genetic information, the psychological impact, stigmatisation and discrimination associated with the use of such information, reproductive and clinical issues and uncertainties associated with gene tests for susceptibilities and complex conditions. It will be interesting to follow modern genetics as it develops because it will undoubtedly have implications for the population's health.

The *Human Genome Project* commenced in 1990 as a 15-year large-scale, international project that involved the US, the UK, France, Canada, Germany, Japan and China. The primary goal was to sequence the entire human genome, with other goals including identifying genes, improvements in technology and data analysis, comparative genomics and the ethical, legal and social implications of such a project. 'From a public health perspective, there is a danger that the enthusiasm for genomics may deflect attention and resources from the important mission of preventing disease in the population' (Schneider 2006 p 211). Genomics is the study of how genes act in the body, and how they interact with environmental influences to cause disease. The fundamental question for public health is the extent to which applying this emerging knowledge will divert resources from the mission of public health, which is to prevent disease in the population.

Diabetes is a good example of the complex interplay of genetic and environmental factors. Consider the following activity on diabetes as an introduction to the nature and impact of a chronic disease on health and wellbeing and the potential role of public health. If you are not familiar with diabetes consider looking at the website located at the back of this chapter to become more familiar with the different characteristics of diabetes. For example, type 1 and type 2 diabetes, their development and prevention and treatment options. Then attempt the activity.

ACTIVITY

Try answering the following questions:
- What is a chronic disease?
- Is diabetes a chronic disease?
- What causes diabetes?
- Is there a genetic contribution?
- Are there different types of diabetes?
- How is the condition managed?
- Can it be prevented?
- How does public health contribute to promotion, prevention, intervention and maintenance of quality of life if a person has diabetes?

REFLECTION

Diabetes mellitus is a condition where the body cannot maintain normal blood glucose levels. There are three types of diabetes: type 1 diabetes, type 2 diabetes and gestational diabetes. A further category of diabetes is not common and accounts for less than 1% of people with diabetes. It includes diabetes caused by a variety of distinct genetic and pathological mechanisms that are generally clearly defined.

Diabetes is caused by resistance to, or deficient production of, the hormone insulin, which helps glucose move from the blood into the cells. When the body does not produce or use enough insulin, the cells cannot use glucose and the blood glucose level rises. This means that the body will instead start to break down its own fat and muscle for energy. Diabetes may lead to severe problems including damage to the heart, blood vessels, eyes, nerves and kidneys (Department of Health and Ageing 2006 website). Diabetes is defined as a chronic disease in Australia. In the United States the definition of a chronic disease is different from the Australian definition. There are some websites listed at the back of the chapter that will help you consider differing definitions of chronic disease. The last section of the activity asks you how public health might contribute to promotion, prevention and rehabilitation of people with diabetes. Think back to what you have learned about the nature of public health, the determinants that contribute to diabetes and what public health strategies might be put in place as prevention and rehabilitation strategies for diabetes.

Biological and behavioural determinants

Biological determinants

Biology refers to the individual's genetic makeup, family history and the physical and mental health problems acquired during life. Ageing, diet, physical activity, smoking, stress, alcohol or illicit drug abuse, injury or violence, or an infectious or toxic agent, may result in illness or disability and can produce a 'new biology' for the individual (Office of Disease Prevention 2007).

Behavioural determinants

Lifestyle or behavioural determinants are multidimensional and they are linked to a number of major health problems. Some health issues share the same determinants such as tobacco, alcohol and nutrition.

Individual health practices are responses or reactions to internal stimuli and external conditions. Both behaviour and biology can have a reciprocal relationship, with each reacting to the other when a person is exposed to a particular health condition. Examples of the reciprocity of the relationship can be seen in the case of a family history of heart disease (biology) which may motivate an individual to add healthy eating behaviours, maintain an active lifestyle and avoid tobacco smoking (behaviours), which may prevent him or her from developing heart disease (biology). Personal choices and the social and physical environments surrounding individuals can shape behaviours. The social and physical environments also include factors that affect the life of individuals, positively or negatively, many of which may not be under their immediate or direct control (Office of Disease Prevention 2007).

ACTIVITY

Select a health issue that is influenced by lifestyle or the behaviours of an individual.
- What lifestyle or behavioural factors make a contribution to the issue?
- Which of these does the individual have some control over?
- Why is it difficult for the individual to have control over their health?
- What are the environmental factors?

REFLECTION

Did you consider any of the following significant factors listed below? What factors may change if an individual could control the determinants of their health? Would it make it easier for them? Would it be more difficult? Does the environment play a role in the health issue you have selected?

Tobacco

Tobacco is clearly responsible for, in part, a worldwide epidemic of coronary heart disease and lung cancer. The work of researchers such as Doll and Hill (1964) clearly linked the smoking patterns of individuals with age and cause of death (Keleher & Murphy 2004). The World Health Organization (WHO) *Global Burden of Disease Study* (Murray & Lopez 1996) reported that by 2020, it was expected that tobacco would account for 12.3% of deaths worldwide.

Alcohol

Alcohol plays an important role in the Australian economy and it also has an important social role. It is a familiar part of traditions and customs in this country and is often used for relaxation, socialisation and celebration. Eighty-three per cent of Australians reported drinking alcohol in 2004. It is a drug that can promote relaxation and feelings of euphoria. It can also lead to intoxication and dependence and a wide-range of associated harms (Ministerial Council on Drug Strategy 2006).

Although the per capita consumption of alcohol in Australia has declined since the 1980s it remains high by world standards. Many of the dangers of alcohol for those who drink, and those around them, are misunderstood, tolerated or ignored. The harms associated with unsafe alcohol use, including drinking to intoxication, are now well documented in the research literature. The *National Alcohol Strategy 2006–2009* (the strategy) is a plan for action developed through collaboration between Australian governments, non-government and industry partners and the broader community. It outlines priority areas for coordinated action to develop drinking cultures that will reduce alcohol-related harm in Australia. The strategy seeks to reflect the *National Drug Strategy: Australia's integrated framework 2004–2009* and build on the previous alcohol strategy (Ministerial Council on Drug Strategy 2006).

Injuries

Injuries result in an estimated 8000 or 6% of deaths each year in Australia and are responsible for an estimated 400,000 hospital admissions annually. Injuries are the principal cause of death in almost half of the people under 45 years of age, and account for a range of physical, cognitive and psychological disabilities that seriously affect the quality of life of injured people and their families. Health costs associated with injury in Australia have been estimated to be $2.6 billion annually.

Injury usually means physical harm to a person's body and the most common types of physical injury are broken bones, cuts, poisoning and burns. Physical injury results from harmful contact between people and objects, substances or other things in their surroundings. Examples are being struck by a car, cut by a knife, bitten by a dog or poisoned by inhaled petrol. Some physical injuries are the intended result of acts by people: harm of one person by another (e.g. assault, homicide) or self-harm (NPHP 2004).

Over recent years, Australia has achieved some significant gains in preventing a number of different types of injuries where concerted efforts have been made. There have been improvements in road safety over the past 25 years. The reduction in road deaths has occurred despite significant growth in the population, vehicle numbers and kilometres travelled. Initiatives such as random breath testing, compulsory seat belts, speed blitzes, car design and safety features (e.g. air bags), better roads, ongoing community education regarding road safety and improved life-saving medical procedures and trauma care have all contributed to the decline in the number of vehicle-related fatalities (NPHP 2004).

Suicide prevention and poisoning

Gains have also been made in the area of suicide prevention and poisoning in children. In the year 2000, the all-ages male death rate from suicide was 19.4 (per 100,000) compared with the 1997 rate of 23.4 per 100,000 (AIHW 2002). Hospital separation rates for poisoning in children aged 0–4 years have dropped from 302 per 100,000 in 1991–92 to 267 per 100,000 in 1999–2000 (AIHW 2002).

Diet and physical activity

A healthy diet and regular, adequate physical activity are major factors in promoting and maintaining good health. Unhealthy diets and physical inactivity are two of the main risk factors for raised blood pressure, raised blood glucose, abnormal blood lipids, overweight/obesity and the major chronic diseases such as cardiovascular diseases, cancer and diabetes. According to the *World Health Report 2002*:

> low intake of fruit and vegetables is estimated to cause about 19% of
> gastrointestinal cancer, and about 31% of ischaemic heart disease and 11% of
> stroke worldwide. Overall, 2.7 million (4.9%) deaths and 26.7 million (1.8%)
> DALYS are attributable to low fruit and vegetable intake.
> (World Health Report 2002 p 60–61)

Globally, physical inactivity is estimated to cause about 10–16% of breast, colon and rectal cancers and diabetes mellitus, and about 22% of ischaemic heart disease. Overall, 1.9 million deaths are attributable to physical inactivity.

A website at the back of this chapter (*Nutrition and Physical Activity*) provides you with further examples of the range of activities that the Australian Government Department of Health and Ageing are involved in to advance healthy diet and physical activity. Consider the range of activities that the government is advocating to promote physical activity and good nutrition.

The following activity asks you to think about the list of *National Health Priority Areas* discussed at the beginning of this chapter. Can you identify those priority areas that have genetic, behavioural or lifestyle determinants associated with them? Use some of the websites listed at the back of this chapter to help you with this exercise.

ACTIVITY
● List the national health priority areas that have genetic or behavioural contributions.
● Discuss each one of the priority health areas you identified in terms of the contribution of each of the determinants listed above.
● What priorities has the federal government set to promote and manage the health issue?

REFLECTION

Remember when we examined the genetic determinants that contributed to a number of health issues earlier in this chapter it became clear to us that many conditions can have both a genetic and a behavioural contribution? In fact, many health issues have multiple causes. Keep this in mind as you consider the environmental determinants of health.

Environmental determinants

An environmental determinant of health can be considered to be any external agent (e.g. biological, chemical, physical, social or cultural) that can be linked to changes in health status. Unfortunately, this definition is far too broad because nearly all changes in health status that are not genetically determined could be considered to result from environmental factors (Soskolne & Sieswerda 2007). As such, the scope of what is an environmental determinant is generally restricted to external physical, chemical and microbiological exposures and processes that impact on individuals and the community at large, and that are beyond their immediate control (they are involuntary) (McMichael et al 2006). For example, exposure to environmental tobacco smoke (passive smoking) is considered to be an environmental determinant, whereas active cigarette smoking is considered to be a physical determinant of health.

There are many ways in which to categorise 'environmental determinants', including in relation to (McMichael et al 2006):

- environmental media (e.g. air, water, food, soil)
- economics (e.g. transportation, land use, energy generation)
- physical scale (e.g. local, regional, global)
- settings (e.g. household, workplace, urban/built environment)
- disease outcomes (e.g. cancers, respiratory conditions, congenital abnormalities).

Figure 5.2 illustrates the relationship between some of these environmental determinants.

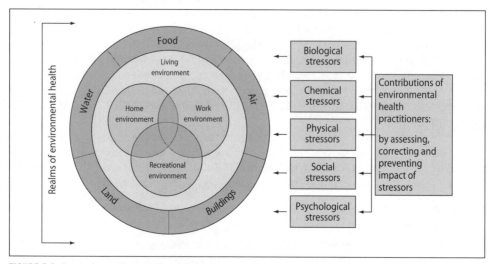

FIGURE 5.2 Human interaction with the environment

(Source: Burke et al 2002, Reproduced under the terms of the Click-Use Licence)

When describing how the environment can impact human health, there are two important underlying considerations that need to be kept in mind (McMichael et al 2006):

1 *Natural variation versus human intervention* – some environmental exposures occur because of natural variation (e.g. seasonal, latitudinal or altitudinal differences in exposure to solar radiation and extremes of heat and cold), whereas much of our effort has been to address human-made environmental hazards. For developed/industrialised countries, much of this effort has been focussed on chemical

contamination of the air, water and food supply, and on urbanisation issues such as noise, traffic injuries, increasing residential density, the so-called 'modern environmental health hazards'. In comparison, developing countries tend to focus on 'traditional environmental health hazards' such as microbiological quality of drinking water and food, the physical safety of housing and workplaces, indoor air pollution and road hazards. Such hazards in developed countries are generally controlled through substantial investment in community infrastructure (e.g. drinking water supply systems, sewage systems and solid waste collection).

2   *Local versus global environmental impacts* – much of our efforts to control environmental impacts on health have focussed on localised exposures (e.g. at a household, community or city level), whereas it is clear that we are now facing much larger scale disruptions of Earth's ecosystems, but unfortunately our understanding of the broader implications of these disruptions is somewhat more limited.

The highly publicised global environmental changes will therefore have a lasting impact on the underlying 'environmental determinants' of human health. The global but local nature and complexity of these changes present unique and unparalleled health risks that have the following key characteristics (Campbell-Lendrum et al 2007):

- The hazards are diverse, global and probably irreversible over human time scales. They range from increased risks of extreme weather events (e.g. storms, floods, heat waves, droughts) to changing patterns of infectious diseases.
- The health impacts are potentially huge, with predicted increases in many of the environmentally-related diseases (e.g. malaria, diarrhoea) as they are highly sensitive to climatic conditions. Worldwide, these diseases are already some of the leading causes of mortality and morbidity.
- The risks are inequitable, in that the greenhouse gases that have caused climate change have predominantly originated from developed countries, but the health risks are concentrated in the poorest countries that have contributed least to the problem.
- Many of the projected health impacts are avoidable, through a combination of short-term public health interventions and long-term strategies to reduce human impacts on climate.

Therefore, the worldwide environmental changes we are currently seeing – and which are predicted to accelerate in coming decades – present, arguably, the greatest challenge we face as a society. The 'environmental determinants' challenge for public health is nicely summarised in the following quote:

> The public health community needs to go beyond reacting to a changing climate. A true preventive strategy needs to ensure the maintenance and development of healthy environments from local to global levels. In the long term, sustainable development and protection of ecosystem services are fundamentally necessary for human health.
>
> (Campbell-Lendrum et al 2007 p 236)

Human interaction with the environment

In order to make an effective contribution to dealing with the global environmental issues introduced in the previous section, it is important for public health practitioners to have an understanding of the complex interactions that occur within natural and man-made environments, and how these interactions impact on human health. The following sections provide an introduction to some of the fundamental ecological process and ecosystem issues and how these can impact on human health.

Up until now we have used the term 'environment' frequently, but a more basic scientific concept is that of an 'ecosystem'. When defining what an 'ecosystem' is, it is important to go back to the core scientific discipline, which is ecology. The term 'ecology' can be traced back to its Greek roots, which literally means 'house-study'. Ecology, therefore, is the study of an organism's home, and is the branch of biology that deals with the inter-relationships between organisms and their environment. There is a range of terminology used to describe ecological processes, and these build on each other in the following way:

Ecology → Ecosystems → Biodiversity → Ecosystem services → Life!

One of the most important developments in the field of ecology during the 20th century was the ecosystem concept. There are multiple meanings and definitions for ecosystems, with the following being a basic definition:

> An ecosystem is a dynamic complex of plant, animal and microorganism communities and the nonliving environment interacting as a functional unit.
> Humans are an integral part of ecosystems. Ecosystems vary enormously in size; a temporary pond in a tree hollow and an ocean basin can both be ecosystems.
> (Alcamo et al 2003 p 3)

Some fundamental concepts relating to ecosystems include the following three interconnected factors that sustain life on earth (Miller 2002):

- There is a one-way flow of high-quality, low-entropy energy from the sun. This flows through materials and living things in their feeding interactions, into the environment as low-quality (high-entropy) energy (mostly through heat dispersal), and eventually back into space as heat.
- The cycling of matter – Earth is closed to significant inputs of matter from space; therefore, all nutrients used by organisms are already present and must be recycled for life to continue.
- Gravity – this keeps atmospheric gases from escaping and draws chemicals downwards in the matter cycles.

Biodiversity is another important concept to consider when discussing ecosystems. Biodiversity is basically the variety of life contained in the various ecosystems, but this layer of living organisms that occupy the land and the seas represent the most complex, dynamic and varied feature of Earth. A more complete definition of biodiversity is:

> The variability among living organisms from all sources including terrestrial, marine and other aquatic ecosystems and the ecological complexes of which they are part; this includes diversity within species, between species and of ecosystems.
> (Millennium Ecosystem Assessment 2005a p 18)

This definition provides some insight into the many dimensions of biodiversity. For example, it recognises that every biota can be characterised by its taxonomic, ecological and genetic diversity, and that the way in which these dimensions vary over space and time is a key feature of biodiversity. In addition to this, biodiversity should not only be considered as relating to unmanaged ecosystems (e.g. wilderness, national parks), but is also equally appropriate for managed/man-made systems. Agricultural and pastoral lands and even urban ecosystems have their own biodiversity. When it is considered that over 24% of Earth's terrestrial surface consists of cultivated land, these ecosystems therefore have enormous impact on biodiversity.

Ecosystem services

Biodiversity is the foundation of ecosystem services to which human health and wellbeing is intimately linked. It is obvious that ecological systems perform essential functions for humans, and these 'ecosystem services' are essential for sustaining human life. In addition to providing goods (e.g. food and medicine), ecosystems provide 'services' such as purification of air and water, accumulation of toxins, decomposition of wastes, mitigation of floods, stabilisation of landscapes and regulation of climate.

We generally take these services for granted, but they are usually on a scale that is so large and complex that we would find it difficult to engineer a substitute for them. There are a range of ecosystem services that can be categorised as follows (Chivian 2002):

- *Cycling and filtration services* – air purification, watershed services, purifying fresh waters, maintaining water quality in estuaries, binding toxic elements, detoxifying sediments and soils and maintaining soil fertility.
- *Stabilisation processes* – controlling potential pest and disease-causing species, migration of floods, stabilising landscapes against erosion, buffering the land against ocean storms and carbon sequestration on land and global climate.
- *Biodiversity preservation* – providing critical habitat, and genetic library function.
- *Translocation processes* – pollinating crops and natural vegetation, and dispersing seeds.
- *Life-fulfilling functions* – recreation and aesthetics.

Ecosystem services and human wellbeing

As described above, ecosystem services are the benefits people obtain from ecosystems. These include provisioning, regulating and cultural services, which directly affect people, and supporting services needed to maintain these other services. The human health impacts of ecosystems are often described within the broader category of 'human wellbeing', with human health being a bottom-line (or integrating) component of wellbeing, since changes in economic, social, political, residential, psychological and behavioural circumstances all have health consequences (Millennium Ecosystem Assessment 2005a). Human wellbeing has been described as having multiple components, including the basic material for a good life, freedom and choice, health, good social relations and security. Changes in ecosystem services therefore impact on each of these components, which are in turn influenced by and have an influence on the freedoms and choices available to people. As such, wellbeing is at the opposite end of a continuum from poverty, which has been defined as a 'pronounced deprivation in wellbeing' (Alcamo et al 2003).

The effects of adverse ecosystem changes on human wellbeing can be classed as direct and indirect. Direct effects occur with some immediacy, through locally identifiable biological or ecological pathways. For example, impairment of the water-cleansing capacity of wetlands may adversely affect those who drink that water. Building dams can increase mosquito breeding and thus increase the transmission of malaria. The deforestation of hillsides can expose downstream communities to the hazards of flooding. Indirect effects take a toll on wellbeing through more complex webs of causation, including through social, economic and political routes. Some may take decades to have an impact (Alcamo et al 2003). For example, where farmlands under irrigation become saline, crop yields are reduced; this, in turn, might affect human nutritional security, child growth and development and susceptibility to infectious diseases.

Ecosystem changes affect human wellbeing in the following ways (Alcamo et al 2003):

- *Security* is affected both by changes in provisioning services, which affect supplies of food and other goods and the likelihood of conflict over declining resources, and by changes in regulating services, which could influence the frequency and magnitude of floods, droughts, landslides or other catastrophes. It can also be affected by changes in cultural services as, for example, when the loss of important ceremonial or spiritual attributes of ecosystems contributes to the weakening of social relations in a community. These changes, in turn, affect material wellbeing, health, freedom and choice, security and good social relations.

- *Access to basic material for a good life* is strongly linked to both provisioning services, such as food and fibre production, and to regulating services, including water purification.
- *Health* is strongly linked to provisioning services, such as food production and regulating services, including those that influence the distribution of disease-transmitting insects and of irritants and pathogens in water and air. Health can also be linked to cultural services through recreational and spiritual benefits.
- *Social relations* are affected by changes to cultural services, which affect the quality of human experience.
- *Freedoms and choice* are largely predicated on the existence of the other components of wellbeing and are thus influenced by changes in provisioning, regulating or cultural services from ecosystems.

The interactions between the ecosystem services (supporting, provisioning, regulating, and cultural) and the constituents of wellbeing (as described above) are diagrammatically represented in Figure 5.3. This highlights in particular that provisioning and regulating services strongly influence wellbeing in the areas of security, basic materials for a good life and health, with each of these also highly mediated by socioeconomic factors. The strength of the links and the potential for mediation do, however, differ for different ecosystems and regions.

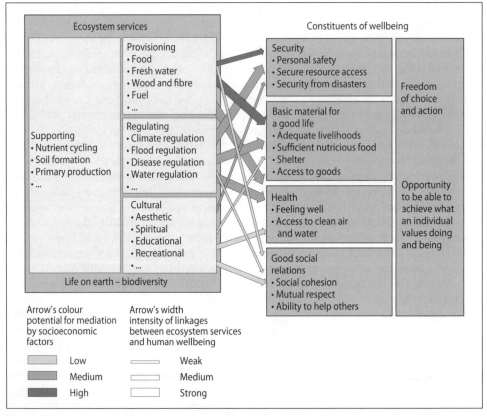

FIGURE 5.3: Links among biodiversity, ecosystem services and human wellbeing

(Source: Reproduced from Millennium Ecosystem Assessment 2005a, World Resources Institute)

Millennium ecosystem assessment

The *Millennium Ecosystem Assessment* (MA) is the most comprehensive assessment that has ever been undertaken into the worldwide impacts of humans on the environment. The goal of the MA was to assess the consequences of ecosystem change for human wellbeing and to establish the scientific basis for actions needed to enhance the conservation and sustainable use of ecosystems and their contributions to human wellbeing.

The MA recognises that interactions exist between people, biodiversity and ecosystems. That is, changing human conditions drive, both directly and indirectly, changes in biodiversity, changes in ecosystems, and ultimately changes in the services ecosystems provide. Thus, biodiversity and human wellbeing are inextricably linked.

The MA also recognises that many other factors independent of changes in biodiversity affect the human condition, and also that many natural forces not associated with humans can influence biodiversity. To assist with directing the assessment, the MA developed a conceptual framework to describe the inter-relationships between biodiversity, ecosystem services, human wellbeing and the drivers for change at the local, regional and global levels. This framework is shown in Figure 5.4. In this figure, changes in drivers that indirectly affect ecosystems, such as population, technology and lifestyle (identified in the upper right corner) can lead to changes in drivers that directly affect ecosystems, such as fisheries, catches or fertiliser application to increase crop yield (identified in the lower right corner). The resulting changes in the ecosystem (lower left corner) cause changes to ecosystem services which then affect human wellbeing. These interactions can take place at more than one scale (e.g. local, regional or global) and can cross scales. For example, a global timber market may lead to regional loss of forest, increasing the magnitude of flooding along a localised stretch of river. These interactions can also take place across different timeframes and strategies and interventions either to respond to negative changes or to enhance positive changes can be taken at almost all points on the framework, except for the direct influence of changes in ecosystem services on human wellbeing (Millennium Ecosystem Assessment 2005b).

The inaugural report of the MA was released in 2005 and the key findings are as follows (Millennium Ecosystem Assessment 2005a):

- Human actions are fundamentally, and to a significant extent irreversibly, changing the diversity of life on Earth, and most of these changes represent a loss of biodiversity. Changes in important components of biological diversity were more rapid in the past 50 years than at any time in human history. Projections and scenarios indicate that these rates will continue, or accelerate, in the future.
- Biodiversity contributes directly (through provisioning, regulating and cultural ecosystem services) and indirectly (through supporting ecosystem services) to many constituents of human wellbeing, including security, basic material for a good life, health, good social relations and freedom of choice and action. Many people have benefited over the past century from the conversion of natural ecosystems to human-dominated ecosystems and the exploitation of biodiversity. At the same time, however, these losses in biodiversity and changes in ecosystem services have caused some people to experience declining wellbeing, with poverty in some social groups being exacerbated.
- Improved valuation techniques and information on ecosystem services tells us that although many individuals benefit from the actions and activities that lead to biodiversity loss and ecosystem change, the costs borne by society of such changes is often higher. Even in instances where our knowledge of benefits and costs is incomplete, using the precautionary approach may be warranted when the costs associated with ecosystem changes may be high or the changes irreversible.

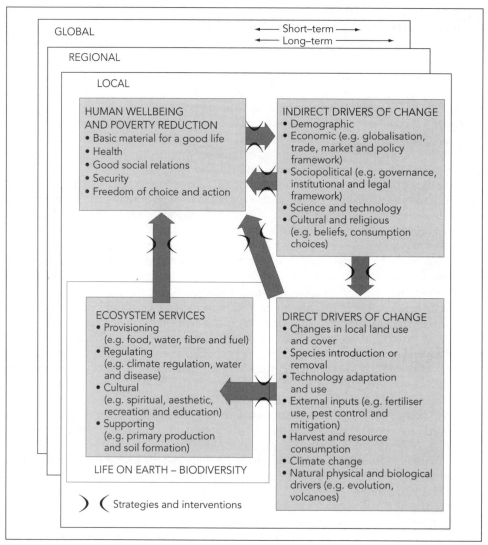

FIGURE 5.4: Millennium Ecosystem Assessment conceptual framework

(Source: Reproduced from Millennium Ecosystem Assessment 2005a, World Resources Institute)

- The drivers of loss of biodiversity and the drivers of changes in ecosystem services are either steady, are showing no evidence of declining over time or are increasing in intensity.
- Many of the actions that have been taken to conserve biodiversity and promote its sustainable use have been successful in limiting biodiversity loss and homogenisation to rates lower than they would otherwise have been in the absence of such actions. However, further significant progress will require a portfolio of actions that build on current initiatives to address important direct and indirect drivers of biodiversity loss and ecosystem service degradation.
- Unprecedented additional efforts would be needed to achieve, by 2010, a significant reduction in the rate of biodiversity loss at all levels.

The findings of the MA are described in more detail in a series of reports, such as *Ecosystems and Human Wellbeing: Biodiversity Synthesis* and *Ecosystems and Human Wellbeing: Health Synthesis*. Further details on the MA project can be obtained from the MA website (see www.millenniumassessment.org).

Case study: Ecosystem changes and human health impacts

A recent example of the many potential impacts of deforestation on human disease comes from the tropical forests of South East Asia and the Amazon. In these areas, widespread logging has impacted on the aquatic habitat of a range of mosquitoes, particularly the *Anopheles* mosquito, which is the vector of malaria. Some indirect impacts of deforestation include removing the overhead trees that acidified standing water through organic acid deposition, which has led to a more neutral pH; removing understorey plants and litter that serve to drain standing water; and increased light and temperatures for the forest floor have accelerated photosynthesis by algae. In addition, deforestation directly disturbs the forest floor by providing depressions that catch and hold water and by creating new breeding sites for the mosquitoes. Taken together these changes have improved the habitat quality for the *Anopheles* larvae which has therefore resulted in a large growth in population for the mosquitoes. As malaria is the most deadly vector-borne disease, killing over 1.2 million people (mainly children) worldwide each year, these ecosystem changes that have led to a proliferation of the malaria vector can only result in increased human health impacts.

(Source: Chivian 2002)

Environmental burden of disease

The previous sections have focussed on fundamental principles related to ecosystems, human impacts on the environment and the relationships between ecosystem services and human health. These sections provide a basis for now discussing the impact of current worldwide environmental conditions on public health status.

In June 2006, WHO released the report *Preventing disease through healthy environments – towards an estimate of the environmental burden of disease* (Pruss-Ustun & Corvalan 2006). This report is the most comprehensive and systematic study ever undertaken on the contribution of environmental hazards to a wide range of diseases and injuries.

The report identifies that as much as 24% of global disease is caused by environmental exposures which can be averted. It estimates that more than 13 million deaths annually are due to preventable environmental causes, with nearly one-third of death and disease in the least developed regions due to environmental causes. Well-targeted interventions are identified as being able to prevent much of this environmental risk, with over 40% of deaths from malaria and an estimated 94% of deaths from diarrhoeal diseases, two of the world's biggest childhood killers, able to be prevented through better environmental management.

The four main diseases influenced by poor environments are diarrhoea, lower respiratory infections, various forms of unintentional injuries and malaria. Measures that could be taken now to reduce this environmental disease burden include promoting safe household water storage and better hygienic measures; the use of cleaner and safer fuels; safer built environment, including a more judicious use and management of toxic substances in the home and workplace; and better water resource management.

Diseases with the largest total annual health burden from environmental factors, in terms of death, illness and disability or 'disability-adjusted life years' (DALYs), are identified as (Pruss-Ustun & Corvalan 2006):

- diarrhoea (58 million DALYS per year; 94% of the diarrhoeal burden of disease), largely from unsafe water, sanitation and hygiene
- lower respiratory infections (37 million DALYs per year; 41% of all cases globally), largely from indoor and outdoor air pollution
- unintentional injuries other than road traffic injuries (21 million DALYs per year; 44 % of all cases globally), with this classification including a wide range of industrial and workplace accidents
- malaria (19 million DALYs per year; 42% of all cases globally), largely as a result of poor water resource, housing and land use management which fails to curb vector populations effectively
- road traffic injuries (15 million DALYS per year; 40% of all cases globally), largely as a result of poor urban design or poor environmental design of transport systems
- chronic obstructive pulmonary disease (COPD) (12 million DALYs per year; 42% of all cases globally), largely as a result of exposures to workplace dusts and fumes and other forms of indoor and outdoor air pollution
- perinatal conditions (11 million DALYS per year; 11% of all cases globally).

Most of the same environmentally triggered diseases also rank as the biggest killers outright – although they rank somewhat differently in order of lethality. Diseases with the largest absolute number of deaths annually from modifiable environmental factors are shown in Figure 5.5.

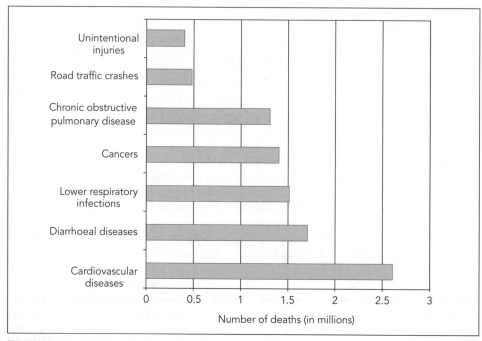

FIGURE 5.5: Annual disease deaths due to modifiable environmental factors

(Source: Pruss-Ustun & Corvalan 2006)

This report shows that in one way or another, the environment significantly affects more than 80% of these major diseases. Further details on the environmental burden of disease can be accessed from the WHO *Quantifying environmental health impacts* website.

Environmental determinants in Australia

Following on from the WHO report described in the previous section, in 2007 WHO released the first ever country-by-country analysis of the impact environmental factors have on the health of residents of individual countries. As expected Australia, along with most of the industrialised countries, fared well in comparison with developing countries. However, this analysis did identify that an estimated 22,000 deaths each year in Australia are due to environmental factors, with this equating to 14% of the total disease burden (WHO 2007a). Specific data for Australia is provided in Table 5.2, with data provided for Angola (a developing nation in Africa) as a comparison.

	AUSTRALIA	ANGOLA
DESCRIPTIVE INFORMATION:		
Population	20.2 m	15.9 m
Gross national income per capita	US$30,610	US$2,210
% urbanisation	88%	53%
% people living in cities with >100,000	72%	20%
<5 years old mortality rate (/1000 live births)	5	260
Life expectancy (years)	81	40
ENVIRONMENTAL BURDEN OF DISEASE FOR SELECTED RISK FACTORS:		
Water, sanitation and hygiene (diarrhoea only): Deaths/year	-	43,500
DALYs/1000/year	0.2	109
Indoor air:		
Deaths/year	-	22,000
DALYs/1000/year	-	57
Outdoor air:		
Deaths/year	700	1800
DALYs/1000/year	0.2	3
ENVIRONMENTAL BURDEN OF DISEASE, PER YEAR:		
DALYs/1000	16	304
Deaths	22,000	116,000
% of total burden	14%	37%
ENVIRONMENTAL BURDEN OF DISEASE, BY DISEASE GROUP (DALYS/1000/YEAR):		
Diarrhoea (range 0.2 to 114)	0.2	114
Respiratory infections (range 0.1 to 56)	0.1	50
Malaria (lowest rate = 0.0, highest rate = 32)	0.0	21
Other vector-borne diseases (range 0.0 to 4.2)	0.0	1.6
Lung cancer (range 0.0 to 2.5)	0.8	0.1
Other cancers (range 0.5 to 4.1)	2.1	1.5
Cardiovascular disease (range 1.3 to 13)	2.4	3.1

	AUSTRALIA	ANGOLA
Chronic obstructive pulmonary disease (range 0.0 to 4.7)	1.5	1.1
Asthma (range 0.3 to 2.4)	1.3	1.2
Musculoskeletal diseases (range 0.5 to 1.5)	0.9	0.6
Road traffic injuries (range 0.3 to 10)	0.4	8.9
Other unintentional injuries (range 0.9 to 19)	2.0	17
Intentional injuries (range 0.1 to 7)	0.6	3.3

TABLE 5.2: Country data on the environmental burden of disease (WHO 2007a)

The information in Table 5.2 indicates that even though Australia and Angola have relatively similar sized populations, on all other measures they are worlds apart. Australia is extremely wealthy, is highly urbanised with people mainly living in big cities, it has a low infant mortality rate and a long life expectancy (double that for residents of Angola). These baseline indicators are then dramatically expressed through the indicators for the environmental burden of disease. For example, over 43,000 people (mainly children) die from diarrhoeal diseases associated with unsafe water and sanitation each year in Angola compared with no deaths in Australia. Furthermore, 22,000 people (mainly women and children) die each year in Angola due to highly polluted indoor air (from using wood, coal and biomass fuels for cooking and heating with inadequate combustion and ventilation systems), whereas this does not rate as an issue in Australia.

It is clear that the environmental burden of disease is significant for developing countries, however, as Table 5.2 indicates, the environmental impacts on health and wellbeing in Australia are surprisingly higher than those which would be expected. To complete the discussion on environmental determinants of health and disease in Australia, the following key environmental determinants have been identified by the AIHW (2006) and each of these will be discussed further in Chapter 11.

Food quality and safety

Despite Australia having one of the safest food supplies in the world, it is estimated that there are between four and seven million cases of gastroenteritis each year in Australia that are due to the consumption of contaminated food (Hall et al 2005).

Case study: Hepatitis A and oysters

In early 1997, a large food-borne illness outbreak occurred across a number of states in Australia that was traced back to the consumption of oysters harvested from Wallis Lake in New South Wales. In total, over 460 cases occurred in NSW with 170 cases in other states. There were 60 hospitalisations and one death due to the outbreak. The pathogen responsible for the outbreak was hepatitis A, which is associated with faecal contamination of water or food, particularly for foods that are not cooked after processing. In this case, in addition to the oysters being consumed raw, oysters are 'filter-feeders' which means they filter nutrients out of the water in which they are growing. Therefore, if the water is contaminated, the oyster will also become contaminated. Even though the oyster processors have sophisticated systems that try to flush out any contamination from the oyster, hepatitis A is particularly difficult to remove. The exact cause of this outbreak was unable to be identified, however, there was evidence of inappropriate sewage disposal from residents and houseboats into the estuary system and the outbreak could have also been triggered by excessive rainfall. In response to the outbreak, a large range of expensive initiatives were implemented such as upgrading sewerage systems, lake-side toilets and waste-disposal practices by houseboats. This outbreak highlights the environmental health links between water contamination, food processing and changed food consumption preferences by the general public.

(Sources: Conaty et al 2000, enHealth Council 2003)

Water quality

Ensuring a safe drinking water supply is fundamental to maintaining good public health, with the quality of the water supply dependent on controlling chemical and microbiological contamination. In Australia, 93% of households are connected to mains water supplies, and over 80% of the population use mains water as their primary source of drinking water. Other important sources of drinking water are rainwater tanks (11% of households), particularly in rural areas, and bottled water (7.6%) (ABS 2005).

Case study: Water fluoridation

Fluoridation of public water supplies is viewed as the most effective public health measure for preventing dental decay, with over two-thirds of Australians living in areas that are supplied with fluoridated mains water. However, the distribution of fluoridated water supplies is unequal, with most of the fluoridated supplies in large cities or capital cities as compared with rural areas, except for Queensland in which Brisbane and most regional centres are currently not fluoridated (this will soon change – with 95% of Queenslanders drinking fluoridated water by 2012). This situation is clearly demonstrated in Table 5.3.

STATE/TERRITORY	% OF POPULATION
New South Wales	89.8
Victoria	75.3
Queensland	4.7
Western Australia	90.1
South Australia	90.2
Tasmania	94.7
Australian Capital Territory	100.0
Northern Territory	84.2

TABLE 5.3: Percentage of population living in areas with fluoride in public water supplies

(Source: AIHW 2006)

Air pollution

Outdoor air quality in Australia is relatively good by international standards, but requires continual monitoring and regulation. Recent studies have found associations between air pollution levels in selected capital cities and mortality and/or hospital admissions, and it is estimated that motor vehicle air pollution accounts for between 900 and 2500 cases of cardiovascular disease, respiratory disease and bronchitis each year, and between 900 and 2000 early deaths.

Example: Health impacts of bushfires

A large number of epidemiological studies have demonstrated a link between exposure to particulate air pollution and respiratory health effects such as reduced pulmonary function, increased respiratory symptoms, increased hospital admissions and emergency department visits and increased mortality. Even though the effects of particulate air pollution on the risk of respiratory diseases are small, the burden of disease may be substantial as the populations exposed are large and detrimental effects have been shown to occur at exposure levels below the current air quality guidelines. Motor vehicles are a primary source for particulate air pollution, but when they occur, bushfires can provide a substantial source of this pollution.

The studies conducted in Australia and overseas that have investigated exposure to particulate pollution from bushfires and respiratory diseases have provided some inconsistent results, but there seems to be general agreement for an association between exposure to bushfire smoke and an increase in respiratory conditions. This includes an increase in asthma symptoms and medication use, increased hospital attendance and admission for respiratory conditions and an exacerbation of symptoms for those with chronic obstructive pulmonary disease. These results highlight the public health need for effectively managing bushfires and controlled burning activities.

(Sources: Chen et al 2006, Johnson et al 2006)

Built environment

With Australia being one of the most urbanised countries in the world, the built environment plays a significant role in the health status of communities. For example, high-density living may create conditions that are favourable to the spread of infectious diseases, while urban sprawl that encourages motor vehicle usage contributes to traffic noise, air pollution and traffic accidents, while deterring physical activity. As we spend the majority of our time indoors (up to 95% in many cases, if car use is included), indoor air quality is also a significant issue within the built environment and can result in health conditions such as 'sick building syndrome'.

Case study: Sick building syndrome

The term 'sick building syndrome' (SBS) is used to describe situations in which building occupants experience acute health and comfort effects that appear to be associated with time spent in a building, but no specific illness or cause can be identified. The complaints may be localised in a particular room or zone, or may be widespread throughout the building. In contrast, the term 'building-related illness' (BRI) is used when symptoms of diagnosable illness are identified and can be attributed directly to airborne building contaminants.

A 1984 World Health Organization Committee report suggested that up to 30% of new and remodelled buildings worldwide may be the subject of excessive complaints related to indoor air quality (IAQ). Often this condition is temporary, but some buildings have long-term problems. Frequently, problems result when a building is operated or maintained in a manner that is inconsistent with its original design or prescribed operating procedures. Sometimes indoor air problems are a result of poor building design or occupant activities. The following have been cited as causes of or contributing factors to SBS:

- *Inadequate ventilation* – building ventilation standards indicate that approximately 15 cubic feet per minute (cfm) of outside air for each occupant is required to be brought into a building by the ventilation system, otherwise the health and comfort of the occupants can be compromised. In addition, some ventilation systems do not effectively distribute air to people in the building and this is also thought to be an important factor in SBS.
- *Chemical contaminants from indoor sources* – most indoor air pollution comes from sources inside the building. For example, adhesives, carpeting, upholstery, manufactured wood products, copy machines, pesticides and cleaning agents may emit volatile organic compounds (VOCs), including formaldehyde. Environmental tobacco smoke contributes high levels of VOCs, other toxic compounds and respirable particulate matter. Research shows that some VOCs can cause chronic and acute health effects at high concentrations, and some are known carcinogens. Low to moderate levels of multiple VOCs may also produce acute reactions.
- *Chemical contaminants from outdoor sources* – the outdoor air that enters a building can be a source of indoor air pollution. For example, pollutants from motor vehicle exhausts, plumbing vents and building exhausts (e.g. from bathrooms and kitchens) can enter the building through poorly located air intake vents, windows and other openings.
- *Biological contaminants* – bacteria, moulds, pollen and viruses are types of biological contaminants. These contaminants may breed in stagnant water that has accumulated in ducts, humidifiers and drain pans, or where water has collected on ceiling tiles, carpeting or insulation. Physical symptoms related to biological contamination include cough, chest tightness, fever, chills, muscle aches and allergic responses such as mucous membrane irritation and upper respiratory congestion. One indoor bacterium, legionella, has caused both legionnaire's disease and Pontiac fever (refer to a case study in Chapter 10 on the largest legionnaire's disease outbreak in Australia).

Even though SBS is a difficult 'condition' to diagnose and attribute causation to in specific cases, at a minimum the above causes/contributing factors can be associated with occupant discomfort and in the worst cases are responsible for adverse health impacts.

(Source: US Environmental Protection Agency)

Global climate change

As discussed in previous sections of this chapter, substantial changes in the world's ecosystems have been identified and Australia is not immune to these changes. It is now widely recognised that much of this change is due to human activities and the implications for Australia of these changes will be discussed in detail in Chapter 11.

A final word

The determinants of health have a profound effect on the health of individuals and communities. An evaluation of such determinants is an important part of developing any strategy to improve health. In this chapter we have covered definitions of determinants of health, the range of factors that might be considered as determinants and discussed their importance in public health planning and implementation.

We have also examined the genetic, physical and environmental determinants of health in some detail. The environmental burden of disease for Australia is at the lower end of the scale, compared with other countries, however at 14%, environmental factors contribute substantially to our overall disease burden.

This chapter provides you with a good understanding of the 'multicausal' role of determinants of health, and the interrelationship of genetic and environmental determinants with physical determinants. In the following chapter we deal with the social and emotional determinants of health.

REVIEW QUESTIONS

1 Define a determinant and describe the range of determinants that impact on health.
2 Describe what is meant by the 'multicausal role' of determinants and how they impact on health.
3 Write a paragraph about the various types of diabetes and how genetic factors impact on environmental determinants to influence the development of the disease.
4 How are environmental determinants defined?
5 What is the relationship between the ecosystem and health?
6 Define 'ecological footprint' and discuss how this impacts on health.

USEFUL WEBSITES

Center for Health and the Global Environment (Harvard Medical School): http://chge.med.harvard.edu/alternate.html
Centers for Disease Control and Prevention – Office of Genomics and Disease Prevention: www.cdc.gov/genomics
Chronic Disease – Home: www.cdc.gov/nccdphp
Chronic Disease – Programs: www.cdc.gov/nccdphp/programs
Department of Health and Ageing – National Chronic Disease Strategy: http://www.health.gov.au/internet/wcms/publishing.nsf/Content/pq-ncds
Department of Health and Ageing – Nutrition and Physical Activity http://www.health.gov.au/internet/wcms/publishing.nsf/content/nutrition%20and%20physical%20activity-1
enHealth Council (Australia): http://enhealth.nphp.gov.au
Human Genome Project – Online Mendelian Inheritance in Man (OMIM): www.ncbi.nih.nlm.gov/omim
Millennium Ecosystem Assessment: www.millenniumassessment.org
National Center for Biotechnology Information (NCBI) Genome sequence: www.ncbi.nlm.nih.gov/genome//seq
National Human Genome Research Institute (NHGRI): www.nhgri.nih.gov
US Department of Energy: www.doegenomes.org
World Health Organization – Chronic Diseases: http://www.who.int/topics/chronic_diseases/en/index.html
World Health Organization – Public Health and Environment homepage: www.who.int/phe/en
World Health Organization – Quantifying environmental health impacts: www.who.int/quantifying_ehimpacts/en
World Resources Institute: www.wri.org
Worldwatch Institute: www.worldwatch.org

REFERENCES

ABS 2005 Environmental issues: people's views and practices. ABS cat. No. 4810.0.55.001. Australian Bureau of Statistics, Canberra
Alcamo J, Hassan R M, Bennett E 2003 Ecosystems and Human Wellbeing: A Framework for Assessment/Millennium Ecosystem Assessment, World Resources Institute, Washington DC

Australian Institute of Health and Welfare 2002 Australia's Health 2002. AGPS, Canberra

Australian Institute of Health and Welfare 2004 Australia's Health 2004. AGPS, Canberra

Australian Institute of Health and Welfare 2006 Australia's Health 2006. AGPS, Canberra

Burke S, Gray I, Paterson K, Meyrick J 2002 Environmental Health 2012: A Key Partner in Delivering the Public Health Agenda, Health Development Agency, London

Campbell-Lendrum D, Corvalan C, Neira M 2007 Global climate change: implications for international public health policy. Bulletin of the World Health Organization 85(3):235–237

Chen L, Verrall K, Tong S 2006 Air particulate pollution due to bushfires and respiratory hospital admissions in Brisbane, Australia International Journal of Environmental Health Research 16(3):181–191

Chivian E (ed) 2002 Biodiversity: Its Importance to Human Health. Center for Health and the Global Environment, Harvard Medical School, Cambridge

Conaty S, Bird P, Bell G et al 2000 Hepatitis A in New South Wales, Australia, from consumption of oysters: the first reported outbreak. Epidemiology and Infection 124:121–130

Doll R, Hill A B 1964 Mortality in relation to smoking: ten years' observations of British doctors. British Medical Journal 1:1399–1467

enHealth Council 2003 Guidelines for Economic Evaluation of Environmental Health Planning and Assessment. Department of Health and Ageing and enHealth Council, Canberra

Europa-European Commission Online 2007. Available: http://europa.eu/documents/comm/index_en.htmHealth and Welfare Canada 1974

Hall G, Kirk M D, Becker N et al and the OzFoodNet Working Group 2005 Estimating foodborne gastroenteritis, Australia. Emerging Infectious Diseases 11(8):1257–1264

Harper A C, Holman C D J, Dawes VP 1994 The Health of Populations: an introduction. Churchill Livingston, Melbourne

Johnston F H, Webby R J, Pilotto L S et al 2006 Vegetation fires, particulate air pollution and asthma: a panel study in the Australian monsoon tropics. International Journal of Environmental Health Research 16(6):391–404

Keleher H, Murphy B 2004 Understanding health: A determinants approach. Oxford University Press, Melbourne

Lalonde M 1974 A new perspective on the health of Canadians. Health and Welfare Canada, Ottawa

McMichael A J, Kjellstrom T, Smith K R 2006 Environmental Health. In: Merson M H, Black R E & Mills A J (eds) International Public Health: Diseases, Programs, Systems, and Policies, 2nd edn. Jones & Bartlett, Sudbury, p 393–443

Marmot M, Wilkinson R G 2006 Social Determinants of Health. Oxford University Press, Oxford

Millennium Ecosystem Assessment 2005a Ecosystems and Human Wellbeing: Biodiversity Synthesis. World Resources Institute, Washington DC

Millennium Ecosystem Assessment 2005b Ecosystems and Human Wellbeing: Health Synthesis. World Resources Institute, Washington DC

Miller G T 2002 Living in the Environment: Principles, Connections, and Solutions. Brooks/Cole, Belmont, pp 70–82

Ministerial Council on Drug Strategy 2006 National Alcohol Strategy 2006–2009. Commonwealth of Australia, Canberra

Murray C J M, Lopez A 1996 The Global Burden of Disease: A Comprehensive Assessment of Mortality and Disability from Disease, Injuries and Risk Factors in 1990 and Projected to 2020. Harvard University Press, Cambridge

National Public Health Partnership (NPHP) 2004 The National Injury Prevention and Safety Promotion Plan: 2004–2014. NPHP, Canberra

Office of Disease Prevention 2007 Healthy People 2010. US Department of Health and Human Services, Washington

Pruss-Ustun A, Corvalan C 2006 Preventing Disease through Healthy Environments: Towards an estimate of the environmental burden of disease, World Health Organization, Geneva

Public Health Agency of Canada 2007 Canadian Health Network. What makes Canadians healthy or unhealthy? Available: http://www.phac-aspc.gc.ca/ph-sp/determinants/determinants.eng.php#culture

Schneider MA 2006 Introduction to Public Health. Jones and Bartlett, Massachusetts

Soskolne C, Sieswerda L E 2007 Environmental determinants of health, Encyclopedia of Public Health. Available: http://www.enotes.com/public-health-encyclopedia/environmental-determinants-health

Turrell G, Stanley L, de Looper M, Oldenburg B 2006 Health inequalities in Australia: morbidity, health behaviours, risk factors and health service use. Queensland University of Technology and AIHW, Canberra

US Environmental Protection Agency Website. Available: http://www.epa.gov/iaq/pubs/sbs.html 7 Feb 2008

World Health Organization 2002 The World Health Report 2002 Reducing risks, promoting healthy life. WHO, Geneva

World Health Organization 2007a Country profiles of environmental burden of disease. Available: http://www.who.int/quantifying_ehimpacts/countryprofiles

World Health Organization 2007b Determinants of Health. Available: http://www.who.int/hia/evidence/doh/en/print.html

World Health Organization 2007c Global Strategy on Diet, Physical Activity and Health. WHO, Geneva

World Health Organization 2007d A safer future: global public health security in the 21st century. WHO, Geneva

CHAPTER 6

Social and emotional determinants of health

Elizabeth Parker

Learning objectives

After reading this chapter you should be able to:

- describe what is meant by socioeconomic differences in health, and the social and emotional determinants of health
- understand how health inequalities are affected by the social and economic circumstances that people experience throughout their lives
- discuss how factors such as living and working conditions, income, place and education can impact on health
- identify actions for public health policymakers that have the potential to make a difference in improving health outcomes within populations
- appreciate the concept of social cohesion and social capital and their role as potential protective factors in health
- understand the conceptual models that can assist in analysing these issues.

Introduction

In Chapter 5, you were introduced to the concept of the determinants of health, with a focus on the physical and environmental determinants of the health of Australians. In this chapter, we extend this discussion and describe the social, economic and emotional determinants of health. After reading both these chapters, you should be able to recognise the importance of this knowledge in providing a deeper understanding of the links between people's physical, environmental, social and emotional circumstances and their health.

In exploring the central theme of why some people are healthy and others are not, Evans et al (1994 p 3) claimed that 'top people live longer'. That is, there are gaps between the health status of those at the top of the socioeconomic scale and those at the bottom (Evans et al 1994). In Australia, there are differences between the health of urban and rural Australians, between Indigenous and non-Indigenous Australians, and between different ethnic groups. Many years later, the observation by Evans et al (1994) regarding the gap in health status between those at the top of the socioeconomic scale and those at the bottom still holds in Australia and in most other countries; furthermore, the gap in health status is widening in many countries.

The Australian Institute of Health and Welfare (AIHW) also claim that people's general background has an influence on their health.

This general background influences the basic levels of security, safety, hygiene, nourishment, technology, information, freedom and morale of societies. It is difficult to put values and quantities on most of these broad factors, let alone measure them and assess their impact precisely. 'However, it is widely agreed that, at least up to a fair degree of societal development, they are a vital determinant of a population's health. They set the background level around which variations then occur between groups and individuals' (AIHW 2006 p 142).

Over the past 20 years, the evidence on health inequalities in populations, both within and between countries, and how these inequalities are linked to socioeconomic position in society, is irrefutable (Evans et al 1994, Kawachi et al 1999, Marmot 2006, Turrell et al 1999). While there is ample research documenting these disparities, the challenge for public health is to translate this research into effective policies and programs that will close this health status gap. This presents a new challenge for public health as it continues its long tradition of analysing the determinants of health in populations, to explain the factors implicated in mortality (death) and morbidity (illness).

Irrespective of your future in the health sciences, knowledge about social and emotional determinants of health can strengthen your understanding of the influence of people's backgrounds, circumstances and the contexts of their everyday lives on their health choices and health opportunities. This perspective will provide you with a depth of understanding as well as sensitivity to the powerful combination of these influences on health. International and national research contributes increasingly to the evidence of these influences on health and provides the public health community with evidence from which to build effective policies and strategies to close the health gap.

This chapter builds on the material presented in Chapter 5 by examining the evidence regarding how social and economic circumstances are linked to differential patterns of health status in societies. We examine several socioeconomic characteristics such as income, work, gender and education, and their relationship to social, emotional and physical health.

Socioeconomic determinants and the health inequalities jigsaw

Health status is influenced by a variety of socioeconomic factors, such as income and employment. The reverse also holds – these factors are influenced by health. The AIHW suggest that the socioeconomic characteristics that influence health include 'education, income, wealth, occupation, marital and family status, labour force participation, housing, ethnic origin and characteristics of the area of residence' (2006 p 153). We will be discussing only some of these. For a comprehensive review of these, see the AIHW website (www.aihw.gov.au). The next section will discuss the evidence regarding the association between socioeconomic characteristics and health inequalities.

Some of the early research in this area began in the UK in the 1830s, when a British epidemiologist, William Farr, observed a relationship between health inequalities and socioeconomic characteristics. In the latter part of the 20th century, this association began to receive the attention it deserved, particularly with the release of the *Black Report* (1980), developed by a working group on health inequalities established in the UK in 1977. The report had three components: a description of differences between occupational classes in mortality, morbidity and use of health services; an analysis of likely explanations and recommendations for further research; and a strategy to reduce health inequalities or their consequences (Macintyre 1997). The findings revealed that there were 'marked differences in mortality rates between occupational classes for both sexes and at all ages, and a class[1] gradient can be observed for most causes of death, a lack of improvement and in some cases deterioration of the health experience of unskilled and semi-skilled manual classes and inequalities exist in the utilisation of health services, especially preventive services' (Townsend et al 1992 p 198).

The general theme of the Townsend et al (1992) findings was echoed in the UK's *Whitehall Study of Civil Servants* that began in 1967 (Langenberg et al 2005). The study examined the 25-year mortality of men (aged 40–69 at the beginning of the study), showing the social gradient[2] by type of occupation within the civil service (Langenberg et al 2005). Marmot (2006) claims that men second from the top of the occupational hierarchy within the civil service had a higher rate of death than men at the top, while those who were third from the top had a higher rate of death than those second from the top. He asks, 'Why among men who are not poor in the usual sense of the word, should the risk of dying be intimately related to where they stand in the social hierarchy?' (Marmot 2006 p 2083). In *Whitehall II*, launched 20 years after the first Whitehall study, the observations were extended to women, and the gradient in mortality applied to most of the major causes of death, especially heart disease. The puzzle is, 'Why there should be social gradient in so many different causes of death?' (Marmot 2006 p 2083).

In the Whitehall study, all the respondents were employed, yet those at the bottom tier of the workforce had the worst health. It makes sense that unemployment would lead to poorer health, because of the lack of funds to enable the purchase of some of the requirements for good health, such as good-quality foods and health care. The reverse may also hold, that is, those who are ill become unemployed or are forced to leave the labour force.

Across and within countries, the evidence of social and economic determinants and health inequalities is compelling, whether the examination is within developed countries such as the UK, the United States, Canada or Australia, within newly developed countries such as Brazil and India or developing countries in Africa. On life expectancy measures alone, an individual's position within society influences his or her health. In other words, while health is multifactorial and influenced by one's genetic make-up and biology (as discussed in Chapter 5), there is a strong correlation between social conditions and a person's position within society, and their health.

As Turrell and Kavanagh (2004) put it:

> While health inequalities often differ in magnitude among these countries
> (reflecting in part differing social, political, economic and cultural systems)
> the overall picture is very similar. Illness and death are patterned in ways that
> indicate that those with the least access to social and economic resources are the
> most disadvantaged in terms of their health.
>
> (Turrell & Kavanagh 2004 p 393)

Marmot (2006) gives an example of these differences in a study on health disparities. There was a large difference in male life expectancy between two suburbs in London even though they were within close proximity of each other (the boroughs of Camden and Hampstead). 'The life expectancy gap between men living in these two areas is 11 years – from 70 years to 81 years for men' (Marmot 2006 p 2086).

Increasingly, then, there is evidence to suggest that people's health is produced and sustained by the social and economic circumstances that they experience differentially throughout their life. 'Those at the lower end of the socioeconomic hierarchy have poorer health partly as a consequence of material disadvantage such as living on a low income or working in a hazardous job, partly as a result of less healthy behaviours, and partly as a result of psycho-social factors such as anxiety, stress, social isolation and feelings of lack of control' (Turrell & Kavanagh 2004 p 392).

ACTIVITY

● Some of the material we're discussing contains various terms and you will find these throughout the literature on this topic. Write down the answers to the following questions: What is meant by a social gradient in health? Find some examples of the work that the early epidemiologist William Farr did in the 1830s. Research further the findings of the *Black Report* and the Whitehall study. Are the findings still relevant? Do you believe less healthy behaviour is more prevalent in circumstances of social and economic disadvantage? If you answered yes to the above, why should that occur, particularly if knowledge about poor behaviour (e.g. tobacco smoking) is widely promoted through television, other media and in local health centres?

REFLECTION

The field of social determinants of health is a challenging one. Did you suggest that a social gradient in health is about the fact that inequalities in population health status are related to inequalities in social status? This presents public health with many challenges, such as where is it optimal to address this issue? Through public policy – remember the various types of public policies from Chapter 3, or through public health campaigns? Can you see the relevance of the work of William Farr in the 1830s and current public health? From your research on the *Black Report* and the Whitehall studies, was less healthy behaviour more prevalent in circumstances of social and economic disadvantage?

How do public health researchers account for these differences within and between societies? In the next section, we discuss various characteristics of socioeconomic position and how these influence the health of individuals and populations. Keep in mind when reading the following section, that although discussed separately, each of these characteristics (particularly income, education and employment status) and their health effects are interrelated.

Socioeconomic characteristics that influence health

Education

Education is an important determinant of health, as it enhances skills, job opportunities and mobility within the workforce. One of the measures of the education level within society is the measure of retention rates in Year 12. Overall, in Australia, the retention rate of students in high school, and therefore their attainment, has increased over the past 25 years. In 1980, 32% of males and 37% of females completed Year 12, compared with 70% of males and 81% of females in 2004 (AIHW 2005a).

So why is education important to health? A study by Erikson (2001), using data from the Swedish Census, showed 'a remarkable social gradient in mortality' (Erikson 2001 p 2084). Erikson discovered that 'men with a PhD had lower mortality rates than those with a master's degree who, in turn, had lower mortality than those with a bachelor's degree' (2001 p 2084). What is it about having an education that has a beneficial effect against behavioural risk factors such as tobacco smoking and overweight; and risk conditions, such as poor and unstable housing, lower income, and fewer work choices? These are sometimes called material circumstances.

A number of authors argue that education provides opportunities for income and job security and gives people a sense of control over their life choices. Dutton et al claimed that 'human capital dimensions of education that link it to health are apparent in its close connections to work and economic circumstances, psychosocial resources and health behaviours' (2005 p 37). Human capital is the value of employees' education, experience and abilities for employers and the economy as a whole (www.answers.com).

ACTIVITY

● Consider your own reasons for study at university, and how having a tertiary education may contribute to your future health – you probably have not thought about this at length! Do you believe a university education offers more life choices? If so, do these life choices provide increased opportunities to be healthy and in what ways? Write down these answers and share them with some fellow students.

REFLECTION

Did you answer that an education provides an increase in life choices through better job opportunities and increased earning capacity? How are these linked to health? Is it because you have easy access to health information and/or better care options through private health insurance? Anything else?

We now introduce income as one of the interrelated socioeconomic characteristics under discussion.

Income

The AIHW (2006 p 154) claim that 'income has been shown to relate strongly to health, especially in lower income countries'. 'Higher incomes can enable the purchase of health-related goods and services such as better food, housing, recreation and health care, and may provide psychological benefits such as a greater sense of control' (AIHW 2006 p 154). This makes intuitive sense, and is borne out in the data in Australia. 'Nineteen percent of the mortality (death) burden for males and 12% for females have been associated with socioeconomic disadvantage' (AIHW 2006 p 154). Wealth or accumulated assets can buffer material living standards, for example in periods of low income (AIHW 2006). The *Household Income and Labour Dynamics in Australia* survey showed that in 2002, the least wealthy 50% of households owned less than 10% of total household wealth, while the wealthiest 10% owned 45% of total household wealth. The challenge for public health researchers, policymakers and planners is to build an evidence base about the interrelationships between income and the other socioeconomic characteristics in order to understand these dynamics and how they influence health.

ACTIVITY

● With some students, write down your thoughts on the following: Does having more income necessarily influence people's health behaviour? Does your answer hold true for alcohol consumption – does it follow that alcohol consumption in the community increases when people have more disposable income? Research this answer, with respect to women and alcohol consumption.

REFLECTION

Think about the fact that while overall incomes in Australia have increased, the disparity in the distribution of income is widening. Does someone on income support have the same health opportunities as a highly paid executive? See the AIHW and ABS websites for further analysis of these issues.

Work and employment status

Although there is a decline in the absolute level of unemployment, 4.5% of Australians are still unemployed and they experience poorer health than the rest of the population. There is continuing evidence that unemployment is linked to health status (AIHW 2006). In the first part of this chapter, the Whitehall study found that those civil servants at the lower end of the employment hierarchy had higher rates of mortality than those at the top end of the occupation scale. Draper et al (2004 in AIHW 2006 p 155) claim that there is evidence of an association between occupation and mortality. Essentially, the authors claim that 'persons employed in manual occupations have higher mortality rates for most causes of death than those employed in clerical or managerial professional occupations'. This could be related to their more hazardous work, for example, in factories where there is potential for workplace injury; or for those with rural occupations, farming, forestry and mining. Research is ongoing into the impact of occupational status, above and beyond those workplace hazards.

ACTIVITY

- Drawing on the initial work conducted in the Whitehall study, find out whether it is a myth or a fact that there is a difference in the prevalence of heart disease between top executives and managers in white-collar organisations and those staff in the less-well-paid jobs in the same type of white-collar organisation. If there is a difference, are the lower paid workers at a greater or lesser risk than executives and managers? What research can you find on the impact of shift work on health?

REFLECTION

With regard to work and employment status, did you consider that the workforce is mobile and that workers' health status may change as they move in and out of jobs and acquire more education and training on the job? Do you think stress is a factor in the workplace? Many Australians work long hours and, as students, many of you are studying and working part time. Is stress distributed across the workforce generally, or does it manifest itself more in specific professions?

We now turn our discussion to the place or location of residence as another piece of the health inequalities 'jigsaw'.

Place (location)

A large body of research has repeatedly shown that where you live is likely to affect your health-related behaviour and health outcomes (Giles-Corti et al 2005). The statistical relationships showing that place and health are significantly connected are known as area effects or *contextual influences* on health and wellbeing (Cummins et al 2007). Area effects refer to trends in Western countries showing that living in a poorer, or lower socio-economic, area means that you are less likely to lead a healthy lifestyle (Kloek et al 2006), and that your chances of morbidity and early mortality are higher (Turrell et al 2007).

For example, in the research into the relationship between place and health-related behaviour, the AIHW (2006) present findings from the Australian Bureau of Statistics *National Health Surveys* for the periods 1989–90, 1995 and 2001 that 'show that persons aged 25–64 years living in socioeconomically disadvantaged areas are more likely to assess their own health as fair or poor, drink alcohol at harmful levels (males), smoke, be obese and have raised blood pressure' (AIHW 2006 p 233). 'These are variously risk factors for a number of major health conditions such as cardiovascular and respiratory diseases, as well as lung and other cancers' (AIHW 2006 p 233). The next section outlines some studies that corroborate these associations.

Giskes et al (2006) followed a group of 404 smokers in 83 areas in the Netherlands, for six years. The authors first gathered initial data on smoking habits and other lifestyle characteristics to ascertain whether their likelihood of quitting smoking was related to the area in which they lived. They concluded that 'living in a deprived area seems to reduce the likelihood of quitting smoking' (Giskes et al 2006 p 485); in other words, the socioeconomic factors of the areas where people live impact on their ability to stop smoking (Giskes et al 2006).

Earlier in the chapter Marmot (2006) introduced us to the differences in mortality between two suburbs in London. So what it is it about 'place/location' (we will use the terms interchangeably) that influences health? Or what is it about living in a poorer neighbourhood that has the potential to influence health? A number of authors have proposed hypotheses regarding this component of the relationship between social determinants and health. For example, a cross-sectional analysis of 4286 women aged 60 to 79 years old from 457 British electoral areas found that the odds of coronary heart disease was 27% greater for those women living in electoral 'wards' (we call them electorates) that are 'deprived' (Lawlor et al 2005). The more deprived an area, the higher the odds of coronary heart disease.

Area effects have been shown to be powerful enough to override what are referred to in this field of literature as *compositional* effects on health. Compositional effects refer to the socioeconomic position of the individuals who live there, and are measured according to a person's income, education level and employment status (Dutton et al 2005). Usually, a person's socioeconomic position or status in society is a reliable predictor of their health-related behavioural patterns and their health outcomes; once again with poorer people being more likely to have higher-risk behaviour and the associated higher levels of morbidity and early mortality (Marmot 2006). However, contextual or area effects have been repeatedly shown to exert a force over compositional effects, to the extent that, from a health perspective, you are better off being poor in a rich area than rich in a poor area. Recent work by JA Carroll and colleagues (personal communication, 4 Feb 2008) corroborate these studies and argue the case for research that examines the area and context in a holistic way so that programs can be planned more effectively to deal with behavioural and lifestyle changes. The authors outline the qualities in poor living contexts that make health a low priority and difficult to pursue and achieve. While researchers have been able to establish the strength of socioeconomic contextual influences on health, they have been less successful at explaining them (JA Carroll, personal communication, 4 Feb 2008). Thus, these puzzling findings demonstrate that neighbourhood and area effects are really powerful in terms of health, but cannot tell us *why*; and have been described by Macintyre et al (2002 p 125), leading researchers in this field, as 'a black box of mysterious influences on health'.

Let us extend this discussion to examine whether area or place makes a difference to the health of the approximately 34% of Australians who live in rural and/or remote communities. One would assume that access to health services such as doctors and hospitals would be an influential factor, but even with that factor taken into account, health profile differences between rural and urban Australians are significant (AIHW 2006). Compared with those Australians living in major cities, those living in rural or remote communities 'are more likely to be smokers; to drink alcohol in hazardous quantities; to be overweight or obese, to be physically inactive' (AIHW 2005b).

ACTIVITY

● With a group of students, write a short summary of the difference between *contextual* and *compositional* factors and their influence on health. Can you speculate as to why living in a disadvantaged area or neighbourhood is linked to poor health? Apart from poor access to health services, including hospitals, health behaviours are poor for many rural and remote Australians. Comment on rural and remoteness as a characteristic of social and economic disadvantage.

REFLECTION

One way to assist your thinking is to search out some of the authors' work on place and health. Remember that public health is about populations. There will be differences in the health status of specific individuals within the population and subpopulations under study, but it is the *overall* population health profile between and among groups that public health is interested in. There are several sources of information concerning rural and remote health, including the AIHW and specific 'rural and remote health' journals to assist your endeavours.

Gender

Gender is another interrelated socioeconomic characteristic and it raises interesting questions about what effects gender has on health. Gender has been used to refer to 'attributes, characteristics, stereotypes, social environments as well as genetic status' (Davidson et al 2006 p 733). There are a number of health disadvantages for women: while women's life expectancy is higher than men's in Australia, women tend to report more physical illness, more psychological distress and more psychiatric symptoms than do men (AIHW 2006). For women living in socioeconomically disadvantaged areas, they 'also reported consulting doctors more often, but dentists less often. Females living in these areas were also less likely to report having had a recent pap smear' (AIHW 2006 p 233). Women are also exposed to more domestic violence.

Are there any predictors of women's self-assessed health? Data on over 20,000 women and men aged 20–59 were analysed from the *British General Household Survey* for 1991 and 1992, and showed the importance of separately analysing educational qualifications, occupational class and employment status for both women and men. Occupational class and employment status are the key structural factors associated with limiting long-standing illness, but educational qualifications are particularly good predictors of women's self-assessed health. In other words, an education enhances both women's sense of self and their self-reported health status. However, men's unemployment has adverse consequences for the health of their wives, due to the family living in disadvantaged material circumstances. Women's participation in employment, and their family role, have undergone substantial changes over the past 30 years, so approaches to measuring inequalities in women's health need to reflect changes in women's employment participation, and changes in marital status and living arrangements (Arber 2002).

There are also specific health issues that affect only men, or have a disproportionate impact on them. Men access health services less than women, indicating poorer health-seeking behaviour, and they have higher rates of smoking – this is unevenly distributed, with higher rates occurring in socioeconomically disadvantaged groups. In addition, there are higher rates of injuries and suicide in these same disadvantaged groups. To expand your knowledge about gender and health, see Doyal (1995), Bird (2008) and Bury & Gabe (2004).

ACTIVITY

● Consolidate your understanding of the above issues by writing a paragraph on the following statement: Research shows undeniably that being socially and economically disadvantaged is hazardous to your health. Find examples from the literature to argue your point.

REFLECTION

If you were the Minister of Health for the state you live in and were shown some of this evidence, what other government departments would you recommend your staff work with to plan public health actions? In thinking this through, what would be the strengths and limitations of such an approach?

The next section tries to unravel the intricacies of the social and emotional determinants of health by examining a number of propositions, and presents frameworks to assist public health in addressing these issues.

A public health framework to address the social determinants of health

Reducing health inequalities

Reducing health inequalities is not an easy task for public health. Turrell and Kavanagh claim that 'meeting this challenge requires will and commitment on the part of politicians, all government departments (not only health), non-government organisations, private sector companies and other groups and organisations' (2004 p 392).

Specific actions to reduce social gradients should include (Oldenburg et al 2000a, 2000b):
- changes to macro-level social and economic policies
- improving living and working conditions
- strengthening communities for health
- improving behavioural risk factors
- empowering individuals and strengthening their social networks
- improving responses form the health care system and associated treatment services.

Frameworks can assist us to order our thinking and when we analyse the extent of social and economic determinants of health across a number of characteristics and risk behaviours, public health is confronted with many options for policies and programs to tackle these inequalities. In this section we present a number of frameworks. Think of these as lenses through which you are trying to analyse complex relationships. They are linked by trying to 'drill-down' and explain conceptual connections. Once these relationships are better understood, policies and programs can be built to ensure health opportunities for all segments of the community. We advance this discussion by presenting a public health framework developed by Turrell et al (1999) as a means of getting you to think about how all the pieces of the health inequalities jigsaw fit together and how public health might move forward in addressing some of the unequal patterning of health in the community. The discussion is accompanied by an explanation of its various features.

The framework has three dominant features: upstream factors, midstream factors and downstream factors. These factors, while discrete, are interconnected. These terms are also presented in the health promotion discussion in Chapter 12.

Upstream factors

Upstream factors (or macro-level) factors include international influences, government policies and the fundamental social, physical, economic and environmental determinants of health. The government policies that can be influential in creating health opportunities are access to housing, transport, economics and welfare (e.g. unemployment benefits and family allowances).

Midstream factors

You can see the range of 'midstream or intermediate level factors' on the framework, for example, health behaviours such as diet/nutrition, smoking, lack of physical activity and the intake of excess alcohol are identified. Other midstream factors could include mental health and depression.

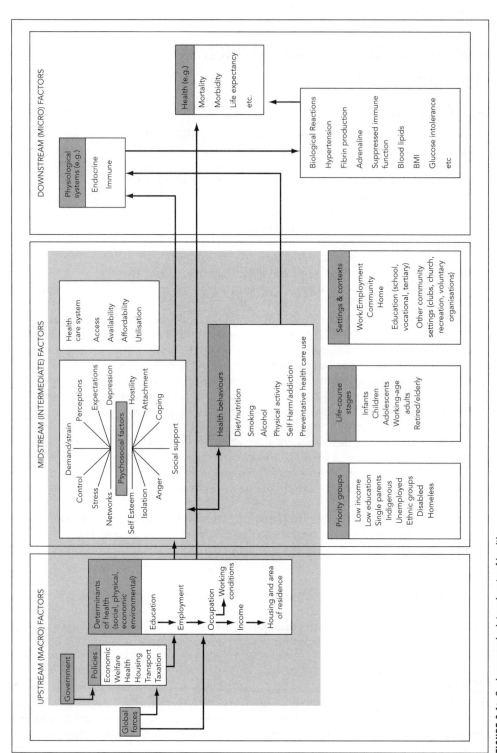

FIGURE 6.1: Socioeconomic determinants of health

(Source: Reproduced from Turrell et al 1999, © Queensland University of Technology, School of Public Health, Centre for Health Research)

Downstream factors

These are the micro-level factors that are influenced by the upstream factors such as global forces, cultural contexts and government policies and the social, physical, economic and environmental determinants of health in the upstream cluster of factors, as well as the midstream factors within the framework such as health behaviour, psychosocial factors and health care access of the mid-stream cluster. The downstream factors include biological and physiological reactions to all these influences, which in turn shape health outcomes such as mortality, morbidity, quality of life and life expectancy.

ACTIVITY

● To consolidate these concepts, complete the following activities. You could do this with a group of students. List two upstream policies that are not identified in the Turrell et al (1999) framework that could potentially have an impact on people's opportunities for health. Some of the midstream (intermediate factors) are 'risky' health behaviours, one of which is physical activity levels. To increase physical activity for those who are inactive, should municipal swimming pools be open free of charge to those who are unemployed or on a pension? Or should municipal swimming pools be made free for everyone? Should there be more publicly funded gyms open free of charge to the public?

REFLECTION

The framework is a lens intended to make sense of these intricacies. What options did you propose for free entry to swimming pools in order to provide accessible physical activity and would it make a difference? Walking paths are 'free', yet not everyone uses them! Working on midstream factors to reduce risky behaviour requires more than a single strategy such as having free entry to pools. In Chapter 12 a range of health promotion success stories are presented. Essentially public health policies and actions have to work across upstream, midstream and downstream factors to make a difference.

Mackenbach and Stronks (2002) argue for a combination of strategies to reduce health inequalities at these three levels. They claim that upstream measures include improving the physical and psychosocial work environment, reducing smoking in lower socioeconomic groups, improving nutrition (preferably through universal measures such as healthier school meals) and reducing childhood poverty. Turrell et al (1999) would view these as midstream under health behaviours. Downstream policies include health care policies that 'improve accessibility for lower socioeconomic groups' (1999 p 104). Turrell et al (1999) would label such policies as upstream policies as they are addressing broad policy initiatives. The point of Mackenbach and Stronks' (2002) argument is that it is a combination of strategies that are needed at these three levels to make a difference.

In Australia, public health policies and programs across each of the clusters are being developed and introduced. For example, there have been reductions in tobacco smoking across the whole population, yet those in the most socioeconomically disadvantaged sectors of the community still have higher rates of smoking than those in the more advantaged sectors. There is greater attention to healthier school food in tuckshops and canteens and health services are available for everyone through Medicare.

The purpose of the following case study is for you to think about how the Turrell et al (2007) model could be used in practice to examine policy and program options to improve health.

Case study: Leila, a refugee

You are a 34-year-old woman called Leila who has arrived in Australia as a refugee with your four children. You are part of a group of refugee women who have arrived in Australia together. Your husbands were killed in a civil war in your country. You had your last child in the refugee camp, where you waited for food trucks each week to deliver food and medical supplies. You have been waiting for three years to be settled somewhere outside your country. You speak three languages, but not English. You have finally been granted refugee status in Australia and now are settled in a suburb with one other family from your country – someone you do not know very well. The local bus goes infrequently during the day to the shopping centre, where the food is totally different from what you know and it is difficult to understand the cooking instructions on the labels. You pick up the children from the local school in the afternoon, a 15-minute walk from your house. On days when you shop, you have to take the bus to the shopping centre, pick up some groceries and time your trips to ensure you are home to pick up your children.

You have decided to make contact with the other family in the suburb – neither of you have a car, but have made telephone contact. Both of you feel stressed and depressed, are homesick and grieving for your husbands. You are both really keen to begin English classes at the local TAFE (Technical and Further Education) college and wonder how you will manage it all. Your family allowance covers some basic essentials, yet you realise that without English it will be difficult to get work. Your children want Australian sporting equipment like a cricket bat and a soccer ball and you know this is important for them to fit in.

ACTIVITY

- What characteristics of disadvantage can you identify in the above case? Can you make any connections between the social and psychosocial determinants of health? Using the Turrell et al (1999) *Framework of Socioeconomic Determinants of Health,* plot the links between each of your identified characteristics so that you get a full picture of the issues. What range of public health policies and programs would you implement to assist Leila and her fellow refugee families?

REFLECTION

Were there connections between the social and psychosocial determinants of health? When you mapped your identified characteristics, could you see how the upstream or macro-level policies, such as transport and access to English language classes, were a potential influence on improving their quality of life? What happens when people who do not speak English seek health care in a local clinic?

So far we have presented the evidence of socioeconomic disadvantage and health, and the impact that these factors have on health. We now turn to a brief examination of the impact of social and economic disadvantage on emotional health and we begin by examining the impact of this disadvantage on the emotional health of children. We introduce a lifecourse approach that has received attention in recent years. It draws its foundation from the persuasive evidence that what happens in terms of differential levels of advantage or disadvantage in childhood has an impact on health in adulthood. This discussion complements the previous identification of the psychosocial factors that are indicated as part of the midstream (intermediate factors) on the Turrell et al (1999) framework. Turn back to the framework and review the midstream factors before reading further. You may well ask what are the links between social and economic disadvantage and emotional health and childhood.

It makes intuitive sense that patterns of health established in childhood would have some bearing on an individual's adult health, through the establishment of good nutrition, exercise, structured and orderly lives, play and emotional security. Moreover, there is an emerging body of research that suggests that parental socioeconomic disadvantage is associated with mental health problems in children (Najman et al 2004). In a large study following mothers and their children at three to five days, six months, five and 14 years, the children from low-income families were 'found to have higher rates of problems with language and reasoning ability, and these were observed at 5 and 14 years of age' (Najman et al 2004 p 1155). The authors conclude that the results of their study were beyond question, that is, 'at ages 5 and 14, children born to mothers in the lowest socio-economic status group have a much greater likelihood of manifesting cognitive development problems, and their mental and emotional health is more likely to be impaired' (Najman et al 2004 p 1156). Teenage maternity was associated with an increased risk of child mental health impairment at five years of age but not necessarily at an older age. The study concludes that socioeconomic disadvantage in the early years of a child's life has the potential to have a deleterious effect on adult health (Najman et al 2004).

The Najman et al (2004) research corroborates a review by Turrell et al (1999) of eight studies that examined the relationship between socioeconomic status (SES) and mental and psychosocial morbidity among children. Children were more likely to experience behavioural disturbances and social problems, and those from lower SES backgrounds were more likely to be diagnosed as autistic. Infants were more likely to experience a shorter duration of breastfeeding or none at all (Turrell et al 1999).

ACTIVITY

● Can you identify what aspects of low income potentially compromise children's health? Research the types of programs that are available to assist families who have children and are under financial and/or housing stress in your local area, for example food banks and children's toy libraries.

REFLECTION

Did you realise that many support programs for families and children are conducted by many government and non-government sectors in the community, such as education, libraries, social and service clubs, parks and recreation? Thus, the health of the community is everybody's business. This reinforces the concept you were introduced to early in the book about public health working across all sectors in the community.

A lifecourse approach traces health outcomes across the lifecycle, and socioeconomic variability in adult disease 'is due to adverse exposure experienced in both early and later life' (Turrell & Kavanagh 2004 p 402). Adolescence is a vulnerable time of transition between the family-determined social status and adulthood, and what that may entail with regard to either continuing the health patterns adopted in childhood or altering these in a more positive or negative direction.

In a study examining the impact of socioeconomic status on adolescent depression and obesity, both of which increase the risk of cardiovascular disease, Goodman et al (2003) analysed a large sample in the US. The attributable risk of depression and obesity in the lowest income households was profound and the authors contend that the impact of socioeconomic status and the social and environmental backgrounds of adolescents as 'risk factors' are often ignored when examining adolescent behavioural choices. In other words, public health efforts need to focus on socioeconomic status in designing programs for adolescents as it is a strong determinant in predicting lifestyle choices.

Keleher et al (2004) pose a number of questions that need to be answered when examining mental health, such as the extent to which literacy and education affect people's mental illness experience, the social supports that are available and the need to have a comprehensive approach that looks at downstream factors such as accessible mental health services, midstream factors that embrace services for early diagnosis of mental illness and upstream factors that provide strong public health policy directions and investment in mental health awareness, such as the national depression initiative.

For our purposes, the evidence of the critical importance of SES and emotional health in childhood and adolescence raises many questions about investments by governments and the need to design early intervention programs.

The following model demonstrates the connections between material disadvantage – poor income, education, limited work opportunities or unemployment – and physical and emotional health, through the early developmental years of childhood through to leaving school. The model provides a glimpse at the pathways to health and the interrelationships between contextual factors such as material disadvantage and physical and emotional health, and how these patterns are connected across the lifecourse. It makes these broad connections explicit and draws together the arguments we have been making in this section. While Turrell et al (1999) provide an overarching framework in which to examine upstream, midstream and downstream factors at the macro or 'big picture level', Graham and Power (2004) focus specifically on the early years of life and how material disadvantage has the potential to effect early childhood development. You can trace the links between cognition (intellectual development) and education, social identity, health behaviour and physical and emotional health, and those patterns potentially linking to poor adult circumstances and poor adult health. Remember that

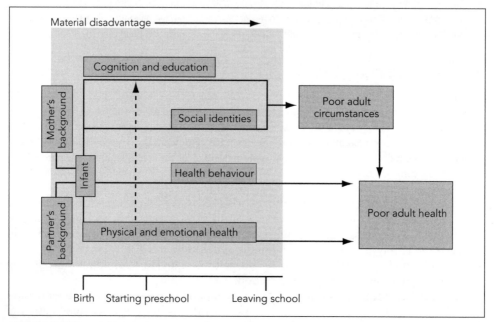

FIGURE 6.2: Lifecourse framework

(Source: Graham & Power 2004. From: Health Development Agency 2004 Childhood disadvantage and adult health: a lifecourse framework. Reproduced by permission)

such frameworks are tools to guide our thinking about complex issues, and they create a lens through which to examine not only evidence about health issues but also strategies to address these issues. See Figure 6.2 for a model illustrating the links between material disadvantage and early childhood development (Graham & Power 2004).

Figure 6.3 shows a model by Mrazek and Heggarty (1994) that illustrates 'both the degree of influence family contexts exert on health outcomes, and the changing nature of developmental milestones and health outcomes' (Nicholson et al 2004 p 22). You can see from this model how important family context is. Parental risk and protective factors such as smoking and drug use, mental health and parental health knowledge and peer influences are also influential on the processes that lead to positive or negative health outcomes. There are specific factors that influence childhood development along the top section of the framework, and for people working in this area this cluster of factors is a useful way of exploring how programs can be designed to address specific issues.

ACTIVITY

● With some other students, identify why you think family income is linked to a child's mental health. What is a lifecourse approach and why is it used? While we have focussed on the early years of life, would a lifecourse approach be useful in addressing health in the middle and later years of life. If you were a public health manager making recommendations in government, what advice would you give about the impact of disadvantage and emotional health, and where public investments to make a difference might occur?

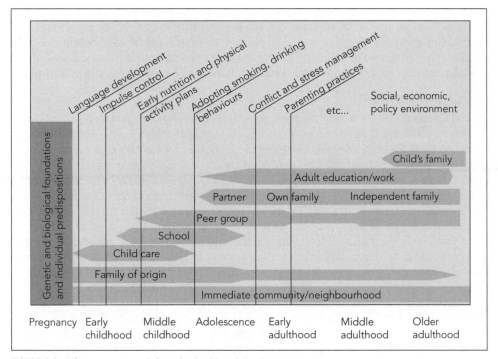

FIGURE 6.3: Lifecourse contexts influencing health and development

(Adapted from Figure 1, Life Course - Social Field Concept. Copyright 1970. Sheppard G. Kellam MD. In: Kellam S G, Branch J D, Agrawal K C, Ensminger M E 1975 Mental Health and Going to School: The Woodlawn Program of Assessment, Early Intervention, and Evaluation. The University of Chicago Press, Chicago, p 22)

REFLECTION

A lifecourse approach can be helpful in mapping policies and programs across the lifespan. In thinking about middle and older adulthood, did you consider that there are many potential public health issues that arise with the ageing of the population such as having adequate recreation and programs to reduce social isolation and loneliness? This last question is a tricky and complex one to answer – did you think about the need for excellent and affordable day care? And parental support programs? These are important and interesting topics to research.

In reviewing all of this material, it is important to note that although poor health and the factors that influence this are more likely to be experienced by socioeconomically disadvantaged groups, health professionals should not inadvertently use these patterns as a basis for stereotyping and labelling individuals from disadvantaged backgrounds (Turrell et al 2004). In the next section we discuss the concepts of social cohesion and social capital as potential mediating factors in health inequalities.

Role of social cohesion and social capital

We have examined the role of social and economic disadvantage in compromising physical and emotional health by using a number of frameworks, including a lifecourse perspective. We did this by reviewing the studies that showed the effects of social disadvantage on children's mental and physical health, and how this potentially compromises long-term health in adulthood for the most disadvantaged.

Is the situation so bleak that the social disadvantages that contribute to health inequalities cannot be improved? There are number of protective factors in this complex web. We are now going to turn our attention to some of these psychosocial midstream factors. Note the psychosocial factors of support, self-esteem and social networks in the Turrell et al (1999) framework. We are going to build on these by examining social cohesion and social capital. The purpose of introducing this material is to provide you with some knowledge of the significance that protective factors such as these can have on health and quality of life.

Social cohesion

Social cohesion can be defined as the connections and relations between societal units, such as individuals, groups and associations, or the glue that holds communities together (AIHW 2005a). Levels of social cohesion are indicated by the fact that the majority of Australians are confident they can rely on their support network in times of crisis, and make contact with family and friends on a weekly basis. A third of Australians engage with the wider community, mostly as volunteers, and three-quarters donate money to charities and non-profit organisations. Markedly smaller percentages are civically engaged, in terms of being regularly involved in the activities of political advocacy or a community organisation. However, less than half of Australians are socially trusting (of less well-known acquaintances and strangers) (AIHW 2005a). Domestic violence and child abuse remain very real for some Australian females and children, and rates of imprisonment increased markedly between 1994 and 2004 (AIHW 2005a).

Interestingly, Marmot (2006) makes the point about the powerful influence of social cohesion on the stability of societies, by pointing to countries like Sri Lanka, Costa Rica and the state of Kerala in India. For example, if we look at the United States, it is the richest country in the world (apart from Luxembourg), but has a similar life expectancy for men as is the case in Costa Rica or Cuba. While the income levels across Costa Rica and Cuba are not high, and the material conditions for good health may not appear evident as people may be relatively poor, the disparity between the highest earning and the lowest earning is relatively narrow; and social cohesion within these societies seems to play some part (Marmot 2006). Social cohesion as social integration is an individual characteristic as well as a characteristic of societies as the examples of the above countries show. Social cohesion incorporates social networks and being engaged with others through these networks.

Being involved in social networks is good for health, as networks can provide social support, trust, friendship and mutual obligations, and there is evidence that social networks are linked to individual health outcomes (Berkman 2000). Social networks and social support include being in supportive families, relationships and organisations, and participating in informal networks through volunteering, playing group sport or participating in group cultural events. The degree to which individuals are embedded in a social network, or the degree to which they belong to a community, is related to health status. Social isolation, often part of being alone in old age, reduces contact with others and reduces the experience of connectedness that is normally gained through a variety of social networks (Berkman 2000). (Note: There are challenges in research on social determinants and health as most of the research is cross-sectional. There is also a need for further cohort-studies to enrich our knowledge. See Chapter 4 on epidemiology.)

Social capital

One of the features of a socially integrated or cohesive society is that it is endowed with stocks of social capital (Berkman 2000). Social capital is a relatively recent term that combines the concept of 'capital', an economic concept, with social concepts such as fairness and trust (Pearce & Davey Smith 2003). Social capital is about people's trust and sense of belonging to networks and communities, and it focuses on strengthening social cohesion within communities. Social capital represents 'social relations of mutual benefit characterised by norms of trust and reciprocity' (Winter 2000 p 1). People's networks, norms, human connections in the form of trust that can be transferred from one social setting to another, as well as community resources and civic engagement are all important for strengthening social ties and opportunities, and hence, health (Putnam 1993).

In a study of 39 states in the US, Kawachi et al (1997) found that membership in voluntary groups and levels of social trust impact positively on mortality data. Mutual trust, a sense of belonging and reciprocity, that is mutual give and take and sharing, are all concepts of social capital. So how can knowing about social cohesion and social capital assist those who are studying in the health sciences? Figure 6.4 depicts the links between (1) the 'State', that is, the government, and its direct effects on health, for example the provision of clean water or Medicare; (2) the links between public policies and the need to build social capital within societies; and (3) that economic equality or inequality in any society is to some extent a consequence of social capital (Kawachi et al 1997 p 670) and for (4) and (5) the direct effects of inequality on health.

Can social capital have a negative effect? Baum (1999) identifies unhealthy and healthy uses of social capital in the *Adelaide Health Development and Social Capital Study*. The healthy uses include many of the elements listed in our discussion: trust, cooperation, understanding, empathy, openness to new ideas and alliances across differences; these are some of the positive elements of social capital. Unhealthy uses of social capital were racism, fear of the unknown, dislike of change and new ideas and an 'us and them mentality' (Baum 1999). Additionally, entrenched norms of behaviour do not necessarily build 'trust and reciprocity' and may militate against advancing health. For example, in some groups violence against women is acceptable (Baum 1999). However, the evidence is increasingly compelling that, in general, social cohesion and social capital are protective factors for health.

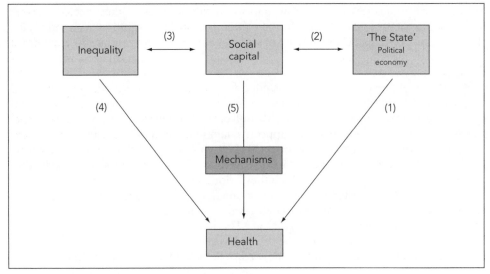

FIGURE 6.4: Interactions between factors impacting on health

(Source: Putman R 2004 Health by association: some comments. International Journal of Epidemiology 33(4):667–671)

For health professionals, social cohesion and social capital are integral to your understanding of factors that can be strengthened to support not only individual health, but also the health of the population. These social forces can be examined as possible avenues and starting points for interventions, programs and policies to redress socioeconomic disadvantage, and improve physical and emotional health.

ACTIVITY

● Find two articles on social cohesion and social capital, and health inequalities. With some students, read and discuss how the concepts could be applied to public health practice.

REFLECTION

Do you believe from your readings that social cohesion and social capital are helpful terms for public health? In your own life, do you have strong social networks of friends, family and neighbours? What were your thoughts on the US study that showed volunteerism as a mechanism for building strong community social cohesion?

A final word

This chapter has introduced you to the social and emotional determinants of health by examining the influence of socioeconomic disadvantage on inequalities in health in populations. This is an introductory overview of this complex work and it is advisable that you read widely to gain a fuller understanding of the dynamic literature that is emerging in this area. We began by describing some of the characteristics of socioeconomic disadvantage and the impact that these *interrelated* factors have on health. A public health framework by Turrell et al (1999) was presented to identify the multilevel and diverse determinants of socioeconomic health inequalities. Frameworks act as lenses through which these complex inter-relationships can be viewed and they give guidance for policy and program investments to improve population health. The links between compromised health in childhood, social and economic disadvantage, poor health behaviours and the potential for poor health across the lifespan were introduced using visual representations of a lifecourse approach. Finally, we introduced the concepts of social cohesion and social capital as potential protective factors for maintaining and promoting health, and what the starting point for public health actions might be. Public health has always faced challenges that reach across all sectors of society, all levels of government and the private and non-government sectors, and the problem of population health inequalities is a significant one. Ongoing international and national research is attempting to unravel the dynamics of inequalities in health and, significantly, the public health actions for all levels of society that can make a difference to improving health.

REVIEW QUESTIONS

1 What do you understand by the term socioeconomic disadvantage?
2 What are the main messages from the *Black Report* and the Whitehall study?
3 Why are education, employment, income, area of residence and gender important characteristics in health inequalities?
4 Low income and its link to potentially poor emotional health in children was introduced. Can you identify some of the risk factors that can affect positive growth over the lifecourse?
5 What do the terms 'downstream', 'midstream' and 'upstream' mean and what are some of their key components?
6 How can social cohesion and social capital be helpful in understanding health inequalities, and what are the healthy and unhealthy uses of these?

ENDNOTES

1 'Class' refers to a social stratum in society whose members share certain economic, social or cultural characteristics. Available: www.answers.com, 21 Feb 2008.
2 'The socioeconomic gradient in health' refers to the worse health of those who are at a lower level of socioeconomic position – whether measured by income, occupational grade or educational attainment – even those who are already in relatively high socioeconomic groups' (Kawachi et al 2002 p 649).
3 Acheson (1998 p 104) made this recommendation based on evidence that these aids double the chance of stopping smoking.

REFERENCES

Acheson D 1998 Independent Inquiry into Inequalities in Health. The Stationery Office, London

Arber S 2002 Comparing Inequalities in women's and men's health: Britain in the 1990s. Social Science and Medicine 44(6):773–787

Australian Bureau of Statistics 2001 Australian social trends 2001. ABS cat no. 4102.0. ABS, Canberra

Australian Bureau of Statistics 2006 Australian social trends 2005 data cube. Table I: Education and training, national summary 2005. ABS cat. no. 4102.0. ABS, Canberra

Australian Institute of Health and Welfare 2005a AIHW cat. No. AUS65. AIHW, Canberra

Australian Institute of Health and Welfare 2005b Rural, regional and remote health – indicators of health. AIHW cat.no. PHE 59. AIHW Canberra

Australian Institute of Health and Welfare 2006 Australia's health 2006. AIHW cat. No. AUS73, AIHW, Canberra

Baum F 1999 The role of social capital in health promotion: Australian perspectives. Health Promotion Journal of Australia 9(3):171–178

Berkman L 2000 Social Support, Social Networks, Social Cohesion and Health. Social Work in Health Care 31(2):3–14

Bird C 2008 Gender and health: the effects of constrained choices and social policies. Cambridge University Press, Cambridge

Black D 1980 Inequalities in health. Report of a research working group. HMSO.

Bury M, Gabe J (eds) 2004 The sociology of health and illness: a reader. Routledge, New York

Cummins S, Curtis S, Diez-Roux A et al 2007 Understanding and representing 'place' in health research: A relational approach. Social Science and Medicine 65(9):1825–1838

Davidson K, Trudeau K, van Roosmalen E et al 2006 Perspective: Gender as a Health Determinant and Implications for Health Education. Health Education and Behavior 33:731

Doyal L 1995 What makes women sick: gender and the political economy of health. Macmillan, London

Draper G, Turrell G, Oldenburg B 2004 Health inequalities in Australia: Mortality. Health Inequalities Monitoring Series No. 1. Cat. No. 55 Queensland University of Technology and the Australian Institute of Health and Welfare, Canberra

Dutton T, Turrell G, Oldenburg B 2005 Measuring socioeconomic position in population health monitoring and health research (Health Inequalities Monitoring Series No.3). Queensland University of Technology, Brisbane

Erikson R 2001 Why do graduates live longer? In: Johnsson J O, Mills C (eds) Cradle to grave: Life-course change in modern Sweden. Sociology Press, Durham

Evans R G, Barer M L, Marmor T R (eds) 1994 Why Are Some People Healthy and Others Not? The Determinants of Health of Populations. De Gruyter, New York

Giles-Corti B, Broomhall M, Knuiman M et al 2005 Increasing walking: How important is distance to, attractiveness, and size of public open space? American Journal of Preventive Medicine, Vol. 28, Issue 2, Supp.2 pp 169–176

Giskes K, van Lenthe F J, Turrell G et al 2006 Smokers living in deprived areas are less likely to quit: a longitudinal follow-up. Tobacco Control 15:485–488

Goodman E, Slap G, Huang B 2003 The Public Health Impact of Socioeconomic Status on Adolescent Depression and Obesity. American Journal of Public Health 93(11):1844–1850

Graham H, Power C 2004 Childhood disadvantage and adult health: a lifecourse framework. Health Development Agency, London. Available: http://www.nice.org.uk/aboutnice/whoweare/aboutthehda/evidencebase/keypapers/papersthatinformandsupporttheevidencebase/childhood_disadvantage_and_adult_health_a_lifecourse_framework.jsp 13 Dec 2007

Kawachi I, Kennedy B P, Lochner K et al 1997 Social capital, income inequality and mortality. American Journal of Public Health 87:1491–1498

Kawachi I, Kennedy B P, Wilkinson R G (eds) 1999 The Society and Population Health Reader, vol. 1: Income Inequality and Health. The New Press, New York

Kawachi I, Subramanian S, Almeida-Filho N 2002 A glossary for health inequalities. Journal of Epidemiology and Community Health 56(9):647–652

Keleher H, Murphy B (eds) 2004 Understanding health: a determinants approach. Oxford University Press, South Melbourne

Kellam S G, Branch J D, Agrawal K C, Ensminger M E 1975 Mental Health and Going to School: The Woodlawn Program of Assessment, Early Intervention, and Evaluation. The University of Chicago Press, Chicago

Kloek G, van Lenthe F, van Nierop P et al 2006 Impact evaluation of a Dutch community intervention to improve health-related behaviour in deprived neighbourhoods. Health & Place 12(4):665–677

Langenberg C, Martin J, Shipley G et al 2005 Adult socioeconomic position and the association between height and coronary heart disease mortality: findings from 33 years of follow-up in the Whitehall Study. American Journal of Public Health 95(4):628–632

Lawlor D, Davey Smith G, Patel R et al 2005 Life-Course Socioeconomic Position, Area Deprivation, and Coronary Heart Disease: Findings form the British Women's Heart and Health Study. American Journal of Public Health January 95(1):91–97

Macintyre S, 1997 The Black Report and Beyond: What are the Issues? Social Science & Medicine 64(6):723–745

Macintyre S, Ellaway A, Cummins S 2002 Place effects on health: how can we conceptualise, operationalise and measure them? Social Science and Medicine 55(1):125–139

Mackenbach J, Stronks K 2002 A strategy for tackling health inequalities in The Netherlands. British Medical Journal 325:1029–1032

Marmot M 2006 Health in an unequal world. The Lancet 368:2081–2096

Mrazek P J, Heggarty R J (eds) 1994 Reducing Risks for Mental Disorders: Frontiers for Preventive Intervention Research. National Academy Press, Washington, D.C. In: Nicholson J, Carroll J-A, Brodie A et al 2004 Child and Youth Health Inequalities in Australia. The status of Australian research 2003. Paper prepared for the Health Inequalities Research Collaboration, Children, Youth and Families Network

Najman J, Aird R, Bor W et al 2004 The generational transmission of socioeconomic inequalities in child cognitive development and emotional health. Social Science & Medicine 58:1147–1158

Nicholson J, Carroll J-A, Brodie A et al 2004 Child and Youth Health Inequalities in Australia. The status of Australian research 2003. Paper prepared for the Health Inequalities Research Collaboration, Children, Youth and Families Network

Oldenburg B, McGuffog I D, Turrell G 2000a Socioeconomic determinants of health in Australia: policy responses and intervention options. Medical Journal of Australia 172: 489–492

Oldenburg B, McGuffog I D, Turrell G 2000b Making a difference to the socioeconomic determinants of health; policy responses and intervention options. Asia Pacific Journal of Public Health 12(suppl.):s51–54

Pearce N, Davey Smith G 2003 Is Social Capital the Key to Inequalities in Health? American Journal of Public Health 93(1):122–128

Putnam R 1993 Making Democracy Work: Civic traditions in modern Italy. Princeton University Press, Princeton

Putnam R 2004 Health by association: some comments. International Journal of Epidemiology 33(4):667–671

Townsend P, Davidson N (eds) 1992 Inequalities in health: The Black Report. Penguin, London

Turrell G, Kavanagh A 2004 Socioeconomic determinants of health: from evidence to policy. In: Moodie R, Hulme A (eds) Hands-on Health Promotion. IP Communications, Melbourne

Turrell G, Oldenburg B, McGuffog I, Dent R 1999 Socioeconomic determinants of health: towards a national research program and a policy and intervention agenda. Queensland University of Technology, School of Public Health and Ausinfo, Canberra

Turrell G, Kavanagh A, Draper G et al 2007 Do places affect the probability of death in Australia: a multi-level study of area-level disadvantage. Journal of Epidemiology and Community Health 61:13–19

Winter I 2000 Major themes and debates in the social capital literature: the Australian connection. In: Winter I (ed). Social capital and public policy in Australia. AIFS, Melbourne

The author would like to thank Julie-Anne Carroll for her contribution to the section on 'Place/location' in this chapter.

Section 3

Ethics, evidence and practice

Introduction

An ethical approach to practice is essential for health workers who see the importance of maintaining a high standard of professional practice in their day-to-day work. Chapter 7 discusses the development of public health ethics and the factors that underpin an ethical approach. It covers key ethical systems and theories and concepts that predicate ethical decision making and then it discusses and applies those to public health practice. Too often health practitioners do not have a clear understanding of ethical practice and an opportunity to explore the range of circumstances that may impact on how they do their job. This chapter explores all of these issues leading from the theoretical to the practical and exploring the range of ways in which ethics applies to public health.

Chapter 8 follows on from the previous chapter in that ethical practice should be based on evidence, not on habit or the practices of those who have come before us. Evidence-based practice began as evidence-based medicine and has evolved and developed into a process that centres on evidence gathering and the limitations of such evidence. It focuses on the 'barriers' and 'facilitators' to identifying and implementing 'best practice'. The chapter also discusses the limitations of evidence-based practice and the potential use of other sources of information to guide practice.

In the final chapter in this section of the book, using an ethical approach to practice and the evidence that should be used to guide practice come together in a discussion of the importance of planning and evaluation to public health practice. Chapter 9 links planning with evaluation and stresses the importance of evaluating the planning and implementation process to ensure that practitioners can decide on what works and what needs to be modified. Evaluation is an essential element in the planning and implementation process because it gives the practitioner an idea of where changes or modifications might need to be made. Chapter 9 also addresses the issue of undertaking a needs assessment to assist in the planning process. Public health plans are based on identifying and assessing needs. In addition, needs can be defined in a variety of different ways. This chapter identifies the variety of ways in which needs can be defined and then discusses the program planning and implementation process. A number of planning models are presented and discussed and the advantages and disadvantages of each are considered. The value of this chapter includes a conversation with the reader about the implications for practice and an understanding of the difficulties associated with the processes of implementing and evaluating a program.

CHAPTER 7

Ethics and public health

Trish Gould

Learning objectives

After reading this chapter you should be able to:

- discuss the concept of ethics and recognise that 'ethics' is often defined and approached in different ways, which can create the potential for conflict in practical situations
- describe the development/underpinnings of public health ethics
- summarise some of the key ethical systems such as liberalism, utilitarianism, and communitarianism and their relevance to public health practice
- outline and critique some codes of ethics, and discuss their application to public health practice
- recognise, communicate and evaluate ethical concerns regarding public health, and apply ethical principles in your practice.

Introduction

This chapter introduces you to the basic ethical principles that underpin public health practice. The themes to be considered in this chapter include the characteristics of 'ethics', the justification for reflecting on ethics and values, the foundations of public health ethics, whether and how we can incorporate ethics and values into our practice and the nature of some of the potential ethical complications of public health practice.

Public health encompasses a wide range of methodologies, requires an extensive combination of knowledge and expertise and is affected by constant changes in technologies, legislation and culture (Fry et al 2004). The beliefs and philosophies that guide practice among people working in a public health-related capacity are intended to promote the health of the population. But until fairly recently, most of the examination of public health ethics that has been undertaken has been concerned with research ethics and responses to infectious diseases (Kenny et al 2006), such as quarantine and/or isolation for SARS (severe acute respiratory syndrome). However, public health ethics deals with more than just communicable disease and research. The primary values of public health ethics emphasise population health, safety and wellbeing; impartiality in service delivery; and acknowledges the rights of both individuals and groups (Gostin 2003). Envisioning ethical values relevant to the extensive scope and complexity of these public health enterprises has been problematic. Thus, there has been little ethics dialogue or an accepted 'framework' for resolving public health ethics problems (Fry et al 2004, Kenny et al 2006).

Moreover, because most ethical analysis has been about individual rights and responsibilities, it is challenging to make the transition from that focus to one that emphasises populations or communities (Bayer et al 2007). It is vital that the fundamental ethical themes, including the 'common good' as well as the principal concerns allied to the core functions of public health, are isolated and explored (Kenny et al 2006). Integrating these competing values is indispensable to a constructive ethical framework (Kenny et al 2006) and a variety of ethical analyses are necessary in order to encapsulate the diversity and depth of public health (Bayer et al 2007).

You may wonder what relevance ethics has to your own practice. Regardless of your particular health-related discipline, all your actions have ethical implications. Health workers are regularly confronted by ethical problems or dilemmas that call for careful consideration and prudent decision making. Frequently, deciding on the correct course of action to undertake when faced with such issues is challenging. For example, as well as yielding improvements in health, an intervention also has the potential to cause harm; for instance, 'justice' may be violated by imposing more of a burden on a subpopulation than on the rest. In addition, it is possible to harm relationships within and between communities (Parker et al 2007). Understanding these risks will help you to practise more thoughtfully and circumspectly.

It is vital that all health professionals explore ethics. This helps to inform their decision making and ensure their motivations and philosophies are apparent – to themselves, their colleagues and their clients. An awareness of the major ethical standpoints relevant to their practice will enable them to better appreciate and defend their own ethical view points and arrive at knowledgeable and insightful decisions about complicated issues (Parker et al 2007). Clarity in the values that motivate and guide our endeavours will enable us to decide whether, and how, research should be undertaken or interventions implemented (Parker et al 2007). Furthermore, examining the place of ethics within your practice will allow you to recognise unconscious biases, reflect on them and develop and apply investigations and programs that abide by a specific ethical stance (Thomas 2003). Since all health workers may be confronted with difficult choices regarding the range of possible options, they need to be familiar with an ethical framework that is in accord with current public health practice.

Your particular occupation may well have a code of ethics to guide your practice; nevertheless, as well as complying with such principles, you will still need to reflect and reason, as such guidelines cannot cover all eventualities. If your profession does not have such a code, then it is even more crucial that you analyse your motives and actions, the ethical implications and the likely outcomes of your actions. Moreover, debates on various cultural, environmental, economic and political issues, which all have the potential to impact on health, regularly raise themes related to ethical and fair conduct, even though these issues may not be overtly identified. This presents another compelling argument for exploring ethics in public health – you will be able to advocate for programs and policies within other sectors that minimise the risks to the population's health.

This chapter does not attempt to give you specific instructions to cover every ethical challenge you may face; rather, it aims to raise your awareness of some of the ethical issues that are bound to confront you in your professional practice, as well as in your more general interactions with the world around you. Additionally, it seeks to provide you with insight regarding the ethical principles that are pertinent to a wide range of professions and an appreciation of the range of perspectives, theories and approaches to any ethical issue or dilemma.

What is your understanding of 'ethics'? Does it have positive, negative or neutral connotations? Do you think your ethical perspective is influenced by your religious, psychological and cultural background? The activity that follows will help you to clarify some of these issues.

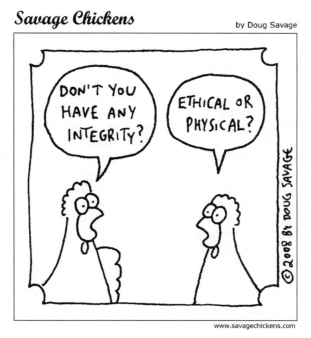

FIGURE 7.1: 'Integrity'
(Source: © 2008 Doug Savage)

ACTIVITY

- Discuss with some of your classmates, friends or family what ethics means to them and how they would define 'ethical practice'. Ask them to imagine some instances of non-ethical conduct within their own particular professions. Write down their answers.

REFLECTION

How do the perceptions of ethics collected from the people you surveyed accord with your own and each other's? Is there an all-embracing theme, one that incorporates all your views, or are there conflicts? Did anyone refer to the issue of religion, society or culture in your discussions, and how do these factors relate to someone's ethical beliefs? Do you think it is possible to work effectively with people whose ethics differ widely from your own? What are the implications of your views, that is, how do your ethical perspectives influence your practice?

The next section summarises some of the background to the study of ethics, so that you have a reasonable grasp of the concepts that are relevant to our discussion.

Ethical theories and concepts

Ethics is one of the disciplines within philosophy; together with logic (learning how to differentiate superior reasoning from inferior); metaphysics (discussions of that which may exist above and beyond our observable physical reality); ontology (the nature of reality and existence); and epistemology (the study of the scope and nature of knowledge and truth) among others. The discipline of ethics enquires into a wide range of concerns: normative ethics tries to ascertain what are good and right actions and motives; meta-ethics analyses the essential nature of ethical principles and whether they can be objectively validated; applied ethics develops methods to bring about a desired ethical outcome in any particular situation; and descriptive ethics explores the ethics people actually believe and/or put into practice.

Given its objective of finding out how to determine what are good and right actions and motives in practice, normative ethics has direct relevance to public health practice. Five of the most common normative ethical positions are outlined here.

1 *Consequentialism* claims that an action's rightness depends on its consequences or outcomes (Cribb & Duncan 2002). One of the most familiar consequentialist theories is utilitarianism (popularised by J Bentham and J S Mill). *Utilitarianism* deems an action to be proper if it brings about the greatest amount of pleasure and the least amount pain, for the maximum number of people. This paradigm, to a large extent, motivates or inspires much of public health practice, for instance, the fluoridation of reticulated water (Parker et al 2007).

2 *Deontology* maintains that every individual has absolute duties and rights – and these should form the basis of ethical decisions. That is, the consequences of actions do not determine whether the action is good or bad, rather, it is other elements (Beauchamp & Childress 2001), such as your intent. One deontological theory is Kant's *Categorical Imperative*, which situates 'morality' within our ability to reason, and maintains that there are incontrovertible moral rules. According to Kant, you should only carry out any action if you would accept that same action as a universal law.

3 *Virtue ethics* gives emphasis to an individual's intrinsic qualities (whatever people agree are desirable personal characteristics, for example bravery, compassion and honesty), in preference to rules or consequences.

4 *Liberalism* – There are many types of liberalism, but its focus is usually rights, equality, freedom and democracy. Such concepts, particularly 'rights' and the 'right' to health, are the basic premise of many influential public health documents (Parker et al 2007). For example, the *Alma-Ata Declaration* states that health '… is a fundamental human right …' (WHO 1978).

5 *Communitarianism* – Communitarians recognise humans as social beings, and therefore emphasise social relationships and common values (Sindall 2002). This perspective requires enforcing limits on individual autonomy for the benefit of the community (Callahan & Jennings 2002). For example, laws that restrict or prohibit smoking in particular areas limit individual autonomy in order to protect the community (Parker et al 2007).

The following example applies each of the five standpoints to demonstrate how different beliefs/theories about ethics have real-world practical impacts.

For example, the time-honoured methods of preventing the spread of infection are quarantine (separating possibly exposed healthy people from non-exposed healthy people) and isolation (separating sick people while they are infectious). During the SARS pandemic the World Health Organization's response was to concentrate on isolation and quarantine; as well as surveillance, contact-tracing and limiting travel (Gostin et al 2007).

A consequentialist may argue that it is right to isolate someone with a highly lethal, infectious disease only because of the consequences of not doing so – a probable epidemic, and subsequent deaths. Contrary to this view, a deontologist could argue that, regardless of the possible outcomes, there is a *duty* to protect people from such a disease, and everyone has a *right* to be protected from disease. A virtue ethicist might defend isolation based on the good intentions of those enforcing it. With its focus on autonomy and freedom, liberalists would be more likely to minimise the use of forced isolation and quarantine, and perhaps argue for education and persuasion to convince infectious people to keep away from other people. Communitarianism, with its focus on communities, may argue that it is justifiable to limit individual freedoms, that is, isolating an infected person, if it benefits the whole community.

Clearly, there are many differences between the various types of normative ethics, for example the divergence between the 'good' of the individual (liberalism) and that of the community (communitarianism). However, there are also commonalities; for example, utilitarianism and communitarianism both tend to favour communal rights and welfare over that of the individual.

The usefulness of these various normative positions can only be realised if their relationships to each other are understood, just as ethics can only be grasped in terms of the relationships between people, groups and their total environment. That is, we cannot have 'stand alone' definitions of these viewpoints, nor employ a one-size-fits-all approach. Nevertheless, we need to agree upon the meanings of the ethical theories and approaches to help us to communicate in our efforts to apply ethics in public health endeavours. Arguably, the SARS example above illustrates that each of the five normative ethical positions offers its own unique perspective on the ethics of any given public health action. Accordingly, taken together, the potential contribution of all the normative positions outlined here should be considered when assessing the ethics of any given public health intervention, research or program.

The next section examines some of the factors that have influenced the development of public health ethics.

The development of ethics in public health

Some authors differentiate between medical ethics and bioethics (Bayer et al 2007, Beauchamp & Childress 2001, Thompson et al 2003). 'Medical ethics' generally refers to a doctor or other health care provider's ethical responsibility towards their (individual) patient or client. Although the category of 'bioethics' sometimes includes 'medical ethics', 'bioethics' more typically encompasses such issues as genetic research, research ethics, genomics and cloning. Bioethics developed in the middle of the 20th century as a discipline separate from medical ethics, and medical ethics' focus on individual autonomy and the right not to be harmed (Bayer et al 2007, Beauchamp & Childress 2001, Thompson et al 2003).

Because bioethics has tended to concentrate on ethical questions relevant to clinical research and practice, it tends to emphasise the interests of individuals – largely patient autonomy (Thompson et al 2003). This is not surprising, in view of the development of bioethics as a reaction to some questionable research practices, such as the *Tuskegee Syphilis Study* (see the activity under 'Research' later in this chapter) and the Nazi 'medical' experiments – brought to the public's awareness through the *Nuremberg Trials*[1] (Beauchamp & Steinbock 1999), that denied patients their rights and humanity.

In the 1970s Beauchamp and Childress (1979) outlined a systematic framework for approaching bioethics and resolving dilemmas (principlism). This consisted of four rules: autonomy, beneficence, non-maleficence and justice. Autonomy is respecting individuals and their rights, beneficence is doing good and ensuring that the benefits of any action outweigh the burdens, non-maleficence is avoiding causing harm and justice means that advantages and burdens should be fairly shared (Beauchamp & Childress 1979). This is the most commonly used system in contemporary medical ethics (Kessel 2003).

In Chapter 2 we discussed the influence of the biomedical perspective on health. Similarly, although frameworks for public health ethics have partially derived from the bioethical tradition, public health ethics is now a distinct, albeit overlapping, discipline, limiting the use of bioethical models to public health practice (Callahan & Jennings 2002, Kass 2001, Thomas et al 2002, Thompson et al 2003).

It is important to distinguish between medical ethics and bioethics, and public health ethics, as there are vital differences. While medical ethics and bioethics primarily focus on the rights of the individual, such an approach is at odds with public health practice, where the emphasis is primarily on the good of whole communities or population groups (Callahan & Jennings 2002, Mann 1997, Thomas et al 2002). Thus, the overarching values of public health often require giving precedence to the needs and rights of the population (many individuals) over those of specific individuals (Bayer & Fairchild 2004). In addition, public health, unlike medicine, focuses more on preventing disease than treating it (Callahan & Jennings 2002, Thomas et al 2002).

Several authors writing about public health have highlighted the need for a satisfactory theoretical model for public health ethics (Kenny et al 2006). The bioethical precepts of beneficence, non-maleficence, justice and autonomy are useful for public health (Parker et al 2007) however, with the emphasis on individual autonomy, fall short of a suitable response to the problems of establishing cooperative public health strategies (Kenny et al 2006). Appropriate public health ethics call for a model that can bridge the gap between the individual and the communal good, illuminate the connection between individual and family health care and public health, acknowledge the vital influence of socioeconomic factors on health (see Ch 6) and the value of improving the conditions of those people who are most at risk (Kenny et al 2006). Moreover, any ethical approach must be sufficiently adaptable to keep up with the constant change in the variety of factors that influence public health (Fry et al 2004).

Related law and human rights discourse

There is an intricate relationship between public health, law, political philosophy and human rights. Although distinct social institutions, ethics and laws are both crucial tools for regulating behaviour, and they work in partnership to provide guidance for public health. Practitioners must use their judgement and sense of responsibility to make decisions within the boundaries of the law. Ethics requires reflection and rationales for public health endeavours, while providing guidance through principles, moral norms, professional codes and examples from earlier situations (Bernheim 2005). Ethics is a reflective procedure best performed with other people and entails investigating and evaluating any proposed strategy, together with giving good reasons for any action – particularly when the law has nothing specific to say about the issue. There are frequently no correct solutions, especially when there is limited scientific data available. Thus, being able to team up with others to pinpoint and reflect on all the potential actions will enable rational and 'justifiable decisions' to be identified (Bernheim 2005 p 102).

Human rights

The key distinction between ethics and human rights is that like law, rights have a legal basis, while ethics do not; both can originate from, and indicate, people's values, however, they are discrete (Leeder 2004). One of the challenges with a rights-based framework is that expressions such as 'the right to equal opportunity' (see below for more on equality and equity) and 'the right to health' are imprecise; they cannot be clarified without straightening out who has a duty to ensure access to each theoretical right (Leeder 2004, O'Neill 2002). In addition, rights often intersect or clash; for example, the right to privacy is in opposition to the right of the public to be protected from infectious disease. Some scholars assert that public health disregards individual rights to liberty, autonomy, privacy and property rights; however, Gostin (2001) rejects this – in the public health paradigm these are still respected, but they often must be overridden by the communal good.

When talking about the 'right to equal opportunity', we also need to compare the concepts of equity and equality. What is equity and how does it differ from equality? Essentially equity is about fairness (WHO 1996). The following quote illustrates the differences between these two concepts:

> Equity in health is not the same as equality in *health status*. Inequalities in
> *health status* between individuals and populations are inevitable consequences
> of genetic differences, of different social and economic conditions, or a result
> of personal *lifestyle* choices. Inequities occur as a consequence of differences in
> opportunity which result, for example, in unequal access to health services, to
> nutritious food, adequate housing and so on. In such cases, inequalities in *health
> status* arise as a consequence of inequities in opportunities in life
>
> (WHO 1998 p 7)

Thus, equity is about having equal opportunities to health-enhancing factors, not equal (health) status. Chapter 8 also discusses the role of 'equity' in public health practice.

Clearly, public health emphasises populations and is concerned with the determinants of health that are primarily outside of the individual's control. Accordingly, a paradigm that articulates values in terms of people's relationships with their social and structural environments may be more appropriate to public health's aims than one that is more individually focussed (Mann 1997). The factors linking public health to human rights can be expressed by three interactions. Public health strategies and procedures can contravene human rights; for example, coercive public health authority can interfere with 'autonomy, bodily integrity, privacy, and liberty' (Gostin 2003 p 182). Second, human rights violations can harm public health; for example, persecuting, torturing or subjecting people to inhuman and demeaning conditions or treatment not only harms the individual, but also the community. Lastly, policies that support both public health and human rights generate constructive, 'mutually reinforcing' effects for individuals and communities (Gostin 2003 p 183). 'There often exists a synergistic relationship between health and human rights, so that one supports the other' (Gostin 2003 p 183).

The basis for human rights 'within the United Nations system is the international Bill of Human Rights comprising the United Nations Charter, the Universal Declaration of Human Rights, and two International Covenants of Human Rights' (Gostin 2003 p 183). The Universal Declaration of Human Rights was proclaimed and adopted in 1948 by the General Assembly of the United Nations. This edict provides a rights-based model for a public health code of ethics. Article 25 states that:

> Everyone has the right to a standard of living adequate for the health and
> wellbeing of himself and of his family, including food, clothing, housing and
> medical care and necessary social services, and the right to security in the event
> of unemployment, sickness, disability, widowhood, old age or other lack of
> livelihood in circumstances beyond his control.
>
> (United Nations General Assembly 1948)

Mann (1997) claims that human rights provide a more practical framework, language and guidance for contemporary public health ethics, rather than a paradigm modified from medical, biomedical or earlier public health ethics, because human rights discourse and law originated completely beyond the health sphere. Thus the language of human rights may be more appropriate for dealing with the determinants of health that are also external to the health sphere, such as housing, education and transport. Furthermore, human rights paradigms look to identify the societal necessities for human wellbeing and therefore address the social determinants of health (Mann 1997). Conversely, Porter (2006) critiques the human rights model for public health as a Western-dominated, consequentialist paradigm. That is, what makes this approach any more valid or desirable than any other ethical model? (Later in the chapter we will be discussing related concepts of cultural relativism and absolutism.)

Gostin (2001) indicates four spheres where ethics can facilitate public health to fulfil its purpose: the first is by helping to define the meaning of 'public health professionalism' and 'ethical practice'; the second is leading dialogue on the moral value of the community's wellbeing; the third is addressing the familiar issues confronting public health practitioners; and lastly, facilitating advocacy to improve the population's health.

Applied ethics

The practitioner not only needs an awareness of their own values, but also the values that are fundamental to public health practice, as these values, whether they are explicit or not, will impact on public health policy and practice. Some scholars even claim that it is the ethical aspects of the public health action itself, rather than the nature of the practitioner, that is more relevant to the application of public health ethics (Gostin 2003). Regardless of which perspective you take, the next section will provide you with more insight by outlining some ethical codes and providing some examples of applying ethical analysis to a range of issues.

Codes of ethics

Many professional and service groups have codes of ethics, albeit often unspoken or implied. A 'code of ethics' is a collection of standards for practitioners and organisations, which dictates certain benchmarks as to their practice and their character while demonstrating their values to the public, as well as the standards of care that the public can expect (Gostin 2003). However, it is not enough to just acquaint yourself with, and implement, the relevant ethical principles; given that there are continuous developments in health technologies, social and political systems, and the determinants of health, the investigation and application of ethics must keep pace.

In the UK and US, there has been increasing debate, research and scholarship regarding the need to define a core code of ethics for public health, and what it should encompass. A number of ethical codes for public health have been proposed or adopted; the three featured here have been selected as they include a variety of ethical perspectives. In 2002, the American Public Health Association (APHA) agreed to a code of ethics for public health practice, comprising 12 tenets:

1 Public health should address principally the fundamental causes of disease and requirements for health, aiming to prevent adverse health outcomes.
2 Public health should achieve community health in a way that respects the rights of individuals in the community.
3 Public health policies, programs and priorities should be developed and evaluated through processes that ensure an opportunity for input from community members.

4 Public health should advocate for, or work for the empowerment of, disenfranchised community members, ensuring that the basic resources and conditions necessary for health are accessible to all people in the community.

5 Public health should seek the information needed to implement effective policies and programs that protect and promote health.

6 Public health institutions should provide communities with the information they have that is needed for decisions on policies or programs and should obtain the community's consent for their implementation.

7 Public health institutions should act in a timely manner on the information they have within the resources and the mandate given to them by the public.

8 Public health programs and policies should incorporate a variety of approaches that anticipate and respect diverse values, beliefs and cultures in the community.

9 Public health programs and policies should be implemented in a manner that most enhances the physical and social environment.

10 Public health institutions should protect the confidentiality of information that can bring harm to an individual or community if made public. Exceptions must be justified on the basis of the high likelihood of significant harm to the individual or others.

11 Public health institutions should ensure the professional competence of their employees.

12 Public health institutions and their employees should engage in collaborations and affiliations in ways that build the public's trust and the institution's effectiveness (Thomas et al 2002 p 1058).

In Australia, as yet there is no code of ethics specifically for public health practitioners, although there are a number of guidelines for ethical conduct in *research* with humans. These include the National Health and Medical Research Council's (NHMRC) *National Statement on Ethical Conduct in Research Involving Humans* (NHMRC 2007) and *Values and Ethics: Guidelines for Ethical Conduct in Aboriginal and Torres Strait Islander Health Research* (NHMRC 2003). All health researchers are obligated to conform to these guidelines. The NHMRC (2003) guidelines emphasise six core values:

1 *spirit and integrity* – the continuity of the cultural heritage of past, present and future generations

2 *reciprocity* – the research must both benefit, and be valued by, the community

3 *respect* – there must be respect for, and acceptance of, dignity and diverse values

4 *equality* – there must be a commitment to justice and equality

5 *survival and protection* – the research and researchers must not harm Aboriginal and Torres Strait Islander cultures, identity or languages

6 *responsibility* – researchers must ensure that they do no damage to Aboriginal and Torres Strait Islander peoples or the things they treasure, and must be accountable to the people (NHMRC 2003).

ACTIVITY

● These guidelines were developed to guide health researchers in their dealings with Aboriginal and Torres Strait Islander peoples; can these same precepts be applied to non-Indigenous populations? What about their more general applicability to any health-related work undertaken with Aboriginal and Torres Strait Islander peoples?

● Do you understand what the principles are trying to communicate, or are they too abstract? How can you determine whether you have complied with these guidelines? Can you see any potential conflicts between the various principles?

REFLECTION

Although devised for health researchers, the guidelines also offer a positive model for implementing a range of programs or interventions with Aboriginal and Torres Strait Islander communities (Parker et al 2007). Additionally, according to Parker et al (2007), the guidelines are applicable in any group with whom you work in partnership, especially different ethnic groups or nations. However, there may be conflicts – for example, the value of respecting Aboriginal and Torres Strait Islander peoples and the things that they treasure. As previously mentioned, the good of the community can often conflict with that of the individual – what benefits the individual could harm the community or vice versa.

First developed in 1993, the *Code of Ethics for Nurses in Australia* was revised in 2002 (Australian Nursing and Midwifery Council 2005). This code of ethics is intended to determine nurses' essential moral obligations, and afford them with a foundation for professional and self-deliberation on ethical actions, function as a model for ethical practice and show the public the principles that nurses should espouse and hold. The code of ethics has six value statements:

1 Nurses respect individuals' needs, values, culture and vulnerability in the provision of nursing care.
2 Nurses accept the rights of individuals to make informed choices in relation to their care.
3 Nurses promote and uphold the provision of quality nursing care for all people.
4 Nurses hold in confidence any information obtained in a professional capacity, use professional judgement where there is a need to share information for the therapeutic benefit and safety of a person and ensure that privacy is safeguarded.
5 Nurses fulfil the accountability and responsibility inherent in their roles.
6 Nurses value environmental ethics and a social, economic and ecologically sustainable environment that promotes health and wellbeing (ANMC 2005 pp 3–5).

ACTIVITY

● Look back over the 12 principles of the *Ethical Practice of Public Health* (APHA 2006) or read the entire nursing code of ethics (five pages – see the website at the end of the chapter). Can you apply either of these codes, in their entirety, to Australian public health practice, or are there some sections that might need to be modified? Which ones and how would you change them?

REFLECTION

All of these value statements in the nursing code of ethics are important and applicable to public health practice, although the code (ANMC 2005) emphasises individuals' rights. This perspective is appropriate for nurses whose practice is oriented to caring for individual patients; however, this is not entirely appropriate for public health practice, where the population or group is generally the focus. For instance, consider the isolation and quarantine example earlier in the chapter – the nursing focus would generally be on the individual patient, caring for their health and wellbeing. A public health perspective, while not actually disregarding the needs of the individual, would tend to emphasise the good of a whole population.

No ethical guidelines can cover every eventuality; however they can assist with further analysis; in addition, it can be advantageous to follow a generic decision-making framework in a step-by-step manner. The model in Box 7.1 may assist you to resolve ethical issues, problems and dilemmas.

Box 7.1: A step-by-step ethical decision-making model

1 *Identify the ethical problem:* Delineate the facts and eliminate assumptions in order to clarify the problem. Decide whether it is in actuality an ethical problem rather than a clinical, professional or legal issue, or a combination of these.

2 *Apply the relevant code of ethics:* Consult your association, organisation or workplace code of ethics for clarification. If there is no such organisation or code of ethics, the issue is more complicated or the code of ethics does not provide sufficient guidance, then you should move on to the next stage in this model.

3 *Establish the nature and size of the problem:* Consider a range of ethical philosophies and precepts. Choose those that are applicable, and decide which take precedence. Confer with colleagues, supervisors and/or the relevant professional organisations. They may notice pertinent issues or viewpoints that you overlooked.

4 *Establish an action plan:* Devise as many strategies as possible, consult with co-workers to generate more ideas.

5 *Appraise the likely consequences:* Assess all the alternatives and reject those that are unlikely to achieve the desired outcomes, or those that may generate additional ethical issues.

6 *Select a possible course of action:* Having rejected any indeterminate and/or possibly harmful strategies, choose the most promising, and least precarious, from those that are left.

7 *Evaluate the selected course of action:* Review the selected course of action to see if it presents any new ethical considerations. If there are problems revisit an appropriate earlier step.

8 *Implement the strategy:* Implement the favoured action, and re-evaluate to judge whether your actions had the predicted outcomes and/or any untoward consequences.

(Sources: Forester-Miller & Davis 1996, Last 1997, Parker et al 2007)

An alternative framework for analysing interventions (specifically in public health) is outlined by Gostin (2003). Under this framework, you need to assess:

- the nature, probability and severity of the risk
- the likelihood that the proposed action will be effective in meeting its objectives
- the economic costs entailed, including opportunity costs
- the burdens on human rights
- the fairness, including a just allocation of benefits and burdens (Gostin 2003 pp 185–6).

Clearly, ethics should underlie all our actions. Some of the conflicts – for example, between the individual and the population, between treatment and prevention – will become more obvious as we examine the examples in the following section that will help you sort out the role of ethics in practice.

Applications – examples of ethics in public health practice

This section gives examples of ethical problems, issues and dilemmas from a range of health domains; this will help you to integrate and apply the theories and precepts to your profession. Moreover it will clarify the relevance of ethics to your practice.

Research

Research is an indispensable element of public health, and research projects require that you obtain ethical approval from at least one institution (e.g. a university or hospital ethical board). However, your ethical responsibility doesn't end there. In addition to your responsibility to safeguard confidentiality and ensure the participants' right to informed consent is respected and so on, there are many other issues, risks and concerns associated with it. These include paying people to participate in a study and the 'implications' for the notion of voluntary consent; research funding and the potential conflict of interest, for example, a fast food company funding research on obesity and 'fast food'; and 'research "add-ons" in studies funded and approved for other purposes' (Fry et al 2004 p 14). The following example raises a number of ethical issues, including the right to informed consent.

ACTIVITY

- The *Tuskegee Syphilis Study* took place between 1932 and 1972 in Tuskegee, Alabama. The 399 participants (and a similar number of controls) were mainly underprivileged African Americans. When the study began in 1932, the accepted treatments for syphilis were not very effective and had toxic side effects. One of the goals of the research was to establish whether outcomes were better if the patients were not treated with these dangerous medications. However by the mid 1940s, penicillin had become the orthodox therapy for syphilis, but instead of terminating the study and administering penicillin to all the study participants, the researchers withheld penicillin and information about it. The study ceased in the early 1970s, when details were disclosed through the press. By this time, many of the participants had died from syphilis, and their families had become infected (CDC website, University of Virginia Health Sciences Library 1996).
- Imagine you are part of the Tuskegee study research team in 1932. What are some of the ethical concerns you might have with regard to the design of the study? From the point of view of the social, cultural and ethical environment of today, are the ethical issues any different? Do you think that the researchers can be absolved, or their actions justified, in light of the change in perspective over the last three-quarters of a century?

REFLECTION

At that time, doctors frequently did not disclose information to patients about their illness – as the medical ethics of that period did not have the rigorous requirements for informed consent that exist today. Research has demonstrated that many African Americans have no confidence in medical and public health authorities as a consequence of this study (CDC website, University of Virginia Health Sciences Library 1996), which can have negative consequences for both the individuals and the population as a whole. As you can see, despite the differences, there is also a large amount of overlap between medical ethics (the physician's duty towards his or her patient), bioethics (medical research ethics) and public health ethics, as you could utilise all these approaches in exploring the above example.

Anthropological research

On 13 September 2007, the United Nations General Assembly adopted the United Nations *Declaration on the Rights of Indigenous Peoples*; four countries voted against the declaration – Canada, New Zealand, the United States and Australia. Article 23 acknowledges the rights of Indigenous peoples to:

> … maintain, control, protect and develop their cultural heritage, traditional knowledge and traditional cultural expressions, as well as *the manifestations of their sciences, technologies and cultures, including human and genetic resources, seeds, medicines, knowledge of the properties of fauna and flora,* [our emphasis]

oral traditions, literatures, designs, sports and traditional games and visual and performing arts. They also have the right to maintain, control, protect and develop their intellectual property over such cultural heritage, traditional knowledge, and traditional cultural expressions.

(OHCHR 2007)

Article 23 states that researchers should not benefit from their research in Indigenous communities, unless the community gets an equivalent or superior advantage. See the following example, which demonstrates some of the downside for Indigenous peoples who are 'researched'.

ACTIVITY

● Supported by *National Geographic* and IBM, the *Genographic Project* commenced in 2005. It is a five-year study of genetic anthropology that aims to collect 100,000 blood samples from Indigenous peoples to investigate human migration in the region. Such research also has the potential to contribute benefits to health for both the populations studied, as well as other populations, as discoveries could, for example, include the genetic foundations of susceptibility to particular diseases. The project quickly ran into opposition from Indigenous groups. 'We know our creation stories and we know who our ancestors are' (Kanehe 2007 p 122).

● Why do you think people would protest about such research? What do you think are the pertinent issues? For the people of the Pacific region, what are the likely advantages and/or disadvantages to participating? Who owns the genes – once the information is acquired who has the intellectual property rights?

REFLECTION

Did you consider the following issues: privacy, autonomy and ownership? There are many potential pitfalls with this project. In many societies, the human body is 'sacred', and must be kept 'whole'; to remove blood or any other body part can be offensive. The peoples' own knowledge of their creation, origins, ancestors, oral histories and languages, and their cultural and spiritual beliefs, may be damaged by the (Western) interpretation of any data acquired (Kanehe 2007). Kanehe claims that such genetic research is 'intrusive and exploitative' (2007 p 125). Furthermore, if the results indicate that some Indigenous peoples did not arrive as early as their own histories indicate, the research could have negative consequences for the land rights of 'traditional owners' (Kanehe 2007). In addition, the researchers have not indicated whether there are any direct benefits (health or other) for the participants. Therefore, a burden is imposed on the people, without the likelihood of receiving any positive return.

Cross-cultural medical research and practice

The stated aim of the following project was to develop a new treatment or cure for people with type 2 diabetes (of course, whoever successfully developed the new treatment stood to make a lot of money out of it!).

ACTIVITY

● People indigenous to the Pacific Islands generally have a raised risk of developing of type 2 diabetes. A New Zealand-based research group wanted to undertake experiments in the Cook Islands into a cure for type 2 diabetes. The research involved transplanting pancreas cells from pigs into people. This type of research was banned in New Zealand in 2001, due to the possibility of humans being infected with the porcine endogenous retrovirus. The Cook Islands' Government eventually decided against allowing the research, after first agreeing, following objections from tribal leaders and the world medical community (Mataiapo 2007).

REFLECTION

If the researchers had been allowed to complete the research, and attained their goal, would that then have been ethical? That is, do the means (transplanting pig cells into humans) justify the ends (a cure for type 2 diabetes)? What about respect for peoples' cultural traditions and beliefs? As stated, in many cultures the human body and spirit is 'sacred' and so to introduce cells from another animal into humans would be 'sacrilegious' or 'polluting' (Mataiapo 2007). Furthermore, there is the issue of carrying out research in a developing country (when you have been refused permission to implement that research in a 'developed' country), because the particular country may not have laws or guidelines to cover such research. Therefore, it has the potential to be exploitative.

Screening

The use and justification of screening will be discussed in Chapter 12. The following example uses screening for prostate cancer to show that screening is a 'double-edged sword', with an array of ethical implications.

ACTIVITY

- In Australia, prostate cancer is the seventh most common cause of mortality in men, causing 2761 deaths in 2004 (AIHW 2006). It is rare before the age of 50, with 96% of deaths occurring after age 60. As with many cancers, if found early, prostate cancer can be treated; however, the treatments have significant and common side effects, including impotence and incontinence. In addition, many prostate cancers are very slow growing and are unlikely to kill the patient. There is screening available for prostate cancer – a blood test for prostate-specific antigen. The limitations of prostate-specific antigen (PSA) screening are the high rate of false positives (where the test falsely indicates the presence of disease) and false negatives (where the test fails to indicate the presence of disease) (Etzioni et al 2002). According to Hoffman (2006), the value of PSA screening is not proven.
- Is it ethical to screen for any particular condition or disease predisposition if there is not always an effective and acceptable treatment, or if the side effects are significant and irreversible? Conversely, is it ethical not to screen, when there is the potential to save lives, whatever the magnitude of that potential?

REFLECTION

Did you consider any of the following issues? Screening carries a risk of 'false positives', which may give the person 'peace of mind' when it is unwarranted; or 'false negatives', which may lead to unnecessary diagnostic tests, and anxiety, for a significant proportion of the screened population? There is also an issue of cost – is it ethically acceptable to spend a large amount of health funds on screening a subpopulation, where the number of 'positives' identified may be minimal? How would you respond if a screening program had the potential to save one life for every 10,000 people tested – should we ignore the life of that one individual, or spend the resources and time?

Disease control

Disease control, which will be considered in depth in Chapter 10, sometimes involves the enforcement of rules and/or control of individuals' behaviour for the good of the population as a whole. Such an approach entails a balance between the rights and welfare of both the individual and the community (Kenny et al 2007). While diseases such as SARS, HIV/AIDS and H5N1 (avian influenza) are important public health problems (McMichael & Butler 2007), they also raise critical ethical issues; for example, should someone who refuses treatment for a virulent disease be detained and/or treated against their will? Consider the following example.

ACTIVITY

● Imagine you are Chief Health Officer in NSW. Having already tried all other avenues to get an individual with active, infective tuberculosis (TB) to comply with a treatment regimen, the patient still refuses, thus posing a health risk to others. You are now required to initiate proceedings to serve a public health order, which will mandate the person's detention and treatment.

● Can you envision any alternatives to the patient's (forced) confinement and treatment; if not is it acceptable to detain and treat them against their will? What, if any, are some of the ethics and/or rights that are in conflict in the above example? If you were responsible for drafting laws or policies to deal with such situations, which options would you support?

REFLECTION

With regard to conflicting rights, did you consider 'the duty to protect the community', 'the collective good' and/or 'the right to privacy and liberty' (Gostin et al 2007 p 261)? If you said 'no' to detaining someone against their will, would you still oppose such a public health order if the patient had a multi-drug resistant form of TB? What if the person also had HIV/AIDS; given that in some countries HIV/AIDS is a significant co-factor for TB. Worldwide, TB is one of the main causes of morbidity in people with HIV (National TB Advisory Committee of CDNA 2002).

In Australia, there is no federal law covering compulsory detention and treatment, with the states having the autonomy to create their own laws, however these generally adhere to federal guidelines. For example, in New South Wales the Chief Health Officer can order the detention and treatment of a patient with an infectious disease for a period of up to 28 days; this applies to non-compliant patients with category 4 diseases, that is, typhoid, SARS and TB, or category 5 diseases, namely HIV/AIDS (Senanayake & Ferson 2004). Clearly, utilising a public health order fails to sort out any ethical tensions, it just allows for the legal confinement of an infectious person who refuses treatment (Senanayake & Ferson 2004). This example raises many other issues. Is it possible, or desirable, to protect people from this type of state intrusion into what are essentially private affairs, that is a person's 'right' to receive or refuse medical treatment as they see fit? What limits to national or state authorities are reasonable? Can you find a balance between the communal and the individual, in a situation such as this, or must the needs of one outweigh the other? If you say that the needs of a population should be put ahead of the group, what sort of ethical theory are you utilising?

Also in Chapter 10, contact tracing is discussed – this entails finding people who may have been in contact with someone who has a communicable or contagious disease; however, these people have not in any way sought diagnosis and treatment, nor given their consent to be contacted. Do these 'contacts' have rights in this instance to privacy/confidentiality? Conversely, do they have a 'right' to be informed of their possible risk status? Which right, if any, should take precedence? What about protecting the public? Unquestionably, one of the core issues for public health ethics is the necessity to use authority to protect the people's health, while also averting the abuse of such power (Thomas et al 2002).

Health promotion

As we will discover in Chapter 12, health professionals undertaking health promotion activities must consider both the societal and the individual responsibility for health. Importantly, they need to recognise that there are numerous, interrelating health determinants, in order to prevent unethical (and unproductive) victim blaming (Kenny et al 2006). Furthermore, interventions have the potential to be patronising and coercive. Another ethical issue with regard to health promotion is that the practitioner's definition of 'health' may not be congruent with the community's (see Chapter 2 for an exploration of 'health'). Therefore, in promoting particular policies, programs or interventions, the health worker may be imposing their own ideas on the population (Parker et al 2007). The following example illustrates some of these issues.

ACTIVITY

- As someone in the field of health promotion, you work in a community that has a high rate of diabetes. You decide the best intervention is to provide information about the role of diet and exercise in controlling diabetes, and establish an exercise group. However, the results are disappointing, as members of the community do not seem very enthusiastic about your project. Those people with diabetes and 'pre-diabetes' (in pre-diabetes blood glucose levels are higher than normal, though not sufficiently high to be labelled diabetes) are not paying more attention to their diets, nor are they exercising more than they were previously.
- What do you think went wrong? Do the people not care, are they lazy, or do they think diabetes is 'no big deal'? Or perhaps it was your approach that was misguided.

REFLECTION

Did you consider what the populace thought was the problem? The members of the community may not consider that diabetes is the most important issue; there could be other problems that they consider to be more urgent. If you decided what the issue was and how to fix it, without consulting the community, not only have you ignored the precepts of good health promotion practice (see Ch 12), you have also disregarded people's autonomy. Perhaps people did want to do something about their health problems but had inadequate access to affordable suitable food, inadequate exercise facilities (e.g. no safe area to walk or run) or no time available. As well as these more practical issues, it also raises problems of meaning – perhaps your idea of 'health' or the meaning of diabetes did not accord with theirs. Some of the ethical issues here would relate to coercion, autonomy and paternalism.

Advocacy

As we have seen in Chapter 6, deprivation and inequality have a strong relationship with ill health, and there is ample published evidence to support the argument that people's social and economic environments impact on their health (Gostin 2003, Wise 2001). This raises the question of whether public health workers have a duty to advocate for equity with regard to direct determinants of health, in addition to the broader determinants, such as housing and employment. WHO (1998 p 5) claims that people in the health professions do have an obligation to 'act as advocates for *health* at all levels in society'. What does it mean to act as an advocate for health? Advocacy is an activity where individuals or groups endeavour to restructure a range of elements, such as institutions, policies and laws (Chapman 2001, Wise 2001). Advocacy for health is actions undertaken by individuals and/or groups that are calculated to achieve 'political commitment, policy support, social acceptance and systems support for a particular health goal or programme' (WHO 1995, in WHO 1998 p 5); and to change some of the factors that shape people's environments and health behaviours (Chapman 2001, Wise 2001). Labonte claims that many public health and health promotion achievements have resulted from advocacy, 'simply because the health of a public often grates against the interests of elites' (2001 p 35); that is, advocates are frequently in conflict with governments or other people in positions of power regarding exactly what the issues or problems are and what should be done about them (Chapman 2001). Furthermore, advocacy is potentially detrimental to professionals and organisations, even more so in societies where people do not have the freedom to express their dissent (Chapman 2001, Labonte 2001, Mail 2006). Any professional working to improve people's health and wellbeing needs sufficient resources and training in order to be able to advocate for improved opportunities and conditions (Wise 2001).

Use the following example to reflect on advocacy and how you can contribute to improving people's living conditions.

ACTIVITY

- Australia funds a range of programs to developing countries, primarily in the Asia–Pacific region. For the period 2007–08, $2.731 billion of the $3.155 billion provided by Australia for development will be managed by the Australian Agency for International Development (AusAID website). AusAID's rules for family planning programs do not permit providing information about either abortion or abortion services to save the life of the woman, even in countries where such services are legal (The AusAID Family Planning Guidelines: the facts ARHA). These guidelines may be amended with the recent change in government.
- Do you think it is wrong for AusAID to provide funding for family planning with 'strings attached'? What, if anything, can you do to change it? If you think it should be changed, what is your justification – is it an equity issue, are 'human rights' more relevant, what about freedom or autonomy? If you think it is fine as it is – can you justify your stance? Is it because you believe that abortion is ethically wrong, foreign aid is unwarranted, or donor countries have the right to say how their money should be spent?

REFLECTION

If you thought the policy should be changed, did you think about lobbying the government or media and information campaigns? Did you consider whether there are any risks to yourself? For example, what happens if your employer does not support your viewpoint, and any public action that you take could risk you your job? Is there any way you can lobby or protest as a 'private individual'? Richards argued that this policy 'seeks to influence practice and values in recipient countries in ways that contravene international human rights' (ARHA).

Can ethical criteria be absolute?

There are a few ethical rules or laws that seem to apply in all human cultures, such as those against murder and theft. These systems or laws enable people to live together (Gostin et al 2007) by minimising conflict. However, different cultures can have very different values and traditions; does this mean that ethics should be analysed from a culturally relativistic perspective? That is, we make the assumption that certain behaviours are acceptable in some cultures but not in others, such as abortion, and must be considered in their specific context (Bayer et al 2007).

ACTIVITY

- In some societies it is not acceptable for women and girls to be seen by non-related males, therefore, they are often denied medical care, because there are no female doctors. Similarly, women in such societies are rarely permitted to attend school: such a lack of education not only impacts on their health and the health of their children, but on the whole population. Does this mean that it is ethical within that particular culture for about half the population to have little or no access to medical care or education? Can you articulate why it is or is not acceptable?

REFLECTION

If you said it is not acceptable, can you say why? On the other hand, if you say that it is acceptable – because that's how it's done in that particular culture and we should respect other people's traditions – what about when people migrate to countries where everyone takes good health care and education for granted? Do the new arrivals have the same rights as they would if they were still in their country of origin, or do they have the same rights as everyone else in their new country of residence? If we accept ethical relativism, we may also have to accept some abhorrent consequences, for example, some groups have beliefs about the worth or 'humanity' of other groups, does that mean that it is ethically reasonable for the former to kill the latter if they think they are not fully human? According to Bayer et al (2007) agreeing to ethical relativism excludes the possibility of condemning or judging the behaviour of other groups. Furthermore, we must discard cultural relativism in order to be able to question the beliefs of other groups as well as our own, and learn from this process (Bayer et al 2007).

Contemporary and future public health

There is a vital need for more research and discussion on public health ethics, especially on the subject of research and practice with vulnerable, disempowered or marginalised populations, including Aboriginal and Torres Strait Islanders, refugees, children and people living below the poverty line. Moreover, health professionals need to consider more than just public health-related ethical concerns, specifically, all the factors that promote or damage health, including the social, environmental, political and economic determinants, and the ethical challenges associated with them. In addition, health professionals undoubtedly have a duty to advocate for all these groups.

Public health ethics, in practice, seems to be based primarily on utilitarian ethics; that is, 'the greatest good for the greatest number' (Gostin 2003). Accordingly, public health ethics emphasise population health and safety as of the utmost importance (Gostin 2003). Nevertheless, it is essential that health professionals not only consider other ethical tenets, such as autonomy and beneficence, but also other normative ethical theories. Health professionals need to question their own moral and ethical underpinnings and how these relate to their practice (Parker et al 2007). Furthermore, a thorough exploration of values and analyses from a range of philosophies will illuminate beliefs and judgements, producing more valuable and equitable public health policies, systems and procedures.

While there has been a recent increase in dialogue on ethical practice in public health, the entire domain is still very underdeveloped. This deficiency is critical, not only for the practitioners and their client populations, but also where politicians, legislators and policymakers look to public health professionals for guidance on important issues. For example, as human populations continue to enter into a global monoculture, with the consequent increase in pandemic and epidemic risks, the decision makers will need help from public health workers to grapple with difficult decisions.

A final word

In this chapter we have considered definitions of ethics and introduced you to a variety of ethical theories that are pertinent to public health ethics. We have examined the role of codes of ethics in health-related practice and outlined a decision-making framework to address ethical problems. We presented a range of practical examples of ethics in action to illustrate some of the dilemmas and issues that confront organisations and professionals in their attempts to protect and promote the health of the public; these include screening, health promotion, research and work with vulnerable groups.

It is evident that there is a case for advancing the discussion and analysis of the ethical aspects of public health. Kessel (2003) maintains that the most effective approach to public health ethics will be a multidisciplinary one that exploits, and is inspired by, not only the philosophical aspects of morality, but also the anthropological, sociological, historical, legal and political.

Ethics provides a theoretical structure and approaches for considering and advancing public health practice (Weed & McKeown 2003); consequently, it should be an ordinary part of our day-to-day public health activities. This chapter has endeavoured to unite ethics and public health to demonstrate that good public health practice is intrinsically ethical. As health professionals your awareness and comprehension of ethical practice is a significant aspect of your professional training. This knowledge and understanding will enable you to anticipate and address any potential ethical issues prior to taking action, and practise in such a way that your motives and values are clearly apparent to others. Anyone working in a public health-related environment should realise that diverse individuals and disciplines might take separate directions in managing similar challenges. There may be more than one correct solution in any given situation or none at all. (All public health actions necessitate weighing up the benefits and harms.) Nevertheless, if you practice systematically through a framework, and reflect on your practice, you can be confident that the approach you take will be the best possible strategy in that particular place and time. Furthermore, you will be able to justify your actions, both to yourself and others.

As we have discussed in this chapter how public health ethics is about identifying, discussing and incorporating 'good' ethics into your practice, the next chapter, 'Evidence-based practice', is concerned with identifying and utilising 'good evidence'.

REVIEW QUESTIONS

You will acquire more knowledge and insight on this topic if you discuss and debate the issues with friends, family or classmates – just as ethical behaviour cannot be considered in isolation, neither can the concepts be fruitfully explored alone.

1   What is the best theoretical approach to public health ethics? For example, consequence- or rule-based? Is there one? Justify your response.
2   Think of an example of a conflict between the principles of autonomy and that of the good of the community. Why is there a conflict, how would you approach it and is there an outcome where both principles can be respected?
3   What, if any, are the differences between public health ethics and bioethics?
4   Do you think it is possible to ethically practise in, or research, a culture or community different to your own? Do you see any likely ethical dilemmas?
5   Find an example of a professional code of ethics within the Australian health sector. Apply the precepts to public health practice. Are there any principles that are particularly applicable to public health? Conversely, are there any that conflict with public health values?
6   What are some of the key contemporary challenges for public health ethics?
7   Revisit some of the earlier chapters and see if you can identify any ethical issues or dilemmas that could potentially occur as a result of public health actions (or lack of action). Explain why they would be problems and outline your solutions. Additionally, you should keep in mind the concepts discussed in this chapter as you read the rest of this book, and also try to identify possible dilemmas and pitfalls.

ENDNOTES

1. The Nuremberg Trials refer to the prosecution of some of the principal leaders of the Nazi movement (World War II) for war crimes and crimes against humanity. The trials were held between 1945 and 1949 in the city of Nuremberg in Germany (Holocaust History Project 2008).

REFERENCES

American Public Health Association 2006 Public Health Code of Ethics. APHA, Washington DC. Available: http://www.apha.org/ 17 Oct 2007

Australian Agency for International Development website. Available: http://www.ausaid.gov.au/default.cfm 3 Feb 2008

Australian Agency for International Development 2002 Family planning and the aid program: a comprehensive guide. Available: http://www.ausaid.gov.au/publications/pdf/fam-plan-guide.pdf 30 Jan 2008

Australian Institute of Health and Welfare 2006 Australia's Health 2006. AIHW cat. no. AUS 73. AIHW, Canberra

Australian Nursing and Midwifery Council 2005 Code of Ethics for Nurses in Australia. Developed under the auspices of Australian Nursing and Midwifery Council, Royal College of Nursing, Australia, Australian Nursing Federation. Published by ANMC July 1993, revised in 2002 reprinted February 2005. Available: www.anmc.org.au 12 Oct 2007

Australian Reproductive Health Alliance Comment on draft international health strategy – AusAID

Australian Reproductive Health Alliance The AusAID Family Planning Guidelines: the facts. ARHA. Available: http://www.arha.org.au/index/AusAID_FP_Guides.pdf 3 Feb 2008

Bayer R, Fairchild A L 2004 The genesis of public health ethics. Bioethics 18(6):473–92

Bayer R, Gostin L O, Jennings B et al (eds) 2007 Public Health Ethics: theory, policy, and practice. Oxford University Press, New York

Beauchamp T L, Childress J F 1979 Principles of Biomedical Ethics. Oxford University Press, New York

Beauchamp T L, Childress J F 2001 Principles of Biomedical Ethics, 5th edn. Oxford University Press, New York

Beauchamp D, Steinbock B (eds) 1999 New Ethics for the Public's Health. Oxford University Press, New York

Bernheim R G 2005 In: Melnick A, Kaplowitz L, Lopez W F et al Public health ethics in action: Flu vaccine and drug allocation strategies. Journal of Law Medicine & Ethics 33(4) Suppl:102–105

Callahan D, Jennings B 2002 Ethics and Public Health: Forging a Strong Relationship. American Journal of Public Health 92:169–176

Chapman S 2001 Advocacy in public health: roles and challenges. International Journal of Epidemiology 30:1226–1232

Centers for Disease Control and Prevention website U.S. Public Health Service Syphilis Study at Tuskegee. Available: http://www.cdc.gov/tuskegee/timeline.htm 14 Nov 2007

Cribb A, Duncan P 2002 Health Promotion and Professional Ethics. Blackwell Science, Oxford

Etzioni R, Penson D F, Legler J M et al 2002 Overdiagnosis Due to Prostate-Specific Antigen Screening: Lessons From U.S. Prostate Cancer Incidence Trends. Journal of the National Cancer Institute, 94(13):981–990

Forester-Miller H, Davis T 1996 A Practitioner's guide to ethical decision making. American Counseling Association

Fry C L, Peerson A, Scully A 2004 Raising the profile of public health ethics in Australia: time for debate. Australian and New Zealand Journal of Public Health 28(1):13–15

Gostin L O 2001 Public health, ethics, and human rights: a tribute to the late Jonathan Mann. The Journal of Law, Medicine and Ethics, 29:121–130

Gostin L O 2003 Public health ethics: Tradition, profession, and values. Acta Bioethica 9(2):177–188

Gostin L O, Bayer R, Fairchild A L 2007 Ethical and legal challenges posed by severe acute respiratory syndrome: implications for the control of severe infectious disease threats. In: Bayer R, Gostin L O, Jennings B et al (eds) Public Health Ethics: theory, policy, and practice. Oxford University Press, New York, pp 261–278

Hoffman R M 2006 Viewpoint: limiting prostate cancer screening. Annals of Internal Medicine 144(6):438–440

Holocaust History Project 2008 The Trial at Nuremberg. Available: http://www.holocaust-history.org/ 29 Jan 08

Kanehe L M 2007 From Kumulipo: I Know Where I Come From An Indigenous Pacific Critique of the Genographic Project. In: Mead A Te Pareake, Ratuva S (eds). Pacific Genes & Life Patents Pacific Indigenous Experiences & Analysis of the Commodification & Ownership of Life. Call of the Earth Llamado de la Tierra and The United Nations University Institute of Advanced Studies, pp 114–127

Kass N E 2001 An ethics framework for public health. American Journal of Public Health 91(11):1776–1782

Kenny N P, Melnychuk R M, Asada A 2006 The Promise of Public Health: Ethical Reflections. Canadian Journal of Public Health 97(5):402–404

Kessel A S 2003 Public health ethics: teaching survey and critical review. Social Science & Medicine 56:1439–1445

Labonte R 2001 Advocacy: From setting the agenda to enabling the actors. Promotion & Education Suppl. 2:35–36

Last J M 1997 Public Health and Human Ecology. Appleton and Lange, Stamford

Leeder S R 2004 Ethics and public health. Internal Medicine Journal 34(7):435–439

McMichael A J, Butler C D 2007 Emerging health issues: the widening challenge for population health promotion. Health Promotion International 21(S1):15–24 doi: 10.1093/heapro/dal047

Mail P 2006 We each have a part to play in public health advocacy Nation's Health, May, Vol. 36 Issue 4:3–3, 1/3p

Mann J M 1997 Medicine and public health, ethics and human rights. The Hastings Center Report 27(3):6–13

Mataiapo Te Tika – Dorice Reid 2007 Pig cell 'guinea pigs' – an experience of 'xenotourism': the proposed Diatranz Experiment in the Cook Islands. In: Mead A Te Pareake, Ratuva S (eds). Pacific Genes & Life Patents Pacific Indigenous Experiences & Analysis of the Commodification & Ownership of Life. Call of the Earth Llamado de la Tierra and The United Nations University Institute of Advanced Studies, pp 82–89

National Health and Medical Research Council 2003 Values and Ethics: Guidelines for Ethical Conduct in Aboriginal and Torres Strait Islander Health Research. NHMRC, Canberra (AUST). Available: http://www.nhmrc.gov.au/publications/synopses/e52syn.htm 29 Nov 2007

National Health and Medical Research Council 2007 National Statement on Ethical Conduct in Research Involving Humans. NHMRC, Canberra. Available: http://www.nhmrc.gov.au/publications/synopses/e72syn.htm 31 Jan 2008

National TB Advisory Committee of Communicable Disease Network Australia (CDNA) 2002 National Strategic Plan for TB Control in Australia Beyond 2000. Available: http://www.health.gov.au/pubhlth/cdi/pubs/tb-plan.htm 6 Nov 2007

Office of the United Nations High Commissioner for Human Rights 2007 United Nations Declaration on the Rights of Indigenous Peoples Available: http://www.ohchr.org/english/issues/indigenous/docs/draftdeclaration.pdf 27 Sep 2007

O'Neill O 2002 Public health or clinical ethics: thinking beyond borders. Ethics & International Affairs 16(2):35–45

Parker E, Gould T, Fleming M L 2007 Ethics in health promotion – reflections in practice. Health Promotion Journal of Australia 18(1):69–72

Porter J D H 2006 Epidemiological reflections of the contribution of anthropology to public health policy and practice. Journal of Biosocial Science 38:133–144

Richards C, Australian Reproductive Health Alliance, Comment on Draft International Health Strategy – AusAID n.d.

Roberts M J, Reich M 2002 Ethical analysis in public health. Lancet 359:1055–1059

Senanayake S N, Ferson M J 2004 Detention for tuberculosis: public health and the law. Medical Journal of Australia 180(11):573–576

Sindall C 2002 Does health promotion need a code of ethics? Health Promotion International 17(3):201–203

Thomas J C 2003 Teaching ethics in schools of public health. Public Health Reports 118: 279–286

Thomas J C, Sage M, Dillenberg J et al 2002 A Code of Ethics for Public Health. American Journal of Public Health 92(7):1057–1059

Thompson A, Robertson A, Upshur R 2003 Public health ethics: Towards a research agenda. Acta Bioethica IX(2):157–163

United Nations General Assembly 1948 Universal Declaration of Human Rights. Adopted and proclaimed by General Assembly resolution 217 A (III) of 10 December 1948. Available: http://www.un.org/Overview/rights.html 10 Oct 2007

University of Virginia Health Sciences Library 1996 Final Report of the Tuskegee Syphilis Study Legacy Committee (20 May 1996). Available: http://www.healthsystem.virginia.edu/internet/library/historical/medical_history/bad_blood/report.cfm 14 Nov 2007

Weed D L, McKeown R E 2003 Science, ethics, and professional public health practice. Journal of epidemiology and community health 57:4–5

Wise M 2001 The role of advocacy in promoting health. Promotion & Education 8(2):69–74

World Health Organization Regional Office for Europe 1978 Declaration of Alma-Ata. International Conference on Primary Health Care; 1978 September 6-12; Alma-Ata, USSR. Available: www.who.int/hpr/NPH/docs/declaration_almaata.pdf 30 Nov 2007

World Health Organization 1995 Report of the Inter-Agency Meeting on Advocacy Strategies for Health and Development: Development Communication in Action. WHO, Geneva

World Health Organization 1996 Equity in health and health care. WHO, Geneva

World Health Organization 1998 Health Promotion Glossary. Geneva, WHO. Available: http://www.who.int/hpr/NPH/docs/hp_glossary_en.pdf 31 Jan 2008

CHAPTER 8

Evidence-based practice

Mary Louise Fleming & Gerry FitzGerald

Learning objectives

After reading this chapter you should be able to:

- define the terms used to describe evidence-based practice
- identify the major challenges and issues associated with evidence-based practice
- describe the need for evidence-based practice and the links between research, practical experience, and evidence-based practice or policy
- appraise the quality of research and evaluate its application to evidence-based practice
- identify the factors that impact on applying research to evidence-based practice or policy.

Introduction

This chapter traces the history of evidence-based practice (EBP) from its roots in evidence-based medicine to contemporary thinking about the usefulness of such an approach to practice. It defines EBP and differentiates it from terms such as evidence-based medicine, evidence-based policy and evidence-based health care. As EBP is concerned with identifying 'good evidence', this chapter will first describe the nature and production of knowledge, as it is important to understand the subjective nature of knowledge and the research process. This chapter considers the necessary skills for EBP, and discusses the processes of attaining the necessary evidence and its limitations. We examine the barriers and facilitators to identifying and implementing 'best practice', and when EBP is appropriate to use. The chapter includes a discussion about the limitations of EBP and the potential use of other sources of information to guide practice, and concludes with applying evidence to guide policy and practice.

The evolution: evidence-based medicine

Health and medical research has always informed the development of clinical practice. However, translating research and innovation into practice has often been prolonged and disjointed. Medical and other health professionals have a proud and determined attachment to the value of experience and the opinions derived from it. Thus, standards of clinical practice were traditionally formulated through a combination of research, analysis and the collective wisdom of the profession, and individual practice was heavily reliant on the individual experience of the clinician.

In 1972, an epidemiologist from the UK, Dr Archie Cochrane, criticised the medical profession for not providing reviews of clinical interventions so that policymakers and organisations could base their practice on empirically proven evidence (Mazurek Melnyk & Fineout-Overholt 2005, Oliver & McDaid 2002).

Similarly, researchers from McMasters University in Canada felt the medical profession were relying on clinical experience and personal judgement, rather than empirically supported evidence (Hamer 2005). It was this group of researchers that first coined the term 'evidence-based medicine', which they defined as 'the conscientious, explicit, and judicious use of current best evidence in making decisions about the care of individual patients' (Sackett et al 1996 p 71). This definition implies an organised process applied to a particular circumstance and recognises the clinicians' expertise. *Conscientious use* of evidence implies a systematic and organised approach to the identification of the evidence. *Judicious use* implies the wise application of the evidence to the particular clinical circumstances and recognises the value and importance of the clinician's cumulative experience, education and skills in applying the evidence to the particulars of the patient.

It was Cochrane's opinion, and that of the McMasters researchers, that 'best evidence' was that which was obtained through rigorously conducted randomised controlled trials (RCT) (Mazurek Melnyk & Fineout-Overholt 2005, Oliver & McDaid 2002). In 1993 The Cochrane Collaboration was launched, which aimed to provide up-to-date systematic reviews of health care interventions and to ensure the accessibility of these reviews by the public globally so that consumers could make informed decisions about their health care (Mazurek Melnyk & Fineout-Overholt 2005).

Box 8.1: The Cochrane Collaboration

Dr Archie Cochrane observed that thousands of low-birth-weight premature infants were dying needlessly. He was able to exemplify his argument for the need for reviews of intervention trials by locating, analysing and synthesising results from several RCTs that tested the effectiveness of corticosteroid therapy to halt premature labour in high-risk women. His systematic review of these trials demonstrated that corticosteroid therapy significantly reduced the likelihood of premature infants dying.

Many would argue that medicine and clinical practice have always been 'evidence based'. The difficulty lies not in the concept but in the practical definition of evidence, access to the evidence and the relevance of the evidence to the particular circumstances of clinical practice.

The impact of evidence-based medicine has been, first, to encourage and develop the means of accumulating the evidence in a systematic manner, analysing the evidence and converting that evidence into clinical pathways, and clinical guideline standards, which translate the often enormous quantities of data available in the literature into an accessible and usable format for clinicians. Figure 8.1 demonstrates that process for clinical guidelines development.

Second, an emphasis on evidence-based medicine has served to reduce the previous reliance on 'opinion' as unqualified 'evidence' in its own right. Opinion, even 'expert opinion', has in the past sometimes relied solely on the accumulated experience of the

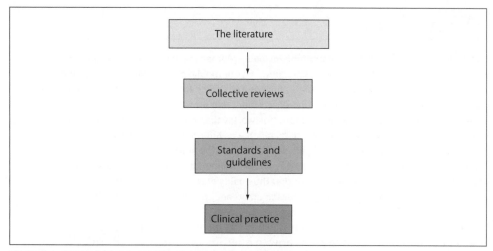

FIGURE 8.1: EXAMPLE OF THE DEVELOPMENT OF CLINICAL GUIDELINE STANDARDS

individual. That experience may be biased, and is often not representative of the broad diversity of experience. Naidoo and Wills (2005) talk about four ways in which decisions have been made, including:

- tradition
- practical experience and practitioner wisdom
- values that influence what should be done
- economic considerations that focus on what the organisation can afford.

Recently, the term has been broadened to evidence-based practice in an effort to spread the concept to all health professionals. The principles have been applied to public health, health policy, health planning and health management (Gerrish 2006). According to Naidoo and Wills 'evidence-based practice and policy has become the new mantra in health care' (Naidoo & Wills 2005 p 45).

The nature of evidence and key concepts of evidence-based practice

What defines evidence? How de we define EBP? Are there other terms that relate to EBP that we should understand? How does EBP fit into the complex nature of public policy, public health and health care? This chapter answers these questions for you.

We are currently living in an 'information age' (Hamer 2005, Mazurek Melnyk & Fineout-Overholt 2005). Technological advancement means increased accessibility to information (Hamer 2005). As an example, the internet brings information from all over the world into our homes. Information is literally at our fingertips.

ACTIVITY

- A family member has read an interview with their favourite celebrity. This celebrity is campaigning against mobile phone towers being placed near school grounds.
- The family member asks you what the health impact of mobile phone towers is, as you are studying for a health degree at university. One way to answer your family member might be to look up some information on the health impact of mobile phone towers.
- What sources might you consult? What sources would you rely upon most? What sources do you think would interest your family member the most?

REFLECTION

There are a range of sources of information including journals, textbooks, newspapers, health magazines, editorials, internet newspapers, news on our mobile phones, lifestyle magazines, Australian telecommunications industry/association's reports and websites, internet blog (opinion) sites run by companies or individuals, and government and private health agencies' websites and reports. Some information sources are more trustworthy than others. Information that is provided by the internet or in news clips may not be as reliable as information that is provided by rigorous scientific studies. There has been a significant increase in the number of research studies being conducted, research papers being published and the number of research journals available. Technological advancements have meant that the quality of research methodologies has improved, and research findings are more easily accessed and readily available (Hamer 2005).

This abundance of information underlies the justification for EBP. With access to so much information we need to know how to interpret information and critically analyse it for its value. Information comes from a variety of sources and provides us with multiple answers to our questions. Research might produce results that bring into question the way in which we practise our profession, or the values or beliefs we hold, or those held by our patients. Is there a single truth? How is knowledge created? Is it neutral or is it influenced by social, economic and political factors?

While we are lucky to have so much more information at our disposal, it does mean that there is more information to sift through to determine what constitutes evidence. In short, information must be sorted, analysed and then given meaning, or moulded into knowledge by describing its practical application in specific settings (Dawes 2005).

This process can be very time consuming. In addition, there are other factors that add to the complexity of identifying and implementing 'best practice', including problems with dissemination and communication of the implications of research, and the methods employed to obtain these results (Courtney 2005). Political pressure might influence what research is conducted, published and used to influence practice, and organisational barriers might hinder health professionals who are implementing EBPs within their organisations.

The nature and scope of knowledge

Underpinning the quest for evidence are questions about the nature of knowledge. This is termed 'epistemology' (Topping 2006). Epistemology is the branch of Western philosophy that is concerned with reality – that is the nature and scope of knowledge and how it is produced (Topping 2006). Over the course of human history different perspectives of reality have dominated. These dominant perspectives or 'world views' are referred to as 'paradigms'. A change in the dominant perspective is referred to as a 'paradigm shift' (Taylor & Roberts 2006).

Professional groups may have different paradigms. What constitutes evidence for one professional group may not be considered so for another profession. Even within health care and health research, individuals may adhere to differing perspectives (Rychetnik & Wise 2004, Taylor & Roberts 2006), and have different views about what forms sound knowledge. Knowledge and evidence is, therefore, socially constructed. Rychetnik and Wise (2004) refer to evidence as 'negotiated phenomena', that is, evidence is constantly being debated and renegotiated by health professionals, managers and consumers.

The prevailing paradigm of a particular health profession can influence both the *content* of the knowledge of that profession and the *processes* used to produce that knowledge (Taylor & Roberts 2006). Research is influenced by assumptions underlying the current paradigm of the profession and individual researchers, and is not an isolated or objective process (Topping 2006). Using 'rigorous' research to guide practice is a requirement of the current scientific paradigm. Corcoran and Vandiver (2004) claim that this approach is now considered the industry standard. Where 'well-established' practices would have once constituted 'evidence', contemporary EBP requires that the efficacy of the intervention is demonstrated in practice (Frommer & Rychetnik 2003 p 60).

The concept of 'rigor' and the methods required for rigorous research are also socially constructed, influenced by the researchers' 'worldviews'. Traditionally, science has taken a positivist approach, believing in absolute and objective truths (Topping 2006). Positivists are concerned about the frequency and distribution of an event or phenomenon, and attempt to use standardised methods and maintain objectivity, primarily through distancing themselves from the subjects under study, to reach a 'truth' (Liamputtong & Ezzy 2005).

However, there has been a growing trend in health research to use qualitative methods. While there are a number of different qualitative approaches, researchers in this field recognise that in order to understand human behaviour, we must gain an understanding of the feelings, values, perspectives and interpretations of individuals and social groups. Qualitative research aims to provide an in-depth, information-rich account of human experience. Qualitative researchers argue that reality is not objective rather it is socially constructed. Therefore, there is no single truth (Topping 2006).

One of the issues we need to be cautious about when considering the use of evidence is that we sometimes think about evidence as only that which is generated by major pieces of quantitative research. However, a more inclusive approach to evidence is advocated by a number of researchers and practitioners (Naidoo & Wills 2005). This broader approach takes into account evidence from government advisers, experts and users. The World Health Assembly advocated such an approach in 1998 when it urged all member states to use an evidence-based approach using the full range of quantitative and qualitative methodologies (WHO 1998).

In Chapter 4 we covered the use of qualitative and quantitative research information and how such information is collected and analysed. In addition Chapter 9 outlines basic research design and discussed the use of qualitative and quantitative data sources and the benefits of mixed methodology when evaluating program implementation.

The activity below should show you how the research process is influenced by the worldview we hold. The perspectives of both the individual researcher, the science and health professions will influence how research is carried out and what is established as 'evidence'. The shift of focus away from quantitative methods to utilising a combination of methods is an example of a paradigm shift (Taylor & Roberts 2006, Topping 2006). Many health researchers argue that using a combination of perspectives and methods can provide a more comprehensive account of the phenomenon under study, and that different methods may be more useful for answering different questions (Topping 2006).

ACTIVITY

- According to Taylor and Roberts (2006) the quantitative paradigm prevails as the dominant perspective in health research. One reason for this, they argue, is its ability to attract more funding from government and private sponsors.
- Why do you think governments are more interested in sponsoring research projects using quantitative research designs as opposed to those using qualitative methods?

REFLECTION

There are a number of reasons for this point of view. It may be that there is a perception that quantitative data is more reliable and draws on large samples to form conclusions. It uses statistical principles to determine reliability and validity. Qualitative methodology on the other hand may be less well understood and there is a perception that the researcher is not adequately distanced from the research activity. At times qualitative data offers a realistic and useful assessment of how practice interventions lead to outcomes (Naidoo & Wills 2005). What other reasons can you think of?

Debating and critically appraising current knowledge and the production of knowledge is important (Rychetnik & Wise 2004). If we had not 'renegotiated' evidence and the processes we used to construct evidence, we might still think that: the world is flat; cigarette smoking is good for our health; disease is a punishment inflicted by God; or that homosexuality is a disease. In some cultures these beliefs and the processes used to establish the 'evidence' to 'prove' such beliefs may not yet be contested and, therefore, still prevail. Can you think of other examples of 'evidence' that have been subsequently falsified over time?

Key concepts of evidence-based practice

EBP was born among a growing concern to improve health care and health outcomes by basing practice on the best available evidence (Rosenthal & Sutcliffe 2002). You will remember that earlier in this chapter we introduced the concept of evidence-based medicine; the origin of this concept can be traced back to 19th century France, and more recently to The Cochrane Collaboration (Rosenthal & Sutcliffe 2002).

EBP should not be confused with 'research utilisation'. Research utilisation refers to using knowledge gained from a single study (Mazurek Melnyk & Fineout-Overholt 2005). While sometimes there may not be sufficient research on a particular topic to conduct a systematic review, there are dangers inherent in using the results of only one study to guide practice. Let us consider the following case study.

Case study: Dangers of 'research utilisation'

Kraaijenhagen et al (2000) reported that a study they had conducted revealed travellers were not at an increased risk from deep vein thrombosis (DVT) compared with the general population. Shortly after, other research studies reported that travellers were at increased risk. In 2001, Scurr et al (2001 p 1485) reported 'symptomless DVT might occur in up to 10% of long-haul airline travellers'. Public opinion was further persuaded by reports of a woman who was travelling by air to Australia and died from a pulmonary embolus.

According to Dawes (2005) several studies published over a six-month period reported conflicting data. Consumers who sought advice from their general practitioner on the health risks of travelling may have received an incomplete picture of the risk, if the health care professional only relied on the first article published.

REFLECTION

Should health professionals use only the results obtained from RCTs to guide their practice? Not all health topics could ethically be tested using a RCT. When there are differences of opinion about an issue in the scientific literature, what information should the health professional use to guide his or her practice? How much evidence should she or he collect before making a decision?

One of the most successful public health interventions of the 20th century led to recognition that smoking was associated with an increased risk of lung cancer. Despite it being widely accepted by the public and health professionals alike, that tobacco use is responsible for many cases of lung cancer, this has not been empirically proven, and it is unlikely that it ever will be. It would be unethical to subject some individuals to tobacco and cigarette smoke and not others, which would be required in order to conduct an RCT.

In some cases there will be no research available at all on a certain topic. In a practice setting it is not feasible to send a client away just because there has been no prior research conducted about his or her problem. Evidence-based practice must also take into consideration the expertise of the health professional, as well as the values and preferences of the client (Mazurek Melnyk & Fineout-Overholt 2005).

In practice, what does an evidence-base mean?

Is it about using strategies that the research suggests are the best means for achieving the stated aims? Is it about changing practice? Is it about a systematic appraisal of the best available evidence? The answer to all of these questions is yes. However, the process is never quite as simple as that. In practice, there is never absolute certainty, as programs that are implemented even in similar circumstances are never quite the same. In addition, research is not always reliable and valid, even if it is available on a particular issue of concern, or there is a reasonable amount of available research information. As Naidoo and Wills (2005) state, 'evidence-based practice is more like a journey towards more effective practice and it is an approach that requires the practitioner to become more open-minded and flexible' (Naidoo & Wills 2005 p 48).

Box 8.2: What is an evidence-based practitioner?

An evidence-based practitioner is one who can use problem-solving skills to determine:

- what it is that you need to know
- if the intervention is effective, acceptable, equitable, implemented consistently and safely, and is cost effective
- if you have the best available evidence
- if the quality of the evidence is good
- if the evidence is appropriate for the population and context in which you will use the evidence.

(Adapted from Naidoo & Wills 2005)

In medicine there have been substantial efforts to make professional practice more based on available good-quality evidence. This process has been through what is termed clinical guidelines. We discussed the development of clinical guidelines early in the chapter. We said that clinical guidelines were designed to make practice more in line with evidence that discusses what works, to ensure comparable standards and reduce variations in practice (Naidoo & Wills 2005). Recommendations are graded according to the strength of the evidence and their feasibility. Therefore, evidence supported by RCTs would be graded more highly than recommendations supported by an expert panel consensus that relies on a lesser quality of evidence.

What is evidence-based practice?

Using evidence to make decisions about practice is very similar to undertaking primary research. There are five steps involved in this process:

1   identifying the problem
2   identifying evidence that relates to the problem under consideration
3   finding the evidence
4   determining how useful the evidence is through critical appraisal
5   synthesising the available evidence into a practical application.

To become an evidence-based practitioner you need to critique the evidence and be willing to change your practice if the evidence suggests this should be the case.

Identifying the problem is the first step in the process of seeking out appropriate evidence. The problem must be defined sufficiently and specifically so that it will be useful for the search for evidence. If it is too specific you may not be able to access the breadth of evidence necessary for you to make an informed decision about your proposed intervention. If it is too general then the problem is that you may not seek out the most appropriate evidence. Look at the example below and consider how we might identify the problem in order to be sure that your focus is on the most appropriate evidence.

ACTIVITY

● You work for Queensland's health department in their Population Health Unit. You are planning to establish a community walking group in a number of suburban areas throughout Brisbane. This group is particularly for people who have had cardiac surgery or who are living with coronary heart disease. Partners and family members are also welcome. How will you do it?

REFLECTION

How did you define the problem? Do you need more information to focus in on the real issues in this example? Try to decide what the focus of your search strategies should be.

Identifying the evidence that relates to the problem is not as easy at it sounds. There are two major issues to be considered when thinking about the evidence that might suggest a particular way of approaching an intervention. The first is what sources should I be looking for as evidence and, second, how should I use evidence to make an informed decision? To answer the first question most EBP relies on primary research from academic or professional journals, text books, published and unpublished reports, conference papers and presentations. The second question is about the range of evidence that might inform practice and that might include how effective the intervention was in meeting its goals, whether there is evidence available on the transferability of the intervention to other settings and with other populations, what the positive and negative effects of the intervention were and what the barriers to implementing the intervention were (Naidoo & Wills 2005).

The scientific model has gained prominence as a quantitatively objective method for *finding the evidence,* and contextual factors such as environment, socioeconomic factors or education are considered as 'confounding variables' and study designs often try to eliminate their effects. RCTs are viewed as the 'gold standard'; however, where populations are concerned it becomes very difficult if not impossible to adopt an RCT methodology

Type 1 evidence	Systematic reviews and meta-analyses including two or more RCTs
Type 2 evidence	Well-designed RCTs
Type 3 evidence	Well-designed controlled trials without randomisation
Type 4 evidence	Well-designed observational studies
Type 5 evidence	Expert opinion, expert panels, views of service users and carers

TABLE 8.1: Hierarchy of evidence

(Source: Naidoo & Wills 2005)

(Naidoo & Wills 2005 p 52). Following this scientific approach, research findings are graded according to an established 'hierarchy of evidence' (see Table 8.1) according to how valid and reliable the methodology for the research is considered to be.

Where do you think public health fits into this notion of a scientific paradigm? How useful is this paradigm when population health research does not fit neatly into an RCT? Does this mean that there is no evidence base for public health? As Naidoo and Wills (2005) point out, a focus on scientific experimental evaluation would ignore a large body of emerging work around public health in community settings and interventions. The authors talk about a more inclusive notion of evidence that enables measuring and validating a range of public health activities. Desirable methodological characteristics of research into the effectiveness of interventions include issues such as:

- the level of detail of an intervention that would enable it to be replicated
- whether the participants who are the target of the intervention are fully described
- whether the size and effect of non-respondents is detailed
- if there are clear outcomes and these outcomes are compared with baseline measurements taken before the intervention commences.

There are a number of ways in which evidence can be sourced. Table 8.2 shows the five characteristics involved in systematic reviews.

THE SYSTEMATIC REVIEW SEARCH SHOULD BE:	
Explicit	Use key terms, record your search, ensure that it is transparent so others can assess value, and it can be replicated
Appropriate	Look where evidence is likely to be
Sensitive	Collecting all information that is relevant to your question
Specific	Collecting only information that is relevant to the question
Comprehensive	Include all available information

TABLE 8.2: Systematic review process

There are a number of other valuable sources of evidence that can be used to guide practice such as bibliographic databases (e.g. Medline and Cinahl) and The Cochrane Collaboration or the Campbell Collaboration. The Cochrane Collaboration focuses on a single disciplinary perspective, while the Campbell Collaboration examines systematic reviews of studies researching the effectiveness of social and behavioural interventions. All searches need to be systematically carried out, using consistent key words or phrases, and they need to be made transparent to ensure that others can gauge their suitability and comprehensiveness

Determining how useful the evidence is is a skilled task and is termed 'critical appraisal'. This process determines the quality of the research process. It is the systematic and structured evaluation of the relevance of the study and the ability to critically appraise a range of study types. In order to undertake this process it is very important to have a good understanding of the epidemiological concepts discussed in Chapter 4, not only to be able to understand the results as they have been presented, but also to be able to have a systematic approach to the appraisal (Guillemin & Gillam 2006 p 65). There are standard checklists available to support the systematic appraisal of different types of study designs. We can use these to determine the validity of the study findings, and determine whether we can generalise the findings to other populations. Critical appraisal, however, has to be pragmatic in that your focus should be on studies that reach a certain standard of rigour and relevance. Pragmatism is important because it is usually possible to identify flaws in published research studies and the ways in which the context of the research and one's own practice differ (Naidoo & Wills 2005).

Both systematic reviews and meta-analyses take primary research studies as their object of investigation. Systematic reviews identify relevant studies and *synthesise the results*. Meta-analyses identify relevant primary research studies and aggregate the results to come up with a quantitative estimate of the overall effect (Naidoo & Wills 2005). The systematic synthesis of qualitative research studies is referred to as meta-ethnography. Here the focus is on the interpretative synthesis of meta-analysis. Meta-ethnography identifies, codes and summarises themes from the literature until no new themes emerge, with the preservation of individual observations where possible (Campbell et al 2003).

Putting evidence into practice – what is working?

Now that you have been introduced to the reasoning behind EBP, and skills for finding, evaluating and translating research evidence, it is important that you consider how the ideal – what you have learnt – compares with reality, in both practice and policy. In this section of the chapter we discuss the evidence–practice gap, and review current research regarding the reasons why research findings are frequently not translated into action. Techniques for analysing barriers to EBP are described, and we also analyse the role of evidence in decision making.

Although you may assume that having the research evidence required will lead to rational practices and policies, this is often not the case. The following three examples demonstrate how the evidence is only slowly incorporated into practice.

Example 1: Advising on smoking cessation in pregnancy

Although evidence from a number of trials strongly suggests that smoking cessation programs can effectively reduce rates of smoking among pregnant women, data showed that 90% of protocols and policies developed and used by antenatal care providers in Australia did not include written advice about smoking cessation (National Institute of Clinical Studies 2003).

Example 2: Measuring glycated haemoglobin in diabetes management

Two major trials have shown that assessing diabetes by glycated haemoglobin (HbA_{1c}) measurement can improve diabetes control. However, the Australian Institute of Health and Welfare estimates that less than one-quarter of people with diabetes have these tests performed as frequently as recommended (National Institute of Clinical Studies 2003).

> **Example 3: Placing infants to sleep on their back to reduce the risk of SIDS**
>
> Although public awareness campaigns have successfully reduced the number of infants being placed on their stomach to sleep (the highest-risk position for sudden infant death syndrome), large numbers of infants, particularly Indigenous infants, are still being placed on their side. Evidence shows that although this position is not as high risk as the stomach, laying infants on their backs provides greater protection from SIDS. Public campaigns need to emphasise the risks of both stomach and side sleeping (National Institute of Clinical Studies 2005).

Why isn't evidence used more in practice? Gaps in the transfer of evidence into practice do not just occur in allied health. For example, studies of medical care in the United States and the Netherlands suggest that 30–40% of patients do not receive care based on current best practice, and up to one quarter of clinical practices are not needed or could be harmful (Grimshaw & Eccles 2004). So what is the problem?

It has been estimated that there is an average delay in conversion of evidence into practice of up to 17 years. We might ask ourselves why there is such a delay. The consequence of this delay is that only a small proportion of clinical practice is in accordance with the latest evidence.

Many of the advances in knowledge occur within research teams whose principal aim is to conduct the research and publish or promulgate the results. These teams are increasingly isolated from the broad scope of clinical practice. Traditionally, exposure of the bulk of the clinical workforce to innovation is often limited to initial education. Clinicians may enhance that initial learning through in-service education and ongoing professional development. However, ongoing development has often been arbitrary and confounded by the alternative communications that face clinicians. In addition, any individual practitioner cannot possibly stay abreast of all the literature available on the full spectrum of their practice. This situation has been aggravated by problems with health workforces, which has resulted in the movement of many 'leading lights' out of traditional teaching roles into research only, or combined clinical and research roles. Thus the diffusion even to new practitioners has been limited.

Why is there a gap between research and practice?

There are many views about the reasons. For example, research may be unrelated to the clinical concerns or clinical situations. For example the research may select proven myocardial infarction cases and determine optimal therapy, but most patients present with undifferentiated chest pain. The research may not apply to the process of clinical decision making. Research is standardised, whereas real practice occurs in diverse settings and circumstances. The research may be inaccessible, confusing and contradictory, and finally, there are practical limitations in a busy practice to keeping up to date.

Tversky and Kahneman (1974, quoted in Jenkins & Carey 2005) suggest that there is a tendency for practitioners to revert to shortcuts or usual ways of behaving when data are meagre or not presented in a way clearly related to the decision-making process. However, the causes of the evidence-practice gap are multiple and vary from setting to setting. One of the simplest models to explain why EBP is not implemented was developed by Michie et al (2005), who propose three overarching groups. Consider the problem of hand washing in hospitals to illustrate these reasons.

Case study: Hand washing in hospitals

Proper washing of hands by personnel in hospitals has been shown to be highly effective in preventing transmission of infection from patient to patient. A number of initiatives have been introduced to increase hand-washing rates, such as increasing the number of sinks and raising awareness of the need for hand washing. However, studies of hand washing reveal hand hygiene is still poor in some departments, particularly between staff consultations (Michie et al 2005).

REFLECTION

A number of reasons could be proposed to explain why staff did not wash their hands appropriately, such as forgetting or not really thinking it is important. Applying the Michie et al (2005) model is useful as it provides a framework to understand the reasons why EBP is not performed, which might suggest avenues to pursue to change the behaviour. In this situation, Michie et al (2005) suggest hand washing is not performed because of:

● resources, facilities and time – these are organisational reasons (reasons at the higher-order, social and systems levels)
● group norms that prioritise patient throughput over hygiene, or view repeated hand washing as obsessive, or beliefs that rates of infection are not linked to hand washing – these are motivational factors (in that they explain why individuals have not yet established an intention to change)
● staff are aware of the need for hand washing but forget to always perform the behaviour – this is action initiation (explains the behaviour of those who are motivated to change).

Viewing behaviour in this way suggests avenues to change behaviour. For example, local cues to action (e.g. reminders) may improve behaviours influenced by action initiation (Michie et al 2005). Alternatively, more in-depth educational campaigns may be needed to re-educate hospital staff if motivational factors are involved.

Another way of understanding why evidence is not implemented into practice is to look at observed and theorised barriers to EBP implementation. A number of surveys of health practitioners have been conducted to assess attitudes to EBP and barriers to its implementation. Although data overwhelmingly suggest practitioners welcome EBP, a number of significant barriers to its implementation have been identified, including:

- reasons relating to the evidence base, such as gaps in the evidence base, or poor quality of evidence
- personal reasons relating to the individual practitioner, such as lack of skills to undertake EBP, or lack of time
- reasons related to the organisation, such as inappropriate or inadequate support for EBP, perceived threat of EBP, lack of understanding of the process, economic constraints, access to evidence, resistance from colleagues (Bristow & Dean 2003), competing agendas, lack of technical support or lack of facilities (Adily & Ward 2005).

Health practitioners may also face challenges relating to using evidence in a group situation, such as group-think syndrome, whereby rather than the team approach enhancing performance, the quality of the group's performance and participation of group members is reduced by group processes (Heinemann et al 1994). Decisions may also be swayed by influential or vocal individuals, or influenced by competing agendas, such as professional rivalry, different perspectives or distrust (Jenkins & Carey 2005).

Studies suggest that although there are gaps in the evidence and other evidence-related reasons and personal barriers, such as a lack of skills, organisational barriers are highly significant in preventing the implementation of EBP (Henderson et al 2006). Reasons seemingly related to the individual practitioner, such as a lack of time or motivation (consider the example of hand washing described above), can also be influenced by organisational factors, as you will now discover.

So what do organisations have to do with EBP? You may ask why health care organisations don't support EBP. The reasons behind this are varied. First, health care practice has evolved over a prolonged period of time, and the role, expectations and environment of the health practitioner have changed dramatically (Dziegielewski & Roberts 2006). A shift to practice based on evidence over experience and judgement in particular represents a fundamental change (Steinberg & Luce 2005). Second, health care is a complex industry, with national, state and local political responsibilities, services and funding, and public and private industry divisions (Corrigan et al 2001). A number of highly differentiated autonomy-seeking groups of professionals are involved in the health industry, and strong leadership is required to implement change (Corrigan et al 2001, Rosenheck 2001).

Organisations in the field of health also frequently have multiple (sometimes conflicting) goals, such as improving health, gaining funding, reducing expenditure, fostering staff development and influencing government and community stakeholders (Rosenheck 2001). This can mean staff groups may have interests incompatible with one another, so that each group becomes focussed on achieving their narrow task, and finds it difficult to achieve larger organisational objectives (e.g. EBP) (Rosenheck 2001). The nature of public health (and other allied health professions) also influences uptake of EBP. Public health is frequently described as a mixture of 'science, art and politics', in that its legitimacy and practice is based on factors such as ideological conviction (e.g. that every individual has a 'right' to health), as well as evidence (United Kingdom Public Health Association 2007). This can lead to debate regarding which practices are 'best', using non-scientific criteria (Rosenheck 2001).

Aspects of organisations themselves also influence uptake of EBP. Consider, for example, the following (hypothetical) examples.

Example 1

Allison is a recent graduate who works as a nutritionist for a private hospital in community A. Unlike most of her colleagues, Allison was taught how to critically appraise research during her university course, and is keen to ensure her practice is based on current evidence. The organisation Allison works for is very busy, and Allison finds she has little time to review journals and keep up to date during her work time. One day when she was reading abstracts online, her supervisor saw what she was doing and told her, 'that's not your job, get back to work'. Allison also finds it difficult to follow EBP as her organisation has limited information resources – few paper copies of journals are available, and the organisation has not subscribed to many journals electronically. After working in the organisation a few months, Allison finds that despite her best intentions, she is largely following the party line and basing her practice on established patterns and information she learnt at university, even though she suspects that new research regarding some practices is probably available.

> ## Example 2
>
> Bianca is another recent graduate who works as a nutritionist for a private hospital (a different hospital). Although most of her colleagues did not receive training in EBP during their university courses, the organisation's CEO believes that the ability to adapt to change is crucial for the organisation's future success, and ongoing training is mandatory. As such, EBP is widely understood and valued. Groups of staff working in various areas also meet monthly to discuss the latest developments in their field, and how these developments can be applied in their practice. Bianca is expected to be familiar with the latest research, and has access to journals online at work. Although her job is very busy, Bianca schedules time in her diary during work hours each week to peruse the evidence and reflect on current practice. Bianca is currently working in conjunction with other hospital staff to identify and overcome potential barriers to changing an aspect of current practice, and feels confident she will be able to implement this change to improve patient outcomes.

REFLECTION

What differences can you see between Allison and Bianca's organisations? One way they clearly differ is in their organisational culture. Schein defines culture as the 'taken-for-granted, shared, tacit ways of perceiving, thinking and reacting' (1996 p 231). A simpler definition might be 'the way we do things around here' (Carson 2005 p 176). Although norms (common ways of behaving, interacting and so on) are visible manifestations of these underlying assumptions, the assumptions are generally never examined or questioned, making them difficult to change (Schein 1996).

Some cultural beliefs that operate in organisations that might make it difficult to introduce new practices include:
- a reluctance to change historical practices (e.g. 'this is how we've always done things')
- a belief that practice is already at a high level
- a lack of preparedness to ask questions (e.g. 'why do we do things this way?') (Henderson et al 2006).

A number of models have been developed to describe organisational cultures. Four of the most common models are highlighted in Box 8.3. As you read about these models, consider how different cultures will respond to, hinder or drive change.

> ## Box 8.3: Models of organisational culture
> ### MECHANISTIC VERSUS ORGANIC
> This model presents two extremes of organisational structure and activities. In reality, most organisations tend to fall somewhere along the continuum between these two extremes. The mechanistic organisation is governed by rules and procedures, generally with extremely hierarchical structures. Communication is most likely to be top-down, and decision making is centralised. The opposite organisation to this is the organic organisation, which is flexible, with few rules and decentralised decision making. Communication can easily occur across the organisation.

ROLE VERSUS TASK

This model again presents a dichotomy, while in reality most organisations fall somewhere between the two model cultures. Role cultures are secure and predictable, with a focus on individuals' roles and responsibilities. These organisations tend towards hierarchy and bureaucracy, as positions of authority are regarded as important. In contrast, task-oriented cultures are project- or job-oriented, enabling flexibility and creativity.

CLUB

This model emphasises personal power. The individual is conceptualised as an entrepreneur, with the organisation providing administrative resources. This can lead to tensions between professional and corporate entities. This model has been common within health care organisations.

LEARNING

The learning culture is characterised by enquiry, autonomy, creativity and entrepreneurship among employees. It most often occurs in flexible, open and pragmatic organisations.

(Source: Carson 2005)

From the example presented above, we might identify Allison's organisation as having a role culture, in that it is clearly focussed on individual responsibilities, yet Bianca's organisation might be considered to be a learning culture, where original thinking and 'out-of-the-box' approaches are valued.

This example also shows the need for organisational infrastructure, such as information resources. Mullen (2004) suggests the following organisational and environmental supports are required for practitioners to apply EBP:

- supportive organisational culture, policies and procedures (e.g. the organisation is open to change, provides information technology supports, opportunities, incentives and funding for EBP)
- external environment of the organisation (e.g. funders, accreditation groups, national/regional/local authorities) must provide similar opportunities and incentives supporting EBP
- organisational procedures to ensure implementation of guidelines and other evidence-based prescriptions for practice
- methods for systematically evaluating the implementation of EBP and providing feedback to stakeholders on practice effectiveness
- staff trained as evidence-based practitioners capable of working in evidence-based organisations.

Another characteristic of organisations that governs, to some degree, the extent to which practitioners can implement EBP relates to organisational structures.

Organisational structures

One of the key features of an organisation's structure is whether the structure is centralised or decentralised. In centralised structures, decision making occurs at the senior level, while employees at lower levels implement the decisions. The opposite of this is the decentralised structure, where decisions are made by employees at the lowest possible level in the organisation (Carson 2005). These are two extremes and in reality most organisations will be more centralised or decentralised; most will not be 'strictly' either.

Centralised structures have the advantages of consistency in their approach, and greater ease in implementing and controlling system-wide change. However, these structures tend to be bureaucratic, with less coordination and flexibility. Decentralised structures encourage creativity and innovation, and the making of decisions at a lower level encourages ownership and motivation. However, it can be difficult to coordinate staff in this situation unless strategic goals are clear (Carson 2005).

You can clearly see the differences in the distribution of power between these models. Practitioners require real power to change practices, so EBP may be easier to implement in a decentralised organisation, where individual practitioners make decisions influencing their practice. However, centralised structures may more easily be able to coordinate system-wide supports, such as the need for funding. Although no one approach is 'better' for EBP, an awareness of the limitations of each may assist you to identify barriers to implementing EBP in your organisation, and possibly advocate for changes to be made.

Finally, although we may expect that, as individuals with new ideas enter an organisation, these ideas will diffuse through the organisation, organisations may display 'defensive routines', or resist new ideas as a way of 'protecting' the way everything has always been done (Schein 1996). Conflict is particularly likely when a proposed change is at odds with existing values and assumptions (Schein 1996).

So what can we do about it? Finding the evidence

Closing evidence–practice gaps requires recognising situations where EBP is not being practised, identifying and addressing barriers to new practices, challenging past beliefs and practices and implementing new practices (National Institute of Clinical Studies 2004). As a trained practitioner who keeps abreast of the latest developments and reflects on current practice, you should be able to recognise when practice is not evidence based. And you are now aware of many of the common barriers to changing practice. The next step involves analysing the barriers to EBP in your particular setting, which is crucial for understanding how to change current practice. A number of different techniques can be used to identify barriers, depending on the setting, available funding, expertise and time, and how rigorous the barrier identification process is designed to be (National Institute of Clinical Studies 2006). A combination of techniques may be useful to overcome biases intrinsic in single research methods; this process is known as triangulation (Liamputtong & Ezzy 2005).

Table 8.3 provides a brief outline of a number of techniques you may use. The appropriate technique for a given situation will depend upon the nature of the organisation or the work undertaken by the organisation, as well as the strengths and limitations of each technique. You are encouraged to investigate techniques thoroughly before applying them, and to seek help from relevant experts when required.

If you are interested in reading more about these techniques, look up the reference for the National Institute of Clinical Studies (2006) at the back of this chapter.

The National Institute of Clinical Studies also suggests five principles should be followed when researching barriers, regardless of the technique that is utilised (National Institute of Clinical Studies 2006). These principles are:

1 *Acceptability* – the degree to which the technique used is acceptable to participants. A technique that encourages participants to express their ideas openly in a manner they find appropriate may assist in increasing enthusiasm of participants in future processes to change practice.

TECHNIQUE	DESCRIPTION	ADVANTAGES	OTHER CONSIDERATIONS
		DISADVANTAGES	
Brainstorming	A group of participants is brought together to stimulate discussion around a specific idea	Relatively fast and easy Generate a wide range of ideas in a short time Involve future participants in change process	Not suitable when cannot organise a group session, or when powerful group members may dominate
		Need skilled moderator Participants may be inhibited in front of others May need incentives for participation	
Case studies	A comprehensive description and analysis of a specific past situation or event	Provides very detailed information May gain insights not seen using other techniques	Not suitable when investigations may influence action or when the group of interest is highly variable
		Requires multiple forms of data collection and analysis Can be time consuming and expensive Findings may be subjectively interpreted, not generalisable	
Key informants	Seeking the views of individuals who have significant insights into a particular problem or situation	Can obtain detailed, in-depth information Can clarify ideas as the investigation continues Relatively fast and inexpensive	Not suitable when require strong evidence
		Requires suitable informants Relationship between investigator and informants can influence information collected Informants' views may not be representative	
Interviews	Discussion between investigator and participants or specific questions asked of participants	Can obtain detailed, in-depth information Participants can express their own views Can explore complex or unanticipated issues	Not suitable when anonymity is required
		Interviewer bias may influence information gained Can be time consuming and expensive Participants may be inhibited Can be difficult to summarise and compare responses	

➡

TECHNIQUE	DESCRIPTION	ADVANTAGES	OTHER CONSIDERATIONS
		DISADVANTAGES	
Focus groups	A facilitated discussion among a group of people in which a moderator uses open-ended questions to encourage discussion of a particular topic or issue	Relatively fast and easy Generate a wide range of ideas in a short time Can obtain detailed, in-depth information Participants can express their own views Involve future participants in change process	Not suitable when group is widely dispersed, when cannot organise a group session, or when powerful group members may dominate
		Participants may be inhibited in front of others Need skilled moderator May need incentives for participation Planning and analysis can be time consuming	
Direct observation	Observing interpersonal interactions, events or activities in a given setting	Can provide direct information and reveal unanticipated outcomes	Observer presence may influence behaviour, not suitable when privacy is required
		May be difficult to obtain agreement for observation Can be time consuming Require skilled observer	
Surveys	Assessment of participants' knowledge, attitudes and/or self-reported behaviour using a standardised set of questions, usually administered via mail	Can send surveys to practitioners or clients anywhere in the country Can gather data from a large number of people in a short amount of time Participants can remain anonymous Relatively inexpensive	Not suitable when responses prone to social desirability bias (practitioners report responses they consider will be judged favourably) Validated questionnaires of perceived barriers to change are available
		Development and testing of questionnaires may be time consuming Cannot ask follow-up questions Individuals may not accurately report their behaviour or factors influencing their behaviour Response rates may be low	

TECHNIQUE	DESCRIPTION	ADVANTAGES	OTHER CONSIDERATIONS
		DISADVANTAGES	
Nominal group technique	Highly structured discussion where ideas of the group are pooled and prioritised	Generate a wide range of ideas in a short time All participants can have input Relatively fast and easy Group consensus can be sought	Not suitable for addressing complex issues, or when cannot organise a group session
		Need skilled moderator May need incentives for participation	
Delphi technique	Information is collected from a group of participants in an iterative process	Participants can remain anonymous Can send surveys to practitioners or clients anywhere in the country	Need continued cooperation and involvement of participants
		Development and testing of questionnaires, and analysis of responses, may be time consuming Response rates may be low	

TABLE 8.3: Techniques to overcome bias in research

(Source: National Institute of Clinical Studies 2006)

2   *Accuracy* – the extent to which the barriers you identify are the barriers influencing practice. For example, if you identify a lack of staff understanding of EBP as a key barrier, training of staff to enhance understanding of EBP should improve practice.

3   *Generalisability* – the extent to which your findings can be generalised to other contexts or settings. This is influenced strongly by the representativeness of your sample.

4   *Reliability* – the dependability or consistency of a research strategy (Liamputtong & Ezzy 2005). For example, a survey of a participant group administered on two or more occasions should yield similar results.

5   *Cost-effectiveness* – you must weigh the cost of investigating barriers to EBP against the possible benefits you may obtain from the knowledge. Barrier analysis is only appropriate if the knowledge obtained can and does subsequently improve practice (National Institute of Clinical Studies 2006).

An example of research into barriers to EBP was completed by Henderson et al (2006) who analysed reports by leaders of projects funded to adopt innovative strategies to close the evidence-practice gap in everyday clinical practice. This group identified eight barriers to the implementation of EBP common to all projects, as shown in Table 8.4. This example demonstrates both key common barriers and some suggestions for improving the change process in organisations.

You should now have a thorough understanding of the barriers to implementing EBP in a workplace and techniques for investigating specific barriers. The final part of this chapter is concerned with the role of evidence in policy development.

THEME	CRITICAL ELEMENTS TO SUCCESSFULLY IMPLEMENTING EVIDENCE INTO PRACTICE	BARRIERS: EXAMPLE CONCEPTS	LESSONS FOR OTHERS
Leadership support	Executives sponsor support within the organisation A steering committee that is committed to a change A 'champion' from the senior staff Support from senior staff	Lack of leadership	Obtain support of executive, professional organisations, influential leaders and senior managers Identify a champion to drive the project
Key stakeholder involvement	Staff acceptance and commitment Multidisciplinary team of major stakeholders Establishing a core group of interested and committed staff and managers to work together	Conflict of interest between different stakeholders Difficulties in gaining key stakeholder engagement or support	Involve key individuals affected by the change in practice Include a multidisciplinary team Invite stakeholders to participate in project prior to commencement of changes
Practice changes	Should be simplified and incrementally implemented Incorporation of practice changes into current processes	Belief that current practice is at a high level Lack of uptake or compliance with project initiative by practitioners Difficulty in acceptance of new practices Resistance to changes in the status quo Lack of experience in uptake of new projects	Implement simple changes first
Communication	Oral presentations to all stakeholder groups Regular written communication A widespread campaign publicising the project to staff	Lack of awareness of project Restricted processes of communication between professional groups Poor intradepartmental communication	Convey the evidence clearly to key staff Use marketing or awareness-raising strategies including regular updates on the progress of change

➡

THEME	CRITICAL ELEMENTS TO SUCCESSFULLY IMPLEMENTING EVIDENCE INTO PRACTICE	BARRIERS: EXAMPLE CONCEPTS	LESSONS FOR OTHERS
Resources	Provide funding to initiate the application of research knowledge	Gaining funding when the project area does not easily fit into one speciality Competing demands of human resources Existing high workloads Time commitments to clinicians involved Insufficient funds to conduct projects Cost effectiveness of project not initially able to be clarified	Provide funding to initiate project to apply the evidence Identify ways to measure multiplicity of effect Allocate a budget for a project officer Allocate a training budget
Staff education	Training of staff in the principles and practice Provide data and examples which demonstrate value of the project Training to know how to rank the quality and generalisability of evidence	Lack of appropriate training for health workers	Commence prior to practice changes being implemented Educate staff on the reasons for making changes
Evaluating outcomes	Effectiveness of practice changes monitored Feedback to doctors by an opinion leader Inclusion of project in a broader quality improvement framework	Weak grasp of the necessity of defining evaluation measures	Establishing continual evaluation of progress with feedback to stakeholders Support evaluation with external review, data audits Evaluate baseline practices
Consumers	Provision of adequate information at point of decision making Ensuring consumer expectations and perceptions about practice are appropriate	Consumer demand for specific (other) options Social barriers to behaviour changes	Involve patients and family in practice changes and as potential agents of change

THEME	CRITICAL ELEMENTS TO SUCCESSFULLY IMPLEMENTING EVIDENCE INTO PRACTICE	BARRIERS: EXAMPLE CONCEPTS	LESSONS FOR OTHERS
	Experiences, beliefs and perception that are based on the available evidence and not obsolete knowledge or anecdote The involvement of patients and their family members in embracing the initiative through discussions about the rationale	Media influences Multiple education brochures on the same topic	Educate patients about benefits of changes in practice

TABLE 8.4: Barriers to implementing EBP
(Source: Henderson A J, Davies J, Willet M R. The experience of Australian project leaders in encouraging practitioners to adopt research evidence in their clinical practice. AHR 2006: 30(4):474–484. ©Copyright 2006. Australian Health Review – reproduced with permission. http://www.aushealthreview.com.au)

Evidence and policy development

Although you may not believe you currently are or will be a policymaker, you are likely to influence policy at some level. Policy may be defined in a number of ways, but may be broadly defined as 'a purposeful plan of action aimed towards solving a problem or issue of concern in the public or private sector' (Cooper et al 2006 p 222). Using this definition, policy can be seen to be made within legislative, judicial or executive arenas, and within both large and small organisations (Cooper et al 2006). Based on what you have read about the barriers to using evidence in organisations, do you believe health policy is likely to be evidence based?

Consider, for example, policy development regarding influenza vaccination. In Australia, the National Health and Medical Research Council recommends vaccination of health care providers and individuals at risk of flu-related complications, including adults aged 65 years and over, Aboriginal and Torres Strait Islander adults aged 50 years and over, women who will be in the second or third trimester of pregnancy during the flu season, and adults and children with chronic illnesses, such as cystic fibrosis or renal dysfunction (Australian Government and Department of Health and Ageing 2004). In the United States, influenza vaccination is also recommended for children aged 6–59 months and adults aged 50–64 years, based on the idea that this will reduce the number of cases, strain on the health care system, absenteeism, mortality and other issues (Jefferson 2006). However, vaccinating healthy individuals is contentious, because vaccine development is expensive and complications from vaccination are possible.

If policy is truly evidence based, we would expect the recommendation that healthy adults and children be vaccinated to be based on evidence that this intervention achieves its aims (e.g. reduced cases and reduced absenteeism). However, evidence for immunisation may be difficult to interpret. First, because influenza is seasonal and the virus varies from year to year, incidence varies greatly over time and place (Jefferson 2006). This makes it difficult to forecast the likely incidence of influenza in the future. Second, most studies that have looked at the impact of influenza have looked at outcomes such as severe illness and death (Jefferson 2006). Although these are important, if we propose extending vaccination based on the aim of reducing the number of cases and absenteeism, we need to judge the vaccination against these outcomes, and the figures are not readily available. Influenza also presents in a similar manner to many other illnesses, and may not be distinguished from them in epidemiological data.

A review of evidence for influenza vaccination identified three central problems in the data currently available. First, there are limitations to the methodological quality of the studies found (Jefferson 2006). For example, few randomised studies exist, limiting interpretations that could be drawn from the data, and many studies suffered from selection bias. Second, evidence surrounding most of the effects promised by the vaccination campaign (e.g. a reduction in absenteeism and the number of cases) was absent, or not convincing (as data sets were very small) (Jefferson 2006). Third, although the review did not point to evidence that annual vaccination of healthy individuals is harmful, it found few studies that considered the safety of the vaccine (Jefferson 2006). The authors of the review thus concluded that there was a large gap between the policy and the evidence.

But, you may ask, why is policy not based on evidence? When you have the skills to find and evaluate evidence, you may expect every decision to be based on a careful consideration of the available data and application to the appropriate context. However, as the Institute of Medicine noted in 1988, decisions regarding health may be based more on 'crises, hot issues, and concerns of organised interest groups' than on an appraisal of the evidence (Institute of Medicine 1988 p 4). In the case of the influenza vaccination, policymakers may have fallen for 'availability creep' – the favouring of doing what is available over doing nothing, even if what is available is imperfect (Jefferson 2006). Policymakers may also have felt that it was better to do something than wait for better data, although this approach may limit the resources that could be used elsewhere.

However, criticism of policymakers must be tempered by an understanding of the complexity of policymaking. Policymaking is not a linear process, and policymakers

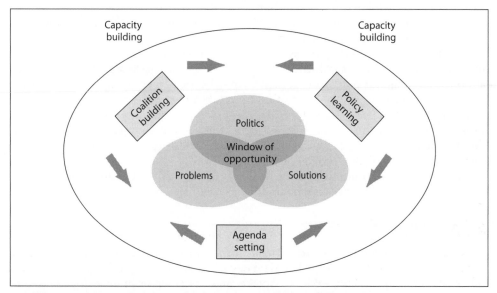

FIGURE 8.2: Theoretical framework for transforming knowledge into policy actions

(Source: Ashford et al 2006, Bulletin of the World Health Organization 84(8):669–672)

may be influenced by information from a variety of sources (not necessarily 'scientific evidence'), other individuals, personal and political agendas and long-standing practices (Ashford et al 2006). The following model developed by the Population Reference Bureau (Ashford et al 2006) describes policy change as a complex interaction of three spheres.

As this model shows, a 'window of opportunity' for policymaking is created only when problems and viable solutions are identified *and* the political environment is favourable (Ashford et al 2006). Activities that may assist in 'opening' the window of opportunity include focussing attention on issues to get them on the political agenda (agenda setting), creating or strengthening coalitions to sustain attention on an issue (coalition building) and increasing policymakers' knowledge about an issue (policy learning). Capacity building, the circle surrounding all other activity spheres, is about providing partners with the tools for policy communication, which assists in the use of data and research for policy change and modification (Ashford et al 2006).

This model explains why, in practice, the release of new research findings alone is frequently insufficient to change policy on a health issue. However, if the research results are accompanied by attention-generating events to place the health issue on the policy agenda, and alliances that push for policy change are fostered, evidence regarding the problem and potential solutions may be used to reform or develop new policy (Ashford et al 2006).

Recognising policymaking as a complex, nonlinear process influenced by competing concerns (e.g. different values, political goals or ways of solving a problem) may assist us to understand why policymaking may not necessarily be evidence based, as we understand it. Lin (2003) suggests health policy is influenced by a set of competing rationalities, or different 'truths' that exist at the same time based on one's viewpoint:

- *technical rationality* – the research evidence regarding the health issue, solutions, etc (these may be difficult for policymakers to interpret, or to translate from the research setting to the local context)
- *cultural rationality* – values, ethics, perceived societal opinions and significance of an issue, which vary across place and time
- *political rationality* – the political imperative, such as the distribution of power, influence of lobbyists, accountability.

The influence of each of these rationalities will depend on the breadth of a policy (e.g. whether it is a broad strategic plan for a government, or a program-level policy for a specific intervention), with research evidence becoming less important as policies become broader and more influenced by political imperatives (Sindall 2003). However, although cultural and political rationalities may be seen to compete with evidence in influencing policy, it must be noted that from a health practitioner perspective, these rationalities are not necessarily to the detriment of the community receiving the policy. Ethical principles such as equity may ensure a policy is written to favour those who are disadvantaged; and health practitioners frequently advocate to raise awareness of a health issue, and influence policy development (Sindall 2003).

Can you think of a health issue in Australia where technical, cultural and political rationalities compete to influence policy?

A final word

This chapter has introduced you to the reality of evidence-practice gaps and why policy is not always based on evidence. We have also described the influence of organisational and other factors in influencing evidence uptake, and described techniques for identifying barriers to change in your workplace. The next chapter will provide guidance in ways to make personal and organisational change to reduce evidence–practice gaps.

REVIEW QUESTIONS

1 What do you understand by the term evidence-based medicine and how does this term differ from evidence-based practice?
2 What are the main elements of evidence-based practice and how might it be useful to you in your day-to-day work?
3 Write down why you think evidence is not used consistently to guide practice.
4 One of the issues you may have identified in the previous question was the organisational context in which a person works. Can you highlight what issues may arise in an organisation that might make it difficult to use evidence-based practice?
5 What are the steps involved in identifying evidence that should guide practice?
6 Is evidence-based practice only guided by high-quality quantitative evidence? What role might qualitative evidence play in making decisions about evidence?
7 From a public health practitioner viewpoint how might you identify and use qualitative evidence to guide your practice?

USEFUL WEBSITES

National Institute of Clinical Studies: www.nhmrc.gov.au/nics
The Cochrane Collaboration: www.cochrane.org

REFERENCES

Adily A, Ward J E 2005 Enhancing evidence-based practice in population health: staff views, barriers and strategies for change. Australian Health Review 29(4):469–477
Ashford L S, Smith R R et al 2006 Creating windows of opportunity for policy change: incorporating evidence into decentralized planning in Kenya. Bulletin of the World Health Organization 84(8):669–672
Australian Government and Department of Health and Ageing 2004 National Health and Medical Research Council recommendations of influenza vaccinatio, Canberra
Bristow I, Dean T 2003 Evidence-based practice – its origins and future in the podiatry profession. British Journal of Podiatry 6(2):43–47
Campbell R, Pound P, Pope C et al 2003 Evaluating Meta-Ethnography: a synthesis of qualitative research on lay experiences of diabetes and diabetes care. Social Science and Medicine 56(4):671–684
Carson S 2005 Organisational change. In: Hamer S, Collinson G (eds) Achieving Evidence-based Practice: a handbook for practitioners. Baillière Tindall for Elsevier, Sydney, pp 175–194
Cooper S R, Trotter Betts V et al 2006 Evidence-Based Practice and Health Policy: a match or a mismatch? In: Malloch K, Porter-O'Grady T (eds) Introduction to Evidence-Based Practice in Nursing and Health Care. Jones and Bartlett Publishers, Boston, pp 221–234
Corcoran K, Vandiver V L 2004 Implementing Best Practice and Expert Consensus Procedures. Im: Roberts A R, Yeager K R (eds) (Evidence-Based Practice Manual: Research and Outcome Measures in Health and Human Services.) Oxford University Press, New York
Corrigan P W, Steiner L et al 2001 Strategies for Disseminating Evidence-Based Practices to Staff who Treat people with serious mental illness. Psychiatric Services 52(12):1598–1606
Courtney M 2005 Evidence for Nursing Practice. Elsevier, Sydney
Dawes M 2005 Evidence-based practice. In: Dawes M, Davies P, Gray A et al (eds) Evidence-based Practice: A primer for health care professionals. Elsevier Churchill Livingstone, Sydney, pp 1–10
Dziegielewski S F, Roberts A R 2006 Health Care Evidence-Based Practice. In: Roberts A R, Yeager K R (eds) Foundations of Evidence-Based Social Work Practice. Oxford University Press, Melbourne, pp 122–129

Frommer M, Rychetnik L 2003 From evidence-based medicine to evidence-based public health. In: Lin V, Gibson B (eds) Evidence Based Health Policy; Problems and Possibilities. Oxford University Press; Melbourne, pp 56–69

Gerrish K 2006 Evidence-based practice. In: Gerrish K, Lacey A (eds) The Research Process in Nursing. Blackwell Publishing, Carlton, Australia, pp 491–505

Grimshaw J M, Eccles M P 2004 Is evidence-based implementation of evidence-based care possible? Medical Journal of Australia 180:S50–S51

Guillemin M, Gillam L 2006 Telling moments: everyday ethics in health care. East IP Communications, Hawthorn

Hamer S 2005 Evidence-based practice. In: Hamer S, Collinson G (eds) Achieving Evidence-based Practice. Baillière Tindall Elsevier, Sydney, pp 3–14

Heinemann G D, Farrell M P et al 1994 Groupthink theory and research: implications for decision making in geriatric health care teams. Educational Gerontology 20(1):71–85

Henderson A J, Davies J, Willet M R 2006 The experience of Australian project leaders in encouraging practitioners to adopt research evidence in their clinical practice. Australian Health Review 30(4):474–484

Institute of Medicine 1988 The Future of Public Health. Committee for the Study of the Future of Public Health; Division of Health Care Services. National Academy Press, Washington DC

Jefferson T 2006 Influenza vaccination: policy versus evidence. British Medical Journal 333: 912–915

Jenkins R A, Carey J W 2005 Decision Making for HIV Prevention planning: organizational considerations and influencing factors. AIDS and Behavior 9(2):S1–S8

Kraaijenhagen R A, Haverkamp D, Koopman M M W et al 2000 Travel and risk of venous thrombosis. The Lancet 356:1492–1493

Liamputtong P, Ezzy D 2005 Qualitative research methods. Oxford University Press, Melbourne

Lin V 2003 Competing Rationalities: evidence-based health policy? In: Lin V, Gibson B (eds) Evidence-based health policy: problems and possibilities. Oxford University Press, Melbourne, p 3–17

Mazurek Melnyk B, Fineout-Overholt E 2005 Creating a Vision: Motivating a Change to Evidence Based Practice in Individuals and Organizations. In: Mazurek Melnyk B, Fineout-Overholt E (eds) Evidence-based Practice in Nursing and Healthcare: a guide to best practice. Lippincott Williams & Wilkins, Sydney, pp 443–456

Michie S, Johnston M et al 2005 Making psychological theory useful for implementing evidence based practice: a consensus approach. Quality & Safety in Health Care 14:26–33

Mullen E J 2004 Facilitating Practitioner Use of Evidence-Based Practice. In: Roberts A R, Yeager K R (eds) Evidence-Based Practice Manual: Research and Outcome Measures in Health and Human Services. Oxford University Press, Oxford, pp 205–209

Naidoo J, Wills J 2005 Public Health and Health Promotion: developing practice. Baillière Tindall, Edinburgh

National Institute of Clinical Studies 2003 Evidence-Practice Gaps Report, Volume 1. Melbourne

National Institute of Clinical Studies 2004 Social program. Melbourne

National Institute of Clinical Studies 2005 Evidence-Practice Gaps Report, Volume 2. Melbourne

National Institute of Clinical Studies 2006 Identifying Barriers to Evidence Uptake. Melbourne

Oliver A, McDaid D 2002 Evidence-Based Health Care: Benefits and Barriers. Social Policy & Society 1(3):183–190

Rosenheck R A 2001 Organizational Process: a missing link between research and practice. Psychiatric Services 52(12):1607–1612

Rosenthal M, Sutcliffe K M (eds) 2002 Medical error: what do we know what do we do. Jossey-Bass, San Francisco

Rychetnik L, Wise M 2004 Advocating evidence-based health promotion: reflections and a way forward. Health Promotion International 19(2), pp 247–257

Sackett D L, Rosenberg W M C, Gray J A M et al 1996 Evidence based medicine: What it is and what it isn't. British Medical Journal 312(7023):71–72

Schein E H 1996 Culture: the missing concept in organizational studies. Administrative Science Quarterly 41(2):229–240

Scurr J, Machin S, Bailey-King S et al 2001 Frequency and prevention of symptomless deep-vein thrombosis in long-haul flights: a randomised trial. The Lancet 357(9267):1485–1489

Sindall C 2003 Health Policy and Normative Analysis: ethics, evidence and politics. Evidence-based Health Policy: problems and possibilities. In: Lin V, Gibson B (eds) Evidence based health policy: problems & possibilities. Oxford University Press, Melbourne, pp 80–94

Steinberg E P, Luce B R 2005 Evidence Based? Caveat Emptor! Health Affairs 24(1):80–92

Taylor B, Roberts K 2006 Research in nursing and health. In: Taylor B, Kermode S, Roberts K (eds) Research in Nursing and Health Care: Evidence for practice. Thomson, South Melbourne, pp 1–32

Topping A 2006 The quantitative-qualitative continuum. In: Gerrish K, Lacey A (eds) The Research Process in Nursing. Blackwell Publishing, Carlton, pp 157–172

United Kingdom Public Health Association UKPHA 2007 Definition of Public Health

World Health Organization 1998 Fifty-First World Health Assembly. Resolution WHA 51.12 on Health promotion. Agenda Item 20, 16 May 1998, WHO, Geneva. Available: http://www.who.int/healthpromotion/wha51-12/en/ 15 Nov 2007

CHAPTER 9

Planning and evaluation

Elizabeth Parker

Learning objectives

After reading this chapter you should be able to:
- identify the importance of planning and evaluation in public health practice
- recognise the links between planning and evaluation through the presentation of models of planning and evaluation
- identify the core concepts of needs assessment in public health
- describe the evaluation cycle and the importance of an evaluation plan
- understand evaluation designs and their application in practice.

Introduction

The core business of public health is to protect and promote health in the population. Public health planning is the means to maximise these aspirations. Health professionals develop plans to address contemporary health priorities as the evidence about changing patterns of mortality and morbidity is presented. Officials are also alert to international trends in patterns of disease that have the potential to affect the health of Australians. Integrated planning and preparation is currently underway involving all emergency health services, hospitals and population health units to ensure Australia's quick and efficient response to any major infectious disease outbreak, such as avian influenza. For example, public health planning to prepare for the Sydney Olympics and Paralympic Games in 2000 took almost three years. 'Its major components included increased surveillance of communicable disease; presentations to sentinel emergency departments; medical encounters at Olympic venues; cruise ship surveillance; environmental and food safety inspections; bioterrorism surveillance and global epidemic intelligence' (Jorm et al 2003 p 102). In other words, the public health plan was developed to ensure food safety, hospital capacity, safe crowd control, protection against infectious diseases and an integrated emergency and disaster plan. We have national and state public health plans for vaccinating children against infectious diseases in childhood; plans to promote dental health for children in schools; and screening programs for cervical, breast and bowel cancer. An effective public health response to a change in the distribution of morbidity and mortality requires planning.

All levels of government plan for the public's health. Local governments (councils) ensure healthy local environments to protect the public's health. They plan parks for recreation, construct traffic-calming devices near schools to prevent childhood accidents, build shade structures and walking paths, and even embed draughs/chess squares in tables for people to sit and play. Environmental health officers ensure food safety in restaurants and measure water quality. These public health measures attempt to promote the quality of life of residents. The federal and state governments produce plans that protect and promote health through various policy and program initiatives and innovations.

To be effective, program plans need to be evaluated. However, building an integrated evaluation plan into a program plan is often forgotten, as planning and evaluation are seen as two distinct entities. Consequently, it is virtually impossible to measure, with any confidence, the extent to which a program has achieved its goals and objectives.

This chapter introduces you to the concepts of public health program planning and evaluation. Case studies and reflection questions are presented to illustrate key points. As various authors use different terminology to describe the same concepts/actions of planning and evaluation, the glossary at the back of this book will help you to clarify the terms used in this chapter.

Planning and evaluation in public health

Planning is described in various ways. Dignan and Carr suggest that 'effective planning requires anticipation of what will be needed along the way towards reaching a goal' (1987 p 4). This statement implies that the goal is defined, as are the necessary steps involved in reaching the goal. Furthermore, it requires an understanding of the steps and how they interrelate. Ideally, planning is a rational activity that assists public health professionals to gauge and reflect on their work to ensure goals are being reached.

As we saw in Chapter 1, the roots of public health planning go back to some of the earliest sanitary control measures; 'these were planned responses to the work of early epidemiology and the mysteries of communicable diseases' (Blum 1974 in Lenihan 2005 p 381). Without good planning, we would not be effective in preventing disease, and promoting and restoring health in the community. Lenihan (2005) claimed there are three models that have typified planning in public health practice. The first is problem/program planning and community assessment. These 'are well established components of health education with a focus on improving the health of defined population groups ...' (Lenihan 2005 p 382). The second is advocacy planning where 'the planner becomes a change agent to raise awareness and mobilise a population group to solve a community problem or develop a program' (Lenihan 2005 p 382). Advocacy planning adds community participation to the planning process, but planners or health professionals often control the process through technical aspects of planning. The third is strategic planning, which connects public health planning practice to current and potential partners needed to meet future challenges (Lenihan 2005); often this happens through senior government officials and politicians, for example, planning to manage potential health emergencies and disasters. Common to each of these models is an identified public health need, adequate financial and human resources to ensure successful program development, implementation, evaluation and sustainability over a numbers of years. Details of strategic planning from a policy perspective at the government level are delineated in Chapter 3. The case study that follows presents an example of program and advocacy planning.

> ## Case study: Primary health care approach to increasing Aboriginal and Torres Strait Islander participation in cervical cancer screening
>
> This project (2002–03) aimed to develop, implement and evaluate an integrated model to increase the participation of Indigenous women in rural/remote North Queensland Cape communities in cervical cancer screening. The project used a community based planning approach that included a consultative process that was inclusive of community women, Aboriginal and Torres Strait Islander health workers and Queensland Health staff in the Cape. A one-day community forum was held in Weipa in December 2002. Thirty-five women from surrounding communities, and service providers from Queensland Health in North Queensland, attended. The results of a presurvey were presented. The participants at the forum proposed a number of innovative service models that included an integrated package of services, such as new venues for screening and an education hub run by women for women (Meiklejohn et al 2004).

ACTIVITY

- Using the public health topic of cervical cancer screening introduced in the case study, discuss with a group of students the differences in the three models of public health planning that Lenihan (2005) proposes, and how these models might be applied and extended to make a difference to the women's health.

REFLECTION

Are there any differences in your approaches and understanding of the models? Can changes in population health occur only through long-term strategic planning at the government level? In the case study, how important was it to engage the community women in the planning of new services?

The next section will summarise some of the key developments in program planning, so that you have an understanding of a number of important concepts and their application.

Models of planning

Planning models help us to organise our thinking. They can be simple or sophisticated in design. Fleming and Parker (2007) identify a diverse number of planning models; Bartholomew et al (2001) developed a planning model called Intervention Mapping. This has been successfully applied to large-scale health promotion programs in communities. Green & Kreuter (1991) developed the PRECEDE model (Predisposing, Reinforcing, Enabling Constructs in Educational/Environmental Diagnosis and Evaluation). This was expanded to PROCEED to include Policy, Regulatory and Organisational Constructs in Education and Environmental Development (2005). The strength of this model is its recognition of various starting points for planning. Each of the models has a focus on rational planning, which is planning that is well informed, addresses a well-defined problem and has adequate resources to ensure a successful outcome. Dignan and Carr (1987) suggest that 'plans should provide answers to three basic questions: What are my goals and objectives, what do I need to do in order to achieve these objectives, and how can I establish whether I have met my objectives?' (Dignan & Carr 1987 p 257 cited in Ewles & Simnett 1999). You can utilise any one of these models or adapt or choose the aspects that are appropriate for your program planning. In the next section, we take one of these models and explain each of the components of program planning in public health.

Ewles and Simnett (1999) propose a seven-stage model that can be used as a template for program planning and action. It is a broad guideline of the steps taken in program planning, and is useful in its simplicity:

1 Identify needs and priorities.
2 Set (goals) and objectives.
3 Decide on the best way of achieving the aims or ultimate outcome (using evidence from the literature and/or focus groups/discussions with providers and the users of your program).
4 Identify the resources needed (staffing, space, transport, financial resources).
5 Plan evaluation methods.
6 Set an action plan.
7 ACTION – implement your plan, including your evaluation (modified from Ewles & Simnett 1999).

You can see from the model that planning and evaluation are integrated. Each of the steps is cyclical, but can be worked on simultaneously. Hence, planning and evaluation are integrated activities, and the evaluation plan should be developed simultaneously when building and progressing the program plan.

Ewles and Simnett (1999) identify needs and priorities as the first step in their seven-step model. We summarise needs assessment next, as it is important knowledge for all program planning endeavours.

Needs assessment and setting priorities

Public health plans are based on identifiying and assessing needs. These needs can be in existence or anticipated. For example, emergency and disaster plans to protect the public are developed in anticipation of events. At the Sydney Olympics, the public health plan was designed to minimise risks and protect the health of patrons, athletes and the public.

And, as public health information becomes more sophisticated and robust, policymakers may have already identified the health issues that need addressing. In Australia, national health policies are based on the evidence of need, and there are numerous sources of data available to assist health professionals to plan robust programs, for example, the Australian Institute of Health and Welfare (AIHW) and the Australian Bureau of Statistics (ABS). See the end of this chapter for their websites.

How are needs identified? Katz et al (2000) identify four different ways of defining needs. This is very similar to the explanations presented by Hawe et al (1990). Bradshaw (1972) in Katz et al (2000) identified a 'taxonomy of needs'; a taxonomy is simply a categorisation. There are commonly four types of need in public health: normative, comparative, expressed and felt. Additionally, there are other ways to gauge needs, such as rapid appraisals and epidemiological evidence.

- *Normative need* – These reflect the views of health professionals and their judgements and standards. For example, 'doctors may define some people's health or behaviour as falling within a "normal" range' (Katz et al 2000 p 262). However, normative standards may change. In nutrition, the norms of healthy food have altered; for example, consuming three or four eggs per week, once implicated in raised cholesterol, is not associated with an increased risk in healthy people (Dietitians Association of Australia website).
- *Comparative need* – Decisions are based on comparing options for program development; for example, if the prevalence of childhood obesity is higher in low socioeconomic areas, should investments and programs be targeted at those

neighbourhoods or across the whole population? Another example comparing options is, should health care resources be moved to outer suburbs or should they remain in more central locations? Comparative needs are often the focus of planning decisions.

• *Expressed needs* – This is about what can be inferred by assessing service use (Hawe et al 1990), or by what people say they need (Katz et al 2000). Long waiting lists are an expressed need that politicians often talk about. All the options regarding the provision of care need to be thoroughly considered. For example, could the long waiting lists be dealt with by community-clinics; and are people using emergency services in hospitals because they cannot find a bulk-billing doctor?

• *Felt need* – These are often the responses to community surveys, based on what people feel they want, or regard as problems worth identifying. Hawe et al caution that people often report solutions to the need, for example, 'more nursing home beds' (1990 p 19), rather than stating the need itself.

• *Rapid appraisals* – Rapid appraisals have increased in popularity in public health in local planning, in both developed and developing countries. They can involve qualitative interviews with health care providers, and consumers or patients, focus group discussions and interviews with key informants. Because rapid appraisals employ both quantitative and qualitative methods to gain insights into needs assessment, processes and gaps, or program use and utility, they are rich sources of information and can be done quickly.

• *Epidemiological evidence* – This is where there is sufficient evidence that an intervention is needed to improve the health of a population or subpopulation.

ACTIVITY

● Write a sentence describing expressed, felt, normative and comparative need. Choose a current public health topic (e.g. skin cancer prevention) and consider how each of these types of need may have influenced a program of action to address the issue. How are the needs identified and by whom? Are the needs based on evidence?

REFLECTION

Did you agree on who defined the need? In practice, planners can propose solutions and programs to inadequately defined needs through political pressure. This means that you need to be aware of the complexities in planning programs when there are competing types of needs.

Beginning the program plan

Once the needs assessment has been completed and priorities established, the next stage of Ewles and Simnett's (1991) model is developing the program plan, writing goals, objectives and strategies, identifying a target group (a population or subpopulation), identifying resources and planning an evaluation. One method to map the components of a program plan is through a program logic model.

Program logic models can be useful to describe the steps in the program plan that will assist you to achieve your goal. A logic model is merely a diagrammatic representation of the logical connections among the elements of a program or initiative, including its goals and objectives, activities, impact and outcomes and its evaluation plan. Ideally, a logic model would involve all the stakeholders. These people are often the funders of the program. They can be government or non-government officials or staff from a granting body (Rootman et al 2001).

Time spent at this stage of program development is wise, because the people involved in developing and funding the program have an interest in the initiatives that they have funded or in programs where they want to see specific health changes. However, various stakeholders can have diverse views of the goals (aims) and objectives of the program, and how the program's success will be measured. A program logic model can be displayed in a flow chart, map or table to portray the sequence of steps leading to program results. See Figure 9.1 for an example of a program logic model.

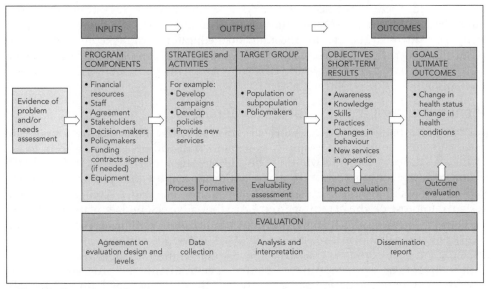

FIGURE 9.1: Program logic model

(Source: Parker 2007 adapted from Taylor-Powell 2005. The UW-Extension Logic Model is owned by the Regents of the University of Wisconsin System doing business as the UW-Extension, Cooperative Extension)

Writing goals and objectives

Goals and objectives need to be written specifically so they can be measured (Hawe et al 1990). A goal is written to describe the desired change in the health or behaviour of a group, for example, the reduction in teenagers who are obese in Years 9 and 10, by 20% over three years.

Objectives are specific and should be linked to the goals, and be realistic and evidence based. This means that you can confidently predict that your objectives are logical and are linked to the evidence base. For example, a goal could be related to nutrition education, for instance, 'the proportion of children who can distinguish healthy foods from overly fatty foods' (Hawe et al 1990 p 43). An aid to writing objectives is that they should be SMART, that is:

- S specific
- M measurable
- A achievable
- R realistic
- T time limited.

Writing strategies

Strategies are the activities you are going to undertake to reach your objectives; in other words, *what* you are going to do. Examples of public health strategies include television campaigns, such as a national skin cancer prevention campaign, websites informing people about how to check their skin, development of new health services, that offer skin checking; and new policies such as those in schools that enforce the 'no hat, no play' rule for students.

Identifying a target group

As public health is about populations, it is common to identify the target group as 'everyone', irrespective of age, socioeconomic status, income or education. The difficulty in designing programs for large population groups is measuring the impact they have had. There is evidence that modifying people's health status through the use of public health campaigns, especially those that use multiple methods (legislative, media campaigns, advocacy, and group and individual education), can take up to five years (Green & Anderson 1986). See Chapter 12 for the discussion on tobacco control in Australia and how diverse strategies, sustained over many years, were used to achieve the goals.

Identifying resources – or program 'inputs'

All programs require resources, and the answers to the following questions will assist in your planning. For example, how many staff will be needed, who is going to manage the program; and will there be a joint planning group that includes staff oversight of the program, staff from another department within your organisation, staff from outside your department, and community members? What are the roles assigned to those on the planning group? Are they advisers, budget planners or web designers? Clarifying the roles for each member of the planning group is critical. Many programs flounder through unstructured 'networks' of people, particularly if the program is not carefully planned. This is where a program logic plan can assist. Will a director or a project officer be hired specifically for the program? Has the development, implementation and evaluation of the program been built into the job description of the staff? Is there a contingency plan if staff leave, and sufficient money available in the budget for printing, computers, transport, telephones, evaluation and writing the evaluation report? Ten per cent of the budget should be allocated for evaluating the program. Again, these resources are often not factored into the development of the resources' plan. A well-crafted budget is necessary for program sustainability.

ACTIVITY

- Why is a program logic model useful in planning public health initiatives?
- What are some of the pitfalls you see in writing goals and objectives for public health programs?
- What sources of evidence would you use in planning a specific public health program?

REFLECTION

In your response to the first question, did you consider that program logic models could be useful in getting everyone to agree on the various components of the program? The 'map' is a useful way for moving a program forwards once the various stakeholders involved have reached agreement. For the second question, often objectives aren't written specifically, so it becomes difficult to evaluate programs (this is discussed in the next section). There are many sources of health data available at national, state and local levels, on health problems. The websites at the end of the chapter can assist you. We now turn our attention to planning the evaluation. This is an important element in program planning.

Plan the evaluation methods

'Evaluation is the process by which we judge the worth or value of something' (Suchman 1967 in Hawe et al 1990 p 6). If you were buying a house, you would have some criteria against which you were judging the 'worth' of the property. Imagine you are 'house hunting' – you wanted a three-bedroom house, and the house you're looking at met this criterion. Originally, you wanted a swimming pool in the garden, but this house doesn't have one, and, with water restrictions in force, this is now not a priority. In other words, you are prioritising the criteria against which you are making your decision. In public health evaluation, the principles are the same. You need criteria against which you would measure the worth or success of your program. Without a comparison of some kind, even if it is only comparison with an imaginary ideal or a purely subjective preference, there can be no evaluation (Fleming & Parker 2007 p 98). Obviously, evaluation must be relevant to the goals and objectives of program activity, and the measurement of these activities needs to be appropriate.

Purposes of evaluation

Essentially, there are two purposes for completing an evaluation: to ensure accountability to stakeholders and to facilitate program improvement. Public accountability for health spending is a top priority for governments as the demand for health services increases. Part of our responsibilities as health professionals is to be consistently improving the quality of the programs we design. Reflecting on practice is about learning to do things better, as well as ensuring that our program judgements are ethically founded. Learning from our evaluations reinforces our professional values to ensure that public health efforts improve the health of populations or specific groups within the population.

The generic goal of evaluation is to provide information to a variety of audiences, including government bodies, funding bodies and professional and client groups, in order to provide accountability and advance practice. Evaluation focuses on systematically collecting and assessing data that provide useful feedback about a program/intervention and is defined by Stufflebeam as a 'study designed and conducted to assist some audiences assess an object's merit or worth' (2001 pp 97–98). It is about generating information to assist in making judgements about a program, service, policy or organisation. Owen (2004) in Fleming and Parker (2007 p 115) refines these points by providing a helpful set of questions. Is the evaluation to determine the way a program is to be implemented; synthesise information to aid program development; clarify a program; improve the implementation of a program; monitor its outcomes; or determine its worth? A clear set of questions about the purpose of the evaluation can set the course for your evaluation plan. Your program logic model will be helpful in this regard, as it sets out all the components of program development and implementation and thus assists you in clarifying your thinking about the kinds of questions you want the evaluation to answer.

You also need to think about the role of the decision makers who are going to use the evaluation. Are the questions they want answered the same as yours? If not, how do you negotiate these differences? For example, if you are conducting a small health promotion program, you might be interested in finding out whether the program is reaching the participants it is intended for; whereas your managers may want to know how effective the program is in making a difference to participants' knowledge about the health problem. One starting point is to develop a list of the questions that each of you want answered. This way both agendas are transparent and the evaluation process becomes a collaborative one, although care has to be taken that the integrity of the evaluation is not compromised.

Now that you have decided on the overall purpose, it is time to put together your evaluation plan. In the following section, we introduce you to a well-known evaluation framework developed by the Center for Disease Control and Prevention (CDC), which is a part of the US Department of Health and Human Services, and adapted from the University of Kansas Community Toolbox (see 'Useful websites'). The steps in the framework (see Fig 9.2) are helpful for planning any public health evaluation, and we will comment on each of the steps and how they can assist your thinking about evaluation.

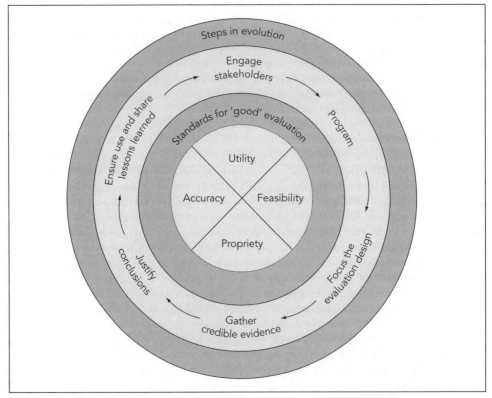

FIGURE 9.2: Evaluation plan and criteria
(Source: CDC 2000)

- *Engage stakeholders* – This extends our previous discussion about the involvement of people or organisations that have something to gain or lose from what will be learned from the evaluation and what will be done with that knowledge. You need to include: those involved in the initiative, such as other staff in your organisation and other organisations involved in the program. These could be community members, your immediate supervisors/directors of programs, or community members; those in the target group such as patients or clients; and intended users of the evaluation, such as those who have funded the program, university researchers and other program staff.
- *Describe the program and its context* – As discussed previously, you need to reflect on the dynamics of the program, particularly by writing a statement of expectations – what are the intended results and what will be the success indicators? What activities are being identified or implemented to bring about change, and what resources are needed? Importantly, identify the initiative's stage of development – how does the planning, implementation and maintenance of the program affect

the goal of the evaluation? What are the dynamics of the program context that could potentially affect it, for example, political, social and economic conditions that may change during the course of the program?

- *Focus the evaluation design* – What will the evaluation of the program address, how will it do so, and how will the findings be used? Include a description of the purpose – what are the goals of the evaluation (these are separate from the goals of the program), and what will be done to accomplish them? For example, evaluation goals can include advancing the knowledge about the program and whether it's working so you can make improvements to quality, and determining the effects and impact of the program. With respect to evaluation questions, what information is important to stakeholders? How well was the program/initiative planned and put into practice? How well has the program met its stated objectives? How much/what kind of difference has the program made in the community as a whole?

Methods

What type of study design will be used to evaluate the effects of the program or initiative? Typical designs include experimental, quasi-experimental and descriptive case studies. You have been introduced to study designs in Chapter 4. This knowledge can be applied to selecting an evaluation design. By what method will data be gathered to help answer the evaluation questions? These methods include documenting and monitoring the way the program has been established and implemented, surveys and interviews with participants in the program, and community-level indicators of the impact of the program on the population.

- *Gather credible evidence* – Decide what evidence is, and what features affect the credibility of the evidence. This includes specifying the criteria used to judge the success of the program and translating this into measures of indicators of success. For example, earlier in the chapter we presented an example of buying a house and the criteria you may establish when buying a house – number of rooms and whether it has a pool. The translation here into measures of indicators of success could be the capacity to deliver services, participation rates in the program, levels of satisfaction, changes in behaviour, community change or new programs, policies and practices and improvements in community-level indicators. Sources of evidence can include interviews/surveys with people, perusal of documents or direct observations. With respect to the quality, this can be done by examining the reliability of the information and how well it relates to the evaluation questions. With regard to the quantity of information, it is important to estimate not only the amount of data required to evaluate effectiveness, but also to know when to stop gathering data.

- *Justify conclusions* – Here, you are analysing and synthesising the methods used to summarise the findings to see if there are any patterns in the evidence; interpreting what the findings mean and how they translate into practical applications. To be precise, you are making judgements about the worth or merit of your findings, and the recommendations for action to consider as a result of the evaluation.

- *Ensure use and share lessons learned* – The final step in the CDC *Evaluation Framework* (1999) is to ensure use and share lessons learned. This is sometimes called disseminating the results of the evaluation. Most often you will write an evaluation report that documents all aspects of your evaluation and recommendations. The report should outline the program's features, particularly its goals and objectives, strategies used and whether these have been achieved. The report should delineate the evaluation design, methods of data collection and analysis, outcomes and recommendations. The recommendations will provide assistance to decision makers, other professionals and policymakers with an interest in the health issue.

Take steps to ensure that the findings will be used appropriately; include the design of the evaluation, such as how the questions, methods and processes were constructed; give feedback to the participants and stakeholders in the evaluation; and communicate the lessons learned to the relevant audiences, such as future users of your evaluation methods and findings. This is an important step in closing the evaluation loop.

Figure 9.2 (CDC 1999) presents a set of standards in the centre of the framework, as the basis for their evaluation actions. These are utility, accuracy, feasibility and propriety. The CDC Evaluation website (noted at the end of this chapter) contains a comprehensive explanation of all of the standards. Each of the standards sets a foundation to guide the conduct of ethical and respectful evaluations. So why are they important? As you learned in Chapter 7, ethical practice is everybody's business and evaluations rest on a foundation of ethical practice. These standards give you a guide to think about the conduct of your evaluation. You can use them as a checklist to tick off whether you have paid attention to each of the standards before you proceed with the evaluation actions. We now introduce you to a summary of them and how they can be used as the basis for thinking about your evaluation.

- *Utility* – The utility standards are intended to ensure that an evaluation will serve the information needs of intended users, in other words that the evaluation is useful. For example, the evaluator should be both trustworthy and competent to perform the evaluation to ensure that the evaluation findings achieve maximum credibility and acceptance. The information collected should be selected to address pertinent questions about the program and be responsive to the needs and interests of clients and specified stakeholders, and the interpretation of the findings should be carefully described. Evaluation reports should clearly describe the program being evaluated, including its context, and the purposes, procedures and findings of the evaluation, so that essential information is provided and easily understood. Evaluation reports should be disseminated to intended users in a timely manner; for example, if decisions need to be made about whether to extend a program or not, and the decision rests on the outcomes of an evaluation, it is vital that the evaluation report be completed on time.
- *Feasibility* – The feasibility standards are intended to ensure that an evaluation will be realistic, prudent, diplomatic and frugal. The evaluation should be practical to keep disruption to a minimum while needed information is obtained. One application in the real world of this standard is to make decisions about when to stop collecting data. The evaluation should be planned and conducted in anticipation of the different positions of various interest groups, so that their cooperation may be obtained, and so that possible attempts by and of these groups to stop aspects of the evaluation or to misapply the results can be averted or counteracted. Questions and decisions need to be asked about cost effectiveness – this does not mean necessarily doing an evaluation on cost effectiveness, but rather the evaluation needs to be efficient and produce information of sufficient value, so that the resources expended can be justified. In summary, utility is about the practical considerations to be thought out prior to embarking on an evaluation.
- *Propriety* – The propriety standards are intended to ensure that an evaluation will be conducted legally, ethically and with due regard for the welfare of those involved in the evaluation, as well as those affected by its results. In other words, propriety deals with correct and appropriate practices (some of which were introduced in Chapter 7); for example, evaluations should be designed and conducted to respect and protect the rights and welfare of human subjects, and that evaluators respect the dignity and worth of others associated with an evaluation, so that participants are not threatened or harmed. Conflict of interest

should be dealt with openly and honestly, so that it does not compromise the evaluation processes and results – again this reinforces the importance of ethical practice. Evaluations should be complete and fair in their examination and recording of the strengths and weaknesses of the program being evaluated, so that the strengths of the program can be built upon and problem areas addressed. It makes sense that the allocation and expenditure of resources for the evaluation be prudent and ethically responsible so that expenditures are accounted for and appropriate.

*   *Accuracy* – The evaluation should convey accurate information about the features that determine the worth or merit of the program being evaluated. Various aspects to think about in applying this standard are that the program is described and documented clearly and accurately, so that the program is clearly identified. The program logic model will assist you in completing this task. Obviously, collecting and analysing valid and reliable information about the program is a 'given', and the accuracy of this information assists in justifying conclusions. This standard also makes clear that when reporting results you should guard against bias and distortions.

ACTIVITY

*   Discuss with some students why the standards for evaluation are an important starting point in planning an evaluation. Write down your reasons. Write a definition of each of the standards to help you understand them. Next, review the first step in the CDC evaluation-planning framework. How would you go about engaging stakeholders in discussing the purpose and procedures in the evaluation? How would you resolve differences among stakeholders if there were any? Describe what you perceive to be the similarities and differences in program and evaluation planning. Share this with other students.

REFLECTION

Were there differences of opinion among your fellow students about the importance of having a set of standards to guide evaluations? If so, what were these? Were you able to understand the meaning of each of the standards? When you are undertaking an evaluation in practice, it is important to be as explicit as possible about the standards of practice for the evaluation and the purpose of the evaluation up front, as agreement on these helps when and if there are any disputes that arise during the evaluation. Did you have ideas about how you might resolve differences among stakeholders if the purpose and procedures in the evaluation vary?

Now that you have a plan for the evaluation, in the next section we are going to explore further the third step in the CDC framework. We will focus on the evaluation design through the presentation of some basic designs and examples.

Evaluation designs in practice

As you would have noted throughout the chapters in this book, the multiple and complex determinants of health indicate the need and possibilities for a wide range of actions for public health; therefore, conceptualising the design and measures in an evaluation cannot be rushed and requires reflection.

There are a number of complete books on program evaluation that can support your knowledge and thinking about evaluation designs, for example, Nutbeam and Bauman (2006), Pawson and Tilley (1997) and Hawe et al (1990).

Nutbeam and Bauman (2006) give guidance on specific designs for evaluation using quantitative and qualitative methods. Pawson and Tilley (1997) give guidance on thinking about the context of the program and how that influences the outcome of the program – remember, context was featured in the second CDC framework step, 'Describing the program'. It can mean the organisational systems and dynamics that support a program, or the social and environmental influences on a health program. We give examples of this type of evaluation in practice in the next section. The book by Hawe et al (1990) is highly regarded and inclusive, and has a specific focus on health promotion evaluation.

We have chosen to describe two approaches to evaluation design: an evaluation using applied research methods, and an evaluation framework for assessing organisational systems and policy. The first is a more traditional evaluation and each of the various levels in the design is most commonly used in public health program evaluation. The second pays particular attention to the 'context' in which the program and evaluation play out.

There are three commonly agreed upon levels of evaluation: process, impact and outcome. Process evaluation covers all aspects of program delivery, its quality and who it is reaching. Impact evaluation measures the immediate effect of the program (does it meet its objectives?). Outcome evaluation measures the long-term effect of the program (does it meet its goals?) (Hawe et al 1990 p 60).

For example, you have planned your program and have reached agreement with your stakeholders about the logic of the program and its components, the standards for the evaluation and steps to be taken from the CDC framework. You are beginning to focus and structure your evaluation. Each of the levels of evaluation described above (process, impact and outcome) is linked as follows.

Process evaluation to measure program strategies and activities

Process evaluation measures the activities of the program, program quality and target audience. It also measures program implementation, and participant satisfaction (are the strategies that have been designed successful?).

Evaluators often try to measure the goals or outcomes of the program without paying attention to the processes or strategies that have been developed to reach the final goal. This can skew results and assume that all the strategies chosen are successful, and that there is a logical connection between the process/impact and outcome evaluation. There are four components within a process evaluation: reach, satisfaction, implementation and quality (Hawe et al 1990). A process evaluation asks whether the strategies are working and how we might determine the reach of a program. In other words, how do we know if the program is reaching its intended audience (or target group as it is sometimes referred to)? If you were working in a clinical setting, one method to find this out would be through the attendance figures from the total number of participants in your program. If you are assessing whether a television campaign had 'reached' its audience, you could conduct a telephone survey of the population to gather this information. For program satisfaction, there are yes/no questionnaires that can be developed to gauge satisfaction. Other ways of measuring satisfaction could be by obtaining feedback from participants regarding the program; the convenience and comfort of the venue and the time of day, cost and adequacy of the facilities; staff sincerity, empathy and approachability; and the content of the materials developed, for example, their relevance, presentation, speed of coverage and depth. To assess program implementation means checking that all aspects of the program are being conducted as you planned, whether all the components of the program work and whether your messages were clearly understood by your target group.

ACTIVITY

● Summarise the measures in a process evaluation. With some classmates, jot down some tools you could use to gather data for each of these measures, for example, how would you gather data on the reach of a television campaign that informs the public about the risks of drink-driving? How could you gather data about the degree of satisfaction with a new service for diabetes patients in a joint allied health-physician centre? How could you gather data about the quality of the materials, such as brochures, or a website you've developed?

REFLECTION

Did you agree with your classmates on mechanisms for data collection? What web-based data collection tools could be available? Could you use online surveys, or chat rooms or blogs that the recipients of your program could use to indicate their levels of program satisfaction? Importantly, the analysis of your process evaluation can help you to change the program if necessary. See the following activity for an example.

ACTIVITY

● You are working in a non-government organisation that is producing a television campaign about sun safety. Your target group is young people aged 18–25 years. The campaign was designed by a marketing company, but not pilot tested with any young people. You perform pilot testing with young people through a series of focus groups to gauge their satisfaction with the design of the TV promotion, the appropriate time of the day the promotion should be aired, the website structure and its content and interactivity. Feedback indicated low levels of satisfaction with the program components and the planners realised that there were many limitations to the concept and the way the program was going to be implemented, so the program was re-adjusted to reach the intended target group more effectively. An effective process evaluation is really important as it can help iron out the bugs prior to the program being launched on a large scale. It also becomes more likely that the program will be more cost effective in reaching its goals and objectives as refinements can be made once a process evaluation is undertaken. The program can then move to the next step, which is evaluability assessment.

Evaluability assessment

To summarise, at the completion of a process evaluation, you will have an accurate picture of what strategies are working, what are not and whether it is appropriate and necessary to make changes to the program. This is an evaluability assessment: where you are ask whether the program elements are working and assess the four components of the process evaluation. Because the program's shape is now more finely tuned, the evaluation itself will be more robust.

An evaluability assessment can satisfy a number of conditions. It assists by eliminating common problems and ensures that you are asking the right questions, in other words, the impact and the outcome of the program can be evaluated. For this to occur, everything needs to be in place; for example, your evaluation design needs to be robust, your measurement tools such as questionnaires need to have been tested or reviewed, your sample size should be large enough in order to be able to make valid judgements. If you are using qualitative methods, your staff should be skilled in interviewing, conducting focus groups, and transcribing and analysis, in order to complete the impact phase of the evaluation. An evaluability assessment is a framework for making decisions about the shape of your evaluation and whether the objectives and goals (impact and outcome levels) of your program can be evaluated.

To assist your thinking about evaluability assessment, turn back to the program logic model and look at where the evaluability assessment sits on the model.

Stage 1 of the evaluability assessment ensures that there are logical links between program planning, development and evaluation; it can reveal assumptions underlying the program by linking objectives (Macaskill et al 2000). Stage 2 involves refining and preparing the program for impact and outcome evaluation. Here it is important to think through facets of the implementation to ensure that it is implemented as intended, and to have a risk management plan in place to allow for contingencies, such as staff resignations, holidays and organisational change. An evaluable program has a rational fit between clearly defined strategies, objectives and goals. In addition, the program will be properly implemented and there will be agreement on which questions should be addressed, how the evaluation should be conducted and what should be measured. Once everything is in place, you will be ready to conduct an impact evaluation.

ACTIVITY

● Consider the following questions with some classmates. Why is an evaluability assessment significant as part of the evaluation process? What are the implications if an evaluability assessment is not conducted? Why would program logic models be useful in evaluability assessment?

REFLECTION

Did you come up with the same answers? Can you think of the messages in some current public health campaigns that you find confusing? How could you find out whether focus groups or other feedback mechanisms were considered in campaign development? We now present a short discussion on impact evaluation.

Impact evaluation to measure program objectives

Impact evaluation focuses on the immediate observable effects of a program, specifically, whether the objectives of the program had been achieved, leading to the intended outcomes of the program goals (Green & Lewis 1986).

Impact evaluation can relate to the risk factors for the health problem you're trying to improve. Risk factors may include awareness, knowledge, attitudes and behaviour related to the health problem, as well as policy, organisational and social factors, that impact on the public health problem. An economic evaluation may also consider the program achievements in relation to program costs; for example, what are the program costs averaged for each life saved through your public health program? Impact evaluation is usually carried out after the program has been implemented or within a short time period after its completion. If the program is ongoing, the evaluation should be conducted at a time when the program strategies have had time to have an effect on the key indicators identified in the objectives. How is an impact evaluation conducted? The selection of impact evaluation instruments depends upon the indicators being measured. If the risk factors usually include awareness, knowledge and attitudes, behaviour, or change to the policy, organisational, physical or social environment, then measurement tools that are appropriate for these factors need to be identified or developed.

Data collection strategies for impact evaluation include questionnaires, qualitative and quantitative interviews or surveys, face-to-face or telephone interviews, focus groups, self-completed questionnaires, journals, observations, document reviews and other data sources. Impact evaluation assesses whether objectives have been achieved.

Outcome evaluation to measure program goals

The outcome evaluation focuses on the ultimate goal and is generally measured in public health by morbidity or mortality statistics in a population. The topics addressed in outcome evaluation are whether it measures program goals, and these goals usually relate to the health issue that the health program is designed to address, so outcome evaluation is concerned with measuring changes to indicators of health. Outcome evaluation is conducted when it is likely that there has been sufficient time for measurable change in the health issue. It may be possible to make some short-term gains in a health issue, for example, reducing violence outside nightclubs by early closing, increased police presence, closing bars earlier, and efficient and safe transport; while cancer or heart disease rates may take many years to be affected by community education and promotion programs, or changes to policy. The next section outlines some evaluation designs that are commonly used to measure impact and outcome.

Evaluation designs for impact and outcome evaluation

Chapter 4 presents some of the designs used in public health research that can be applied to an evaluation; the books by Hawe et al (1990) and Nutbeam and Bauman (2006) are excellent resources for guidance on what type of design to choose for your evaluations.

As introduced previously, evaluation design decisions need to be made at the outset of your program, and especially during the evaluability assessment phase. The design will depend on the nature of the intervention and its goals and objectives. Some common designs include: a post-test, self-reported questionnaire for participants if no pre-evaluation test has been undertaken; a single group, pre-test/post-test design administered to the participants; and a time-series design.

Whether any changes have occurred in health status and quality of life could be determined by an outcome evaluation.

ACTIVITY

● Write down the differences between impact and outcome evaluation. Research two of the evaluation designs suggested above and compare their applications with measuring an impact and an outcome evaluation. You could do this by searching out an article in the literature that contains both types of evaluations.

REFLECTION

Were you able to discern the differences between impact and outcome? One clue is that an impact evaluation measures the immediate impact of your program in making a difference to a population's awareness or knowledge or a change in attitude or change in practice in a service while an outcome evaluation usually measures the long-term impact of a program on the population's health.

Evaluations can also be designed to measure broader aspects of a program, for example, measuring an organisation's system and its policies and what impact these have on the delivery and outcomes of a program. Programs are not implemented in a vacuum and we present an explanation to make this clearer.

Stufflebeam and Shinkfield's (2007) CIPP model for evaluation is used for the following case study, as it is particularly useful when evaluating organisational systems and policy development. Four elements are proposed in this evaluation model: context, input, process and product.

Context evaluation defines the environment in which change is to occur. Input evaluation determines how one can utilise resources to meet program goals by identifying capabilities of the organisation in implementing a program. *Process evaluation* is an ongoing evaluation of the program's implementation while *product evaluation* measures, interprets and judges the effectiveness of a program or policy (O'Connor-Fleming & Parker 2001 p 106). The following case study demonstrates how CIPP was used by the authors to compare a diabetes prevention pilot initiative in two different health services.

Case study: Evaluation of a diabetes prevention pilot initiative

Diabetes is a national health priority (see Ch 3). It is estimated that 7.6% of the Australian population (approximately 1 million people) have diabetes, with approximately 90% having type 2 diabetes (AIHW 2006). Studies show that type 2 diabetes can be prevented or delayed through pharmacological interventions and, more efficaciously, through lifestyle interventions. The *Diabetes Prevention Pilot Initiative (DPPI) Evaluation Project* aimed to evaluate two projects that were funded by the Commonwealth Department of Health and Ageing in 2003.

The projects needed to develop and conduct innovative community-based projects to test methods of implementing the National Health and Medical Research Council's (NHMRC 2001) *National Evidenced Based Guidelines for the Management of Type 2 Diabetes Mellitus: Primary Prevention*. Projects were required to increase physical activity, improve diet and achieve a healthy weight for people at risk of developing diabetes. One project was linked to a university department in a rural area where participants were recruited through general practitioners; the other project was conducted through a regional health service in a medium-sized town, where patients were recruited through the local community health service.

Stufflebeam's (2003) CIPP model was used to evaluate the program. It ensured that common aspects of both projects were considered. The similarities and differences between the two projects were able to be synthesised and analysed using the four constructs of the CIPP in a comparative analysis. Context evaluation assessed the needs, assets and problems within the defined environments. Input evaluation assessed the work plans and budgets of the selected approaches in the two trials. Process evaluations assessed the program's activities and product evaluation included an impact evaluation of (1) the program's engagement of the targeted audience as outlined in the NHMRC guidelines (2001) for case detection and assessment; (2) an effectiveness evaluation that assessed the quality and significance of the program's outcomes; and (3) a sustainability evaluation that included the extent to which the program's contributions could be successfully institutionalised and continued over time. Economic evaluation examined the costs and potential health benefits of the programs. Stufflebeam's CIPP model provided a lens through which the components of each of the programs could be analysed and compared.

(Source: Queensland University of Technology 2007. Case study approved November 2007)

Table 9.1 presents a checklist to be used as a guide to assist your thoughts on planning and evaluation.

STAGE	ACTION
Problem analysis and needs assessment	
	Getting started – what issues do I need to consider in the planning and evaluation cycle?
	Engage stakeholders – who are they, and what are their values/expectations/concerns?
	Determine program objectives/mission – hierarchy of outcomes to guide action, and to link strategies and evaluation
	Pilot testing – how many participants?
Program planning and implementation	
	Select/describe strategies and methods – selection is linked to objectives
	Implementation process – needs to be managed in detail; suggested implementation and evaluation plan
	Evaluation procedures – qualitative, quantitative, or elements of both
	Data collection – what, when, and how to measure (pre-intervention testing – otherwise there is no basis for doing a reasonable evaluation, and post testing)
	Analysis of data – how much and what should be analysed?
	Costs, and what resources (human, financial, time) are available to meet the planned actions
	Using external evaluators – costs, expertise and independence of the evaluation?
Evaluation and dissemination	
	Evaluation management
	Dealing with all the players in the evaluation process and their individual expectations about program outcomes
	Participant burden be aware of over-evaluating participants – the tyranny of evaluation
	Process, impact, outcome levels – how do you make these judgements and what are the implications for broader applications of the evaluation beyond the program?
	Investment in evaluation – money, time, personnel
	Evaluation outcomes – what did I learn and how can I use that information for the future?
	Dissemination of the results, to whom and for what purpose?

TABLE 9.1: Planning and evaluation checklist: evaluation and dissemination

(Source: O'Connor-Fleming et al 2006 A framework for evaluating health promotion programs. Health Promotion Journal of Australia 17(1):61–66)

A final word

This chapter has exposed you to public health planning and evaluation and its importance and place in addressing public health issues. Program, advocacy and strategic planning and the integration of evaluation with planning were introduced. Program logic models can depict the steps and links between program components, including inputs and outcomes.

They provide a graphic overview that needs to be agreed upon by all involved. Various aspects of needs assessment were introduced to ensure that your programs are based on evidence. The CDC framework is a starting point for developing an evaluation plan and its standards set a foundation for ethical practice as an evaluator. Levels of evaluation and evaluability assessment were discussed. A model for assessing organisational dynamics and policy development was considered. The significance of a comprehensive evaluation report to disseminate evaluation findings concluded this chapter.

REVIEW QUESTIONS

1 Why are planning and evaluation important practices in public health?
2 How are planning and evaluation linked, and why should these be integrated activities?
3 What are the types of needs assessments that can be used to build effective programs and what are their differences?
4 What are the steps in the CDC *Evaluation Framework* and how can it be used?
5 What are three evaluation designs that could be used in an impact and outcome evaluation?

USEFUL WEBSITES

Australian Bureau of Statistics: www.abs.gov.au
Australian Institute of Health and Welfare: www.aihw.gov.au
United States Center for Disease Control and Prevention: www.cdc.gov
University of Kansas Community Toolbox: http://ctb.edu/tools/en/tools_toc.htm
University of Toronto Centre for Health Promotion: www.utoronto.ca/chp

REFERENCES

Australian Institute of Health and Welfare 2006 Australia's Health 2006 AIHW cat. No. AUS 73. AIHW, Canberra
Bartholomew K, Parcel G S, Kok G et al 2001 Intervention Mapping: Designing Theory and Evidence-based Health Promotion Programs. Mayfield, Mountain View
Bradshaw J 1972 The concept of social need. New Society, 19:640–643. In: Katz J, Peberdy A, Douglas J (eds) 2000 Promoting health: knowledge and practice. The Open University, London
Blum H L 1974 Planning for Health: Development and Application of Social Change Theory. New York: Human Sciences Press. In: Lenihan P 2005 MAPP and the Evolution of Planning in Public Health practice. Journal of Public Health Management and Practice 11(5):381–386
Centers for Disease Control and Prevention. Available: http://www.cdc.gov/prc/program-evaluation/ 9 Nov 2007
Centers for Disease Control and Prevention 1999 Framework for Program Evaluation in Public Health. MMWR 48(RR-11). Available: http://www.cdc.gov/eval/framework.htm 9 Nov 2007
Centers for Disease Control and Prevention 2000 Evaluation Working Group. Practical evaluation of public health programs. Available: http://www.cdc.gov/eval/workbook.PDF 5 Dec 2007
Dietitians Association of Australia website. Available: http://www.daa.asn.au/index.asp?PageID =2145847413 12 Nov 2007
Dignan M B, Carr P A 1987 Program Planning for Health Education and Health Promotion. Lea & Febiger, Philadelphia
Ewles L, Simnett I 1999 Promoting health: a practical guide. Ballière Tindall, London
Fleming M L, Parker E 2007 Health Promotion: Principles and Practice in the Australian Context. Allen & Unwin, Sydney
Green L W, Lewis F M 1986 Measurement and evaluation in health education and health promotion. Mayfield, Palo Alto

Green L W, Anderson CL 1986 Community Health Planning. Times Mirror/Mosby College, St Louis

Green L W, Kreuter M 1991 Health promotion planning: An educational and environmental approach, 2nd edn. Mayfield, Mountain View

Green L W, Kreuter M 2005 Health promotion planning: An educational and ecological approach. 4th edn. McGraw-Hill, New York

Hawe P, Degeling D, Hall J 1990 Evaluating Health Promotion. MacLennan & Petty, Sydney

Jorm L, Thackway S, Churches T et al 2003 Watching the Games: public health surveillance for the Sydney 2000 Olympic Games. Journal of Epidemiology and Community Health 57:102–108

Katz J, Peberdy A, Douglas J (eds) 2000 Promoting health: Knowledge and practice, 2nd edn. The Open University, London

Lenihan P 2005 MAPP (Mobilizing for action through planning and partnerships) and the evolution of planning in public health practice. Journal of Public Health Management and Practice 11(5):381–386

Macaskill L, Dwyer J M J, Uetrecht C et al 2000 An evaluability assessment to develop a restaurant health promotion program in Canada. Health Promotion International 15(1): 57–69

Meiklejohn B, Parker E, Scott M 2004 Report on a Primary Health Care approach to increasing Aboriginal and Torres Strait Islander Women's participation in cervical cancer screening. For Queensland Health. Queensland University of Technology, Brisbane

National Health and Medical Research Council 2001 National Evidence Based Guidelines for the Management of Type 2 Diabetes Mellitus: Primary Prevention. NHMRC

Nutbeam D, Bauman A 2006 Evaluation in a Nutshell. McGraw-Hill, Sydney

O'Connor-Fleming M, Parker E 2001 Health Promotion: principles and practice in the Australian context. Allen and Unwin, Sydney

O'Connor-Fleming M, Parker E, Higgins H et al 2006 A framework for evaluating health promotion programs. Health Promotion Journal of Australia 17(1):61–66

Pawson R, Tilley N 1997 Realistic Evaluation. Sage Publications, Thousand Oaks

Queensland University of Technology 2007 Diabetes Prevention Pilot Initiative: Evaluation Project. Final Report for the Australian Government Department of Health and Ageing. Case Study approved November 2007

Rootman I, Goodstadt M, Hyndman B et al 2001 Evaluation in health promotion: principles and perspectives. WHO Regional Publications, European series, No. 92 Copenhagen

Stufflebeam D L 2001 Evaluation Models: New Directions for Evaluation 89:7–98

Stufflebeam D L 2003 The CIPP model for evaluation: An update, a review of the model's development, a checklist to guide implementation. Presented at the 2003 Annual Conference of the Oregon Program Evaluators Network (OPEN) Portland, Oregon

Stufflebeam D L, Shinkfield A J 2007 Evaluation theory, models and applications. Jossey-Bass, San Francisco

Suchman E A 1967 Evaluative Research. Russell Sage Foundation, New York

Taylor-Powell, E 2005 Logic Models: A framework for program planning and evaluation. University of Wisconsin-Extension-Cooperative Extension. University of Wisconsin-Extension, Madison

University of Kansas Community Toolbox n.d. Based on the USA CDC Evaluation Working Group Resource Practical evaluation of public Health Programs', prepared by the University of Texas Health Sciences Centre, School of Public Health and the Texas Department of Health. Available: http://ctb.edu/tools/en/tools_toc.htm 12 Nov 2007

Section 4

Public health interventions

Introduction

The three chapters that make up this section of the book centre on the concept of intervention along a continuum from health advancement and the promotion of health-to-health protection, and disease prevention and control.

Public health activity has always focussed on a continuum of care from prevention to treatment and rehabilitation. Along this continuum are a range of strategies and intervention activities that provide the population or subpopulations with appropriate interventions to meet their needs.

The first of the three chapters, Chapter 10, addresses public health's role in the prevention and control of chronic and communicable diseases. The focus for public health is clearly on chronic disease prevention in the first instance and then the management and control of the condition once a chronic disease has developed. Over three million Australians, or nearly one in seven, suffer from chronic disease and the problem is likely to be one of the great health challenges for Australia and the world in the 21st century.

Chronic diseases and conditions are generally defined as those that are long term (lasting more than six months), non-communicable, involving some functional impairment or disability and are usually incurable. They can affect people of all ages and contribute to the disease burden in our society.

Chronic diseases, such as diabetes, cancer, cardiovascular disease, asthma and certain mental health conditions are among the most significant contributors to morbidity and mortality in Australia and as such have been recognised as National Health Priority Areas. Public health has an important role to play in preventing and managing these conditions. Just as we discussed in the earlier section on risk and determinants, these health conditions are complex and multifaceted. Strategies to prevent and deal with the health consequences also need to be multidisciplinary and diverse. Chapter 10 presents you with a good introduction to both chronic and communicable diseases prevention and control. Communicable diseases are a common and significant contributor to ill health throughout the world, particularly so in developing countries. Illness and death from infectious diseases can in most cases be avoided at an affordable cost. Chapter 10 examines both examples of infectious diseases and zoonotic diseases; it covers the concept of immunity and explores the range of public health strategies that can be put into place to deal with infectious disease prevention and treatment.

Chapter 11 examines how the environment can impact on human health. It discusses the definition of environmental health and how human health can be protected from environmental hazards as well as exploring the key environmental health issues and how they might be managed through a range of public health strategies. The other fundamental issue facing the planet is the question of environmental sustainability and the importance of managing our environment to protect human health. Chapter 11 discusses the range of management tools including legislation and risk assessment as mechanisms for controlling environmental hazards and protecting the population's health.

The final chapter in this section, Chapter 12, looks at the concept of promoting health and protecting people from illness through health education and promotion strategies. Education and promotion are an important part of public health activity as the future will need to see far more attention placed on promotion and prevention if governments are going to manage health care costs. The costs of living with chronic disease, as an example, far outweigh the cost of promoting health and preventing the development of such diseases. Chapter 12 takes the reader on an exploration of the history of health education and health promotion and the emergence of the 'new public health'. It explores the *Ottawa Charter for Health Promotion* and examines a range of health promotion strategies in a variety of settings.

CHAPTER 10

Disease prevention and control

Thomas Tenkate, Mary Louise Fleming & Gerry FitzGerald

Learning objectives

After reading this chapter you should be able to:

- define chronic disease
- understand the differences in definitions of chronic disease between the World Health Organization and the Australian Government
- describe an integrated approach to chronic disease management, and what the elements of that approach might be
- understand the broad nature and causes of communicable and infectious diseases
- identify the public health principles used to prevent, treat and manage communicable diseases
- identify, by working through a number of case study examples, the principles of disease control and prevention.

Introduction

Globally, the main contributors to morbidity and mortality are chronic diseases, including cardiovascular disease and diabetes. Chronic diseases are costly and partially avoidable, with around 60% of deaths and nearly 50% of the global disease burden attributable to these conditions. By 2020, chronic illnesses will likely be the leading cause of disability worldwide. Existing health care systems, both national and international, that focus on acute episodic health conditions, cannot address the worldwide transition to chronic illness; nor are they appropriate for the ongoing care and management of those already afflicted with chronic diseases. As such, approaches to chronic diseases require integrated approaches that incorporate interventions targeted at both individuals and populations, and emphasise the shared risk factors of different conditions. International and Australian strategic planning documents articulate similar elements to manage chronic disease, including the need for aligning sectoral policies for health, forming partnerships and engaging communities in decision making.

Communicable diseases are also a common and significant contributor to ill health throughout the world. In many countries, this impact has been minimised by the combined efforts of preventative health measures and improved treatment of infectious diseases. However, in underdeveloped nations, communicable diseases continue to contribute significantly to the burden of disease. According to the latest World Health Organization (WHO) estimates, infectious diseases caused 14.7 million deaths worldwide in 2001 and accounted for 26% of global mortality. The following diseases were responsible for about 78% of the total disease burden in 2001 (Kindhauser 2003):

- respiratory infections (3.9 million deaths)
- AIDS (2.9 million deaths)
- diarrhoeal diseases (1.9 million deaths)
- tuberculosis (1.6 million deaths)
- malaria (1.1 million deaths).

In addition to this high level of mortality, infectious/communicable diseases disable many hundreds of millions of people each year, mainly in developing countries, with the global burden of disease from communicable diseases being estimated to be around 450 million DALYs (disability-adjusted life years) in 2001 (Lopez et al 2006, WHO 1999).

The aim of this chapter is to outline the impact that communicable and chronic, non-communicable diseases have on the health of the community, the public health strategies that are used to reduce the burden of those diseases and the historic and emerging risks to public health from infectious diseases. This chapter, therefore, examines the comprehensive approaches implemented to prevent non-communicable, chronic diseases and communicable diseases, and manage and care for the population with these conditions. It analyses models of care in the context of need, service delivery options and the potential to prevent or manage early intervention for chronic and communicable diseases. Many of the communicable disease concepts introduced in this chapter are further illustrated in Chapter 14, which discusses the new disease epidemics faced by our global community.

Defining chronic disease

Chronic diseases are those involving a long course in their development or their symptoms. They account for a high proportion of deaths, disability and illness and are a major health problem in all developed countries. Yet many of these diseases are preventable, or their onset can be delayed, by relatively simple measures.

For a number of reasons, including the fact that people are living to older age, chronic diseases have increased in prevalence over the past century and today they affect one in four Australians. Most chronic diseases are generally not cured completely. Some can be immediately life threatening, such as heart attack and stroke; others are often serious, including various cancers, depression and diabetes. However, they all persist in an individual through life. They are however, not always the cause of death. Chronic diseases are listed as the top 10 causes of the burden of disease in Australia. These diseases alone account for nearly 43% of the total disease burden in Australia (see Fig 10.1) (AIHW 2008).

There are a number of behaviours that can prevent or delay the development of many chronic diseases such as controlling body weight, eating nutritious foods, avoiding tobacco use, controlling alcohol consumption and increasing physical activity. Figure 10.2 illustrates a number of risk factors that contribute to the onset, maintenance and prognosis of many chronic diseases. In this figure these are classified as 'behavioural risk factors', 'biomedical risk factors' and 'other factors'.

Most of the chronic diseases have multiple risk factors and are considered to be 'adult' behaviours and conditions, however the situations that lead to their initiation often begin early in life, or even in the womb. It is therefore important to have a lifecourse

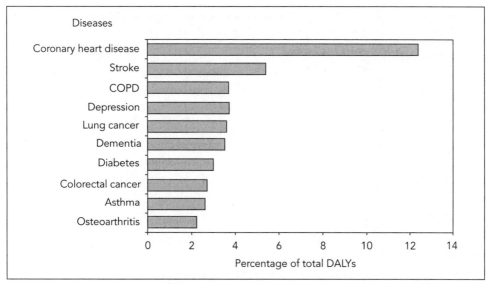

FIGURE 10.1: Top 10 leading causes of disease burden in DALYs* terms, Australia, 1996
Note: *DALYs counts equivalent years of 'healthy' life lost due to poor health or disability and potential years of life lost due to premature death.
(Source: AIHW 2005)

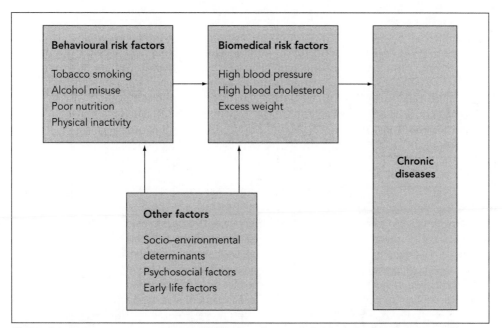

FIGURE 10.2: Behavioural risk factors, biomedical risk factors and other factors contributing to chronic disease
(Source: AIHW 2002)

perspective of chronic diseases and their risk factors that recognises the interactive and cumulative impact of social and biological influences throughout life. Table 10.1 examines the relationship between risk factors and chronic diseases in Australia. It clearly points out the strong relationship between a range of behavioural and biomedical risk factors and chronic diseases (AIHW 2008).

DISEASE/CONDITION	RISK FACTOR						
	BEHAVIOURAL				BIOMEDICAL		
	POOR DIET	PHYSICAL INACTIVITY	TOBACCO	ALCOHOL MISUSE	EXCESS WEIGHT	HIGH BLOOD PRESSURE	HIGH BLOOD CHOLESTEROL
Coronary heart disease	✓	✓	✓	✓	✓	✓	✓
Stroke	✓	✓	✓	✓	✓	✓	✓
Lung cancer			✓				
Colorectal cancer	✓	✓		✓	✓		
Depression		✓		✓	✓		
Diabetes	✓	✓			✓		
Asthma			✓		✓		
COPD			✓				
Chronic kidney disease	✓				✓	✓	
Oral diseases	✓		✓	✓			
Osteoarthritis		✓			✓		
Osteoporosis	✓	✓	✓	✓			
Excess weight	✓	✓					
High blood pressure	✓	✓		✓	✓		
High blood cholesterol	✓	✓			✓		

TABLE 10.1: Relationships between various chronic diseases, conditions and risk factors

(Source: AIHW 2002)

Chronic diseases, including cardiovascular disease (CVD), cancer, respiratory conditions and diabetes, are the major cause of death and disability worldwide (WHO 2005a, Yach et al 2004). Specifically, around 60% of deaths are attributable to non-communicable chronic diseases, and nearly half of the global disease burden is attributable to these conditions (WHO 2003a, WHO 2003b). With the exception of Sub-Saharan Africa, chronic diseases are responsible for more mortality than other causes worldwide (Le Gales-Camus 2005).

The success of public health initiatives, in part, mean that people are living longer (WHO 2002, National Health Priority Action Council (NHPAC) 2006) and this increased life span allows more time for chronic illness to develop (AIHW 2002, Centers for Disease Control and Prevention (CDC) 2003, NHPAC 2006, National Health and Medical Research Council (NHMRC) 2001, National Public Health Partnerships (NPHP) 2001). Chronic conditions place an extra burden on health care systems and by the year 2020 it is predicted that chronic conditions will be the leading cause of disability in the world, with over 70% of the global burden of illness mainly attributable to CVD, cancer, diabetes and chronic respiratory diseases, as well as mental health problems, injuries and violence (AIHW 2002, CDC 2003, NHPAC 2006, NHMRC 2001, NPHP 2001, WHO 2002, WHO 2005b).

In Australia, chronic, non-communicable diseases are responsible for around 80% of the total burden of disease and injury (AIHW 2006, Department of Health and Ageing (DoHA) 2006). Moreover, nearly 50% of all deaths in 2004 were due to chronic disease – arthritis, asthma, CVD, chronic obstructive pulmonary disease (COPD), colorectal and lung cancer, diabetes and osteoporosis (AIHW 2006). The Australian position on chronic disease is that a definition includes only non-communicable diseases; these include CVD (coronary heart disease and stroke), diabetes, some cancers, respiratory diseases (COPD and asthma) and musculoskeletal disorders (osteoarthritis, rheumatoid arthritis and osteoporosis) (NHPAC 2001, NHMRC 2001, NPHP 2001). WHO regards the expected increase in non-communicable diseases as one of the key health challenges for the 21st century (WHO 2000). Similar to WHO, Australia acknowledges chronic disease as a major health challenge (Australian Chronic Disease Prevention Alliance (ACDPA) 2004, AIHW 2006).

Continuum of care/integrated approach to chronic disease

In 2005 the NHPAC (2006) reviewed the national and international evidence for strategies for preventing and managing chronic disease and endorsed the *National Chronic Disease Strategy* (NCDS). The NCDS concentrates on four key areas for improving outcomes for people with chronic diseases: prevention across the continuum, early detection and treatment, integrated and coordinated care and self-management (NHPAC 2006). Such a comprehensive approach incorporates the entire population continuum, from the 'healthy', to those with risk factors, through to people suffering from chronic conditions and their complications. Supporting this approach is the amendment, and relaxation of qualification criteria, for the *Chronic Disease Management Plan* (formerly the *Enhanced Primary Care Plan*) that provides funding for a more multidisciplinary management plan for patients with chronic conditions and/or complex care needs and more preventive care for older Australians (DoHA 2006).

Chronic disease management and care is often seen as primarily the role of medical and allied health workers and the public health and health promotion role as a preventative one; however, due to their broad perspective on health and health determinants, the public health workforce also has the potential to make a significant contribution to this area. Furthermore, public health has a place in managing chronic diseases, as there are two main types of prevention – avoiding the development of chronic disease and delaying the expected complications of existing chronic diseases through good-quality treatment and management (WHO 2005c).

Public health and health promotion embrace an inclusive model, one that incorporates a population health perspective that views disease prevention and health promotion as a continuum (Pruitt & Epping-Jordan 2005). This position accentuates the whole scope of care, from primary prevention for healthy populations to early detection and intervention for subgroups considered at risk, through to management, tertiary prevention, rehabilitation and palliative care for people with established disease (AIHW 2002, NHPAC 2006, Pruitt & Epping-Jordan 2005, WHO 2005c). For example, the timely detection and treatment of diabetes is a valuable measure towards precluding or at least postponing the onset of CVD. Such an approach requires integration across all sectors (including hospital and community care) and treatments that are uninterrupted between different sites and providers, and coordinated over the person's lifetime (Pruitt & Epping-Jordan 2005).

Disease management programs

Disease management programs are a comprehensive approach to enhancing the quality of care for people with chronic diseases (Velasco-Garrido et al 2003). They use evidence-based criteria of care, coordinate care through multicomponent and multidisciplinary programs, and focus on the entire path of chronic conditions. Although there is no generic model suitable for all conditions, Velasco-Garrido et al (from Kesteloot 1999) identify seven major components of chronic disease management:

1 comprehensive care (multiprofessional, multidisciplinary, acute care, prevention and health promotion)
2 integrated care, care continuum, coordination of the different components
3 population orientation (defined by a specific condition)
4 active client/patient management tools (health education, empowerment, self-care)
5 evidence-based guidelines, protocols, care pathways
6 information technology, system solutions
7 continuous quality improvement.

Within Australia, there are now a variety of programs addressing the management and prevention of chronic diseases; these are outlined under the NCDS's four action areas for preventing and reducing the burden of chronic disease (NHPAC 2006). It should be noted that many of these interventions are multifaceted and, therefore, could be categorised in two or more of the action areas that follow.

Early detection and early treatment

Early detection and treatment can reduce complications, comorbidities and mortality. In Australia only about half of the people with diabetes have been diagnosed and treated (NHPAC 2006). There are two primary approaches to early detection and treatment: population-based screening and opportunistic screening by health workers for risk factors and/or early signs and symptoms (NHPAC 2006). Examples of the former include mammography for women aged 50–69, and bowel cancer screening, while the latter includes, for example, the Victorian 'Go for your life' program. This program, in part, aims to detect people with pre-diabetes (impaired glucose tolerance and impaired fasting glucose) and provide support for lifestyle changes to decrease the risk of diabetes developing (Department of Human Services 2006).

Integration and continuity of prevention and care

Integration and continuity of prevention and care includes care planning and coordination through a range of providers and settings (NHPAC 2006). An example of this is the chronic disease management (CDM) items available through Medicare for patients with chronic conditions and complex care needs; these include diabetes, heart disease and other chronic conditions (DoHA 2006). The CDM items cover a range of allied health workers, including exercise physiologists, diabetes educators, nutritionists, Aboriginal health workers and podiatrists (DoHA 2006).

Self-management

Self-management entails a person's active involvement in his or her own health care. An important component of self-management is cooperation between the person, their family, health service providers and the health care system (Holman & Lorig 2000, Lorig et al 2001, NHPAC 2006, WHO 2005c).

Case study: Example of self-management

One example of a self-management program is the federal Department of Health and Ageing's *Sharing Health Care Initiative* (SHCI) demonstration projects, aimed at evaluating different approaches to chronic disease self-management. Through grant funding, the SHCI aims to enhance the quality of life for people with chronic diseases and their communities; to improve care providers' appreciation of the advantages of self-management and advance collaboration between care providers, people with chronic conditions and their families; and to improve the effectiveness of health service utilisation. Initial outcomes include a decline in depression, pain and general distress; improved symptom management; and a fall in general practitioner visits and hospitalisations (Department of Health and Ageing 2005). An example of the SHCI is the *Pika Wiya Health Service*, a chronic condition self-management project for diabetes, in South Australia. A camp for Aboriginal people introduced education on medication, nutrition, exercise, podiatry, renal disease and palliative care. Many Aboriginal people in this area also have other chronic diseases, such as heart disease, renal disease and asthma (DoHA 2005).

REFLECTION

The SHCI draws on the Flinders Model, which has developed instruments and processes to facilitate the evaluation of self-management behaviours, the collaborative identification of problems and establishing targets, and allowing strategies to be tailored to the individual (Flinders Human Behaviour and Health Research Unit 2005).

Chronic disease prevention and management – some issues

As indicated previously, health care systems generally focus on responding to acute episodic health conditions, consequently, they are inadequate for the ongoing care and management of those with chronic health problems (Glasgow et al 1999, NHPAC 2006,

NHMRC 2001, NPHP 2001, Weeramanthri et al 2003, WHO 2002). Furthermore, a large proportion of funding for chronic disease management is directed at programs that target comparatively restricted categories of populations, diseases or risk factors; therefore, managers of comprehensive chronic disease programs need to ensure that programs are integrated to reduce unnecessary duplication (CDC 2003).

Chronic diseases are often not seen as emergencies, as the benefits to the population or subpopulation may take a long time to become apparent (Brownson & Bright 2004, Yach et al 2004). In addition, there may be a lack of risk-factor information and data around needs for specific communities or populations, and inadequate resources pledged to chronic disease management programs (Brownson & Bright 2004). Both communities and individuals may also be more concerned about involuntary risk exposure, for example toxic waste, than voluntary risk exposure, such as insufficient exercise (Brownson & Bright 2004).

Clearly, it is essential to coordinate realistic and comprehensive strategies to advance the Australian health system's ability to provide comprehensive chronic disease prevention and management.

Defining communicable diseases

Communicable diseases are a common and significant contributor to ill health throughout the world, particularly for developing countries. The importance of communicable diseases is summarised in the following quotes from the previous Director General of WHO, Dr Gro Harlem Brundtland:

> One out of every two people in low-income countries dies at an early age from an infectious disease. Most of these deaths should have been prevented. How can families, communities and countries reach their dreams with this burden? Healthy development removes these obstacles and helps individuals and countries achieve their full potential. If the world invests in priority strategies to fight infectious diseases, much of this death and suffering could be prevented.
>
> (WHO 1999 p i)
>
> Illness and death from infectious diseases can in most cases be avoided at an affordable cost. It is in the interest of all that these obstacles to development be removed. Because of drug resistance, increased travel and the emergence of new diseases, there may only be limited time in which to make rapid progress.
>
> (WHO 1999 p 68)

Unfortunately there is some inconsistency in the language used in regard to communicable diseases, and there is value in using the following simple (plain-English) approach to describe the various key terms.

A communicable (or contagious) disease is one that can spread from one individual to another. Infectious diseases are diseases caused by pathogenic microorganisms, such as bacteria, viruses, parasites or fungi. Zoonotic diseases are infectious diseases of animals that can cause disease when transmitted to humans (WHO 1999).

Most communicable diseases are infectious diseases, but not all. For example, some chemically induced diseases, such as organophosphate poisoning, can be spread from one individual to another and could be described as 'communicable'. Most infectious diseases (but not all) can be communicated from one individual to another. Some can only be transmitted by an inert life stage (e.g. tetanus spores) or via a vector (e.g. malaria transmitted by mosquitoes).

Infectious diseases occur commonly in all communities and may be said to be 'endemic' in those communities. When a new disease occurs or an existing disease suddenly becomes more common, the disease may be considered to have 'broken out' out in that community. Such a situation is described variously as an outbreak or an epidemic. The simultaneous outbreak of an infectious disease in a number of communities is called a pandemic.

Infectious diseases are very common and generally do not cause significant pathology. For example, some of the most common infectious diseases such as the common cold, dental caries and acne vulgaris have a highly significant economic and social impact, but do not have significant individual morbidity or mortality, although dental caries have been shown to increase the rate of myocardial infarction (refer to Box 10.1). However, from a statistical perspective, there are around 125,000 communicable disease case notifications made each year in Australia (Owen et al 2007), with infectious and parasitic diseases contributing to 1.7% of the total burden of disease, acute respiratory diseases accounting for 1.3%, and oral health contributing 0.9% (almost all of which is caused by dental caries) (Begg et al 2007).

Box 10.1: Common infectious diseases

Acne (or pimples) is a hormonally induced condition that is often complicated by infection. It causes considerable social impact in a particularly vulnerable age group and at times causes residual scarring, which has long-term personal and social impacts.

Dental caries is associated with infection of the teeth and surrounding soft tissues. Caries is the most common infectious disease that, if untreated, may lead to long-term poor dental health with significant dietary, social and health consequences. Prevention through fluoridated water supplies and good dental hygiene can reduce the impact of this disease.

Influenza is another and more serious common infectious disease. Most people when they say they 'have the flu' mean they have a common cold. Influenza is a more serious upper respiratory tract disease that is commonly associated with consequential pneumonia. Annual outbreaks of influenza cause a significant number of deaths, particularly among the young and the elderly. The virus is very changeable and annual 'flu shots' are recommended for those most at risk.

Medical microbiology

Medical microbiology describes the study of microbes that cause diseases in humans (Irving et al 2005). Humans and other large multicellular animals co-exist with microorganisms in the environment. This relationship does not always result in harm; it may be either:

- a commensal relationship in which the microorganism and the human co-exist for mutual benefit; for example, microorganisms live in the large intestine of humans where they protect us against invasion by pathogenic organisms and in turn have a ready supply of food for their own survival and reproduction
- a neutral relationship in which the organisms and the humans live in harmony without any adverse or mutual beneficial effects (our skin is colonised by microorganisms that cause no problems unless our defence mechanisms are breached)
- a pathogenic relationship in which the microorganism causes disease in the larger organism.

The concept of disease is multidimensional and includes: the interaction of the body part/s with the pathogen, the interactions between various body parts, and the interactions between the body and the various environments within which we live. Thus, for any disease state, there are always three elements (Hurster 1997):

1   the *person* or *host* who is the target of the disease, and who may succumb to it
2   the *agent*, which is either the direct cause of disease or a contributing or predisposing factor to its onset
3   the *environment*, which may influence the existence of the agent, exposure of the host to the agent, or the susceptibility of the host.

These interactions are commonly described in terms of two models of infectious diseases: the 'agent-host-environment triangle', which is also known as the 'epidemiologic triad', and the 'chain of infection' model (refer to figures 10.3 and 10.4).

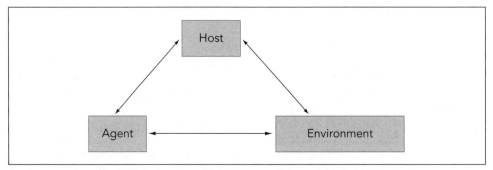

FIGURE 10.3: Triangle model of infectious diseases

(Redrawn from: Weber & Rutala 2001 p 4, adapted from APIC 1996 p 12)

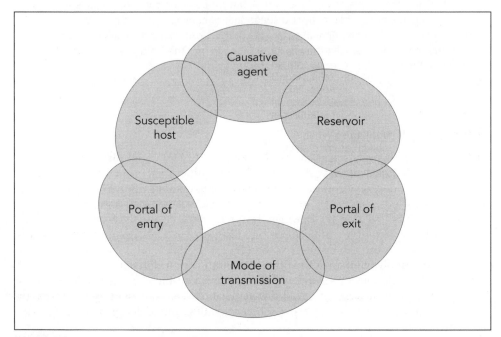

FIGURE 10.4: Chain model of infectious diseases

(Redrawn from: Weber & Rutala 2001 p 4, adapted from APIC 1996 p 18)

For the chain model of infectious diseases, the following elements must apply (Weber & Rutala 2001):

- *Susceptible host* – despite living in a sea of microbes, people are generally healthy due to intrinsic and specific host defences. Susceptibility includes the host being immuno-compromised, or other defects in the host's defences.
- *Infectious agent* – an agent must be present and capable of causing infection (e.g. virus, bacteria, fungi, protozoa).
- *Reservoir* – the agent needs a reservoir where it can propagate (that is, live, reproduce and die in the natural state). This includes humans, animals and the environment.
- *Portal of exit* from reservoir and *portal of entry* into a susceptible host – examples include the respiratory tract, the GI (gastrointestinal) tract, skin and mucous membranes.
- *Transmission* – the agent needs to be transmitted, directly or indirectly, from one place to another.

Microorganisms

Microorganisms are all pervasive. No drop of water, grain of soil or skin surface is free of microscopic organisms. These organisms may be characterised broadly in several categories (Irving et al 2005).

Eukaryotic organisms

Eukaryotic organisms are those with a 'proper' cellular structure, often with complex cellular structures. These include larger complex organisms such as parasites (worms and insects) and fungi (moulds and yeasts) or single cellular organisms such as protozoa. For example, helminths are parasitic worms. The three main groupings are roundworms, tapeworms and flukes. Once they enter the body, they lodge in the intestines or tissues, and go through their life cycle (i.e. unfertilised egg, egg, larva, adult). Even though infestation of the host does not always produce observable signs of disease, the helminth is robbing the host of food, and may be releasing toxins into the host's body, which may cause damage, so in time the effects of infestation become apparent. These effects include weight loss; swelling of the legs, scrotum and breasts; anaemia; and muscular pain. Diseases include hookworm, ascariasis, trichinosis, beef tapeworm and pork tapeworm.

Arthropods

Arthropods are another example of parasites that live on the surface of the host's body. The main parasites that affect humans are lice, fleas, ticks and mites. They may play a direct or an indirect role in causing disease. In a direct role, they create skin eruptions. When they serve as a vector (or carrier) for disease transmission, they are considered to be having an indirect role in causing disease. For example head lice cause direct skin irritation (a direct role), while ticks can transmit diseases such as Q fever or Lyme disease (an indirect role).

Fungi

Fungi are single- or multi-celled plants that lack chlorophyll and are generally characterised as moulds or yeasts. Many, but not all, forms of fungi are pathogenic to humans. The diseases that they produce are collectively known as *mycoses*. Superficial mycoses include ringworm and athlete's foot, while deep-seated (or systematic) mycoses include infections of the mucous membranes and lungs, such as moniliasis.

Protozoa

Protozoa are one-celled microscopic animals that are parasitic in nature and exist in either an active stage (called a trophozoite) or an inactive stage called a cyst. During the trophozoite stage the protozoa cause infection in the host. In the cyst stage, the protozoa lodge in the host's body and do not create disease, with the host then becoming a carrier and potential transmitter of the protozoa to another host. The two main groups of protozoa are intestinal, oral and genital protozoa, which cause diseases such as amoebic dysentery and giardiasis; and the blood and tissue protozoa such as *Plasmodium*, which causes malaria. Parasitic organisms may rely on a larger host for their survival. These 'parasites' may always need a host in order to survive (obligate parasites) or they may simply 'hitch a ride' when convenient (opportunistic parasites).

Prokaryotic organisms

Collectively known as bacteria, prokaryotic organisms are single cell organisms with no nucleus, but still with the capability of independent life and reproduction. Bacteria can occur either as a ball or sphere, called *Coccus* (e.g. S*taphylococcus* and S*treptococcus*); a rod, called *Bacillus* (e.g. responsible for diseases such as diphtheria, tuberculosis, botulism, salmonellosis and cholera), and a spiral, called *Spirochete* (e.g. responsible for syphilis and Lyme disease) (Hurster 1997).

Some bacteria, such as rickettsia or chlamydia, are not capable of independent life and are thus considered atypical bacteria. Rickettsia are closely related morphologically to bacteria. However, unlike bacteria, they require an insect vector to complete the disease transmission cycle. Therefore, rickettsia are associated with diseases in which ticks, fleas and body lice act as an intermediary between the host (man) and the animal reservoir on which it was living and from which it obtained the rickettsia. Examples of rickettsial diseases are typhus, Rocky Mountain spotted fever and Q fever (Hurster 1997).

Non-cellular organisms

Non-cellular organisms include viruses and prions. Viruses, from the Latin noun *virus*, meaning toxin or poison, consist simply of genetic material (RNA or DNA) and other protective components such as proteins. Viruses are incapable of independent life or reproduction and must invade a cell in order that the virus's genetic material can become incorporated into the cell's genetic material resulting in the production of new viruses. Some viruses can invade and damage bacteria. These are known as bacteriophages (or simply phages).

Prions are protein molecules of only a few nanometres in size, which cause *Bovine spongiform encephalitis* ('mad cow disease'). Prions act in a way similar to viruses by invading cells so that they influence the cell to produce more prions, which in turn are released from the cell to continue the process of infection.

Pathogens

A disease-producing microorganism is known as a pathogen. Pathogens vary in their capacity to cause disease; even within the same species of microorganisms. Terms used to describe the capacity of any particular microorganisms to cause disease include:
*   *virulence* – this refers to the strength or power of the pathogen to produce disease
*   *infectivity* – this is the ability of the pathogen to lodge or gain a foothold in the body, and represents the first step in the disease-producing process
*   *pathogenicity* – this is the pathogen's ability to multiply and spread, which are further steps in the disease-producing process (Hurster 1997)
*   *antigenicity* – this is the ability of the pathogen to stimulate the production of antibodies.

Mechanism of infectious disease

A microorganism can cause disease via several mechanisms. Organisms can cause direct cellular injury as occurs when the organisms invade healthy cells to enable replication or to provide nutrients to the organisms. The result is the death of the cell, and the clinical or symptomatic consequences of cellular injury and death depend on the number of cells affected and the body organ or system affected. Microorganisms that invade and grow in the body can cause symptoms or disease by releasing a toxin, which in turn causes injury to cells and resultant symptoms. For example, *Clostridium tetani* may invade small breaches in the skin and cause a minor infection, which may be unnoticed. However, the toxin released by the cells causes widespread neurological injury and death, resulting in the characteristic symptoms and signs of tetanus.

Microorganisms can also cause disease by affecting the body's own protective responses. Human immunodeficiency virus (HIV) invades the body's immunological response mechanisms and thus leads to acquired immunodeficiency syndrome (AIDS), which limits the body's ability to mount a normal immunological response to certain diseases. Thus the mortality and morbidity is related to the presence of other diseases, which cannot be resisted. Microorganisms can also cause long-term low-grade infections that can predispose the patient to other diseases. For example, human papilloma virus causes a low-grade (often asymptomatic) infection of the uterine cervix, which increases the rate of cervical cancer. Similarly, *Helicobacter pylori* infection of the stomach has been shown to predispose patients to acute peptic ulcers and higher rates of stomach cancer. Finally, organisms can act in concert to cause illness. For example the hepatitis viruses D and E have been shown to predispose people to infection by other hepatitis viruses, such as C and B, with more significant pathology.

Any particular organism can have a range of effects, from causing no disease or can cause mild or severe illness. The extent of the impact of microorganisms on the patient is dependent on the organism, host or environmental factors. An organism with a relatively low pathogenicity can cause severe illness in a host whose defences have been weakened by malnutrition or immune suppression.

Most microorganisms, particularly viruses, vary considerably from time to time or location to location in their structure, and thus their potency and recognition. For example, influenza viruses vary from year to year hence vaccines from one year are not necessarily effective in following years. Some years the influenza viruses are highly pathogenic, in other years they cause relatively mild illnesses. Variations in the protein coat of the virus will change the infectivity and pathogenicity of the virus.

Host defences

The body has a range of protective mechanisms in place to prevent infection. These include:
- physical barriers designed to prevent the organisms entering the body (the most obvious is the skin, where a thick layer of keratin normally prevents the entry of organisms into the underlying tissues)
- immunological responses including (a) *cellular immunity* in which specially designed cells will recognise the entry of foreign particles and seek to destroy those particles; and (b) *humeral immunity* in which the body produces antibodies to foreign particles that combine with and deactivate or destroy the foreign material, bacteria or virus.

However, the body's defence mechanisms must be able to gain access to the invading organisms in order to prevent infection. Thus infection may be more likely and more difficult to treat in circumstances where the blood supply is restricted (e.g. in gangrene) or when the organisms are sheltered from the body's defences by foreign bodies, such as contaminants or surgical implants.

Therefore, symptomatic infection occurs when a microorganism is able to break through the body's defences and reproduce in sufficient numbers so as to cause damage to living tissues. This process of contagion and reproduction takes some time and this period between contact and symptomatic disease is commonly referred to as the incubation period of the disease. It is during this period that the disease is difficult to detect and may easily be spread to other people before symptoms are evident. The gap between the contact and infectivity of the patients is termed the 'latent period'. Patients with infection are potentially infectious to others for a period of time, which varies with the particular illness. This often predates the onset of symptoms but may cease before the symptoms cease. It is during this period before the onset of symptoms, and when the patient is infective, that the risk of transmission to others is very high.

Environmental factors

Environmental factors also affect the expression or transmission of the pathogenic microorganisms. Organisms need an environment that facilitates their protection and growth. Microorganisms generally need an environment in which they can survive or replicate. Thus, outside of a larger organism, most organisms require either a moist environment with nutrients, or they must adopt an inactive form such as spores (e.g. tetanus).

Most organisms are particularly vulnerable to environmental factors such as sunlight, soaps and many chemicals. Thus organisms need to survive in an environment that is sustaining. Viruses will survive provided they can be protected in water droplets or other secretions. Bacteria and other more complex organisms require an ongoing source of energy, and thus require a food source to remain alive. Therefore, most organisms are vulnerable to simple cleaning measures and their transmission can be interrupted by clean environments. However, some organisms can transform themselves into resilient forms such as spores, which withstand survival outside of a host. For example, the tetanus-causing organism, *Clostridium tetani,* forms itself into spores that can survive in soil or other protective environments for considerable periods of time.

Spreading disease

In order to survive and replicate, organisms need to be able to spread from host to host, and therefore they require the close proximity of hosts to each other, or vectors (e.g. mosquitoes), which can transmit the organism from one host to another. The ability of an infected patient to cause further infection is determined by the infectivity of the organisms, that is, its capacity to cause disease and the exposure to suitable hosts. This infectivity or R factor describes the number of other individuals an infected person may infect. The R factor is dependent on the virulence of the organism and the community environment, for example, overcrowding. The mode of transmission of diseases varies with the disease, and some infectious diseases can only spread from one person to another via an intermediate host or vector.

The mechanism of the spread of organisms from one animal to another is determined by a range of factors, and is ultimately different for each organism and the disease it can cause. Therefore, knowledge of the characteristics of an organism is essential to determine the particular circumstances of each disease. However, in general, organisms must be released by one individual and be introduced into another via one of the following pathways.

- Microorganisms may be excreted via body fluids or wastes, such as faeces, urine, semen, saliva or sputum. These excretions may then pass by direct contact, or via contaminated food or water, to another individual who may ingest or inhale the organism or the organisms may invade directly through breaches in the body's physical barriers.
- Microorganisms may be passed from individual to individual via blood that may be exchanged during intimate contact, through blood transfusion or shared needles.
- Microorganisms may be passed from individual to individual via a third-party organism (vector). This often involves insects, but may involve large animals as occurs with rabies. For example, the mosquito is instrumental in spreading malaria from one individual to another. The mosquito bites an infected individual and draws blood, which contains the flagellate. The microorganism undergoes reproduction in the mosquito that then can transmit the new organisms to another person when it injects the saliva required to prevent coagulation and allow it to draw blood. Vectors can be an essential step in disease transmission as occurs with the mosquito and malaria, or it may be simply a means of transferring the live organisms from one person to another.

In addition, other animals may also play a role in transmitting disease between humans. Those animals may directly transmit the disease (as occurs with bites from animals, particularly animals with rabies), or other animals may act as a reservoir (vector) for the organism and carry the pathogen. For example, the rat is a reservoir for plague and in this case the organism lives in the rat and is transferred by the rat from one location to another. Finally, in some circumstances the animal may be a host to related organisms, which can then mutate within the animal and result in a more pathogenic organism. This is of particular concern with influenza viruses, in which it is possible for the avian influenza virus and the human influenza viruses to infect a large animal, such as a pig, and then mutate into a more lethal and infective form.

Therefore, the mode of transmission describes the way in which an infectious disease may be spread from one source to another. Transmission may occur between people, between humans and animals, and between humans and plants.

Diagnosis of infectious disease

To adequately define/classify a disease as being communicable, four criteria should be met (Hurster 1997):

1 the presence of a host
2 the presence of a disease-producing agent/pathogen
3 a mode of transmission
4 a mode of entry.

Managing any particular disease or outbreak of disease depends on accurately identifying the disease. Diagnoses can be made in several ways. Many diseases, such as measles, present with classic signs and symptoms, which in some cases are unmistakeable. Clinical diagnosis is not always reliable, particularly when the expression of the disease is incomplete, or symptoms and signs may reflect any number of other diseases. However, in the case of disease outbreaks, clinical diagnoses will be most common.

Direct identification of the causative organism can be used to diagnose particular diseases where the organism is characteristic. For example, microscopy can be used to identify malaria on blood smears, or tuberculosis in sputum. Direct microscopy requires considerable skill and usually special staining mechanisms. Specimens from an infected person can be introduced into cultures to try and grow the microorganism, which enables a more accurate identification of the organisms, either by direct microscopy or by the characteristics that organisms display in particular chemical or other environments. Some diseases have particular, and often characteristic, effects on the pattern of cells in the patient's blood. For example, viral illnesses produce larger numbers of lymphocytes while bacterial organisms produce more granulocytes. Infectious mononucleosis ('glandular fever') produces a classic pattern of high levels of lymphocytes. Specific tests seek to identify the presence of specific antigens (proteins derived from the organism) or antibodies (the body's defences). These tests are generally highly specific to the particular organism and can now be available for immediate testing.

Accurate diagnostic capacity is an essential element of the public health infrastructure. That capacity is indispensable for closely monitoring the patterns of disease in the community, and thus provides a mechanism to alert authorities to potential new diseases or outbreaks. For example, this infrastructure is utilised to observe influenza strains, so as to inform vaccination strategies. Similarly, international cooperation to monitor the avian influenza strains enables authorities to monitor the potential for the virus to mutate into a form that may be readily transmitted between humans.

Infectious disease management

Managing infectious diseases in society is reliant on a range of complementary strategies, which together aim to prevent, monitor or treat disease. These strategies include those targeted at disease prevention, those involved with surveillance and early detection and strategies aimed at managing disease when it occurs. This approach is equivalent to primary, secondary and tertiary prevention. This text focuses on the public health aspects of disease prevention and not on managing individual patients with disease, which is rightly the domain of medical practitioners. Accordingly, the three key aspects of managing infectious diseases are: disease prevention; surveillance, early recognition and early intervention; and the management of a disease outbreak. These are the essential pillars of the public health management of infectious diseases.

Disease prevention

The prevention of infectious diseases is achieved through a combination of individual and population strategies, as detailed below.

Societal and environmental structures

Because infectious diseases require close proximity in order to spread, one of the most significant factors involved in disease prevention in developed countries is the social isolation that results from increased living standards. We live in small population groups, often nuclear families at most, in large or at least separate, well-constructed homes that are often designed to exclude disease vectors (e.g. screens that keep out mosquitoes). Properly constructed houses permit easy cleaning of surfaces to reduce person-to-person transmission. Added to this is the capacity to use chemical and physical barriers to disease entry.

Our societal systems and structures are designed to minimise the risks of disease transmission. We have laws and regulations to provide access to safe drinking water; clean, safe food; and hygienic waste disposal. A long-established, but now rarely used social prevention measure is that of quarantine (i.e. forced isolation of individuals).

In Australia we value our personal space. Thus, we tend to maintain social separation, except with intimate contacts. We often travel alone in individual vehicles. We have rules and standards of social conduct, which help limit disease transmission. We expect people to cover their mouths when sneezing, not to spit in public and to wash their hands after toileting. All these aspects of our social norms contribute to reducing infectious diseases being easily transmitted.

Immunisation

Immunisation is credited with dramatically reducing morbidity and mortality from communicable diseases during the 20th century. The significant public health success of immunisation is clearly demonstrated in Table 10.2.

DISEASE	BASELINE 20TH CENTURY ANNUAL MORBIDITY*	2003 MORBIDITY	% DECREASE
Smallpox	48,164	0	100
Diphtheria	175,885	1	99.99
Pertussis	147,271	8067	94.52
Tetanus	1314	14	98.93
Poliomyelitis	16,316	0	100
Measles	503,282	42	99.99
Mumps	152,209	194	99.87
Rubella	47,745	8	99.98

TABLE 10.2: Vaccine preventable disease data for the United States

(Source: Orenstein et al 2005)

*These are representative figures, for example, for smallpox, this figure represents the average annual number of cases during 1900–1904, and for diphtheria, this figure represents the average annual number of reported cases during 1920–1922, three years before vaccine development. Also note that the decline in the absolute number of cases occurred despite considerable population growth.

All societies have active immunisation programs for disease for which vaccines are readily available. Our public vaccination programs are strongly supported through public and professional awareness campaigns, and through free access to the vaccines. We support this program through schools and employment programs, and through monitoring community vaccination status. Approved vaccines are provided free of charge to the patients through government funding programs. The scope and range of vaccination programs is articulated in the *Australian Immunisation Handbook* (NHMRC 2003).

From birth, and particularly during infancy and early childhood, humans are exposed to countless foreign antigens and infectious agents in the environment. Responding to these stimuli helps the immune system to develop and mature. Compared with exposure to the natural environment, vaccines provide specific stimulation to a small number of antigens.

Often the terms 'immunisation' and 'vaccination' are used interchangeably; however, more narrowly defined, vaccination is the process of administering a vaccine (i.e. actually administering the injection), whereas immunisation is the process of administering a vaccine and the development of a specific immune response (i.e. becoming immune to a disease due to being vaccinated). Immunity is the ability of the human body to protect itself from infectious disease. There are two main mechanisms for conveying immunity (Salisbury et al 2006):

- *innate or non-specific immunity* – this is present from birth and includes the physical barriers (e.g. intact skin and mucous membranes), chemical barriers (e.g. gastric acid, digestive enzymes and bacteriostatic fatty acids of the skin), phagocytic cells and the complement system
- *acquired immunity* – this is generally specific to a single organism or group of organisms and is acquired through either active or passive mechanisms.

The human can 'acquire' immunity through either natural or artificial means. The most common natural means of acquiring immunity is through exposure to the disease, either by contracting the disease personally or by coming into contact with someone who has the disease. In response the body produces 'antibodies' to the 'antigens' that are contained in the organisms that produce the disease. Vaccination programs aim to replicate this naturally acquired immunity through artificial means, which avoid the risks of the disease itself. Acquired immunity can thus be achieved by either active or passive immunisation.

Active immunity

Active immunity is produced by a person's own immune system and is usually long lasting. This type of immunity generally involves cellular responses, serum antibodies or a combination, acting against one or more antigens on the infecting organism. Vaccines produce a protective effect by inducing active immunity and providing immunological memory. Immunological memory allows the immune system to recognise and respond rapidly to exposure to natural infection at a later date, and, therefore, prevent or modify the disease. Thus a vaccine administered to a patient who was previously not exposed will stimulate the body to produce antibodies to the antigen. This initial reaction takes some time and is, therefore, not fast enough to produce sufficient antibodies to prevent infection. However, following this exposure the body will record the previous exposure and maintain cells, which can readily recognise the antigen again and produce a more rapid antibody response. Thus, most vaccination programs recommend two or more vaccinations to obtain maximum protection and regular boosters to maintain the body's immune responsiveness.

The principal types of vaccines are inactivated vaccines, which are produced generally by reproducing the antigen of the organism that initiates the antibody response. This can be achieved either by killing the organisms and extracting the elements that produce the antibody response, or by manufacturing the antigen using recombinant technology, which involves modifying microorganisms to produce the antigen. Live attenuated vaccines are created by modifying the disease-causing organism, so that it produces the antibody response without producing the disease. Live vaccines are still used, but there is a small risk that the patient may acquire the actual disease because of poor immunity or other factors. Recent approaches have involved the development of DNA vaccines, which are produced by directly injecting DNA into the animal so that the animal produces the foreign antigen itself. This approach is likely to be extremely safe as is does not involve administering foreign material, and should be relatively cheaper than other vaccines.

Passive immunity

Passive immunity is the protection that is provided by the transfer of antibodies derived from immune people. The most common source of passive immunity is that acquired by newborn infants from their mother. However, passive immunisation is used to provide 'post-exposure' protection such as may occur following contact with rabies or hepatitis, or for protection against toxins such as snake venom. Unfortunately, passive immunity is temporary (that is, from a few weeks to months) because the protection provided is due to an antibody produced by a different host.

The role of immunisation

The primary aim of immunisation is to protect the individual who receives the vaccine, with vaccinated individuals also less likely to be a source of infection for others. Therefore, this reduces the risk of unvaccinated individuals being exposed to infection. This means that individuals who cannot be vaccinated will still benefit and this concept is known as 'population immunity' or 'herd immunity'. When vaccination coverage is high enough to produce high levels of population immunity, infections can be eliminated from a community. However, if vaccination coverage is not maintained, it is possible for these diseases to return. Consequently, health agencies are extremely concerned with vaccine coverage levels in their community and encourage the widespread uptake of immunisation. In Australia, the *Australian Immunisation Handbook* (NHMRC 2003) provides the vaccination standards that form the basis for the government's schedule of free or subsidised vaccines outlined in the *Australian Immunisation Program Schedule* (see the Immunise Australia website). In 1997, as part of the *Immunise Australia* program, a number of incentives were introduced to improve vaccination coverage including incentives for parents to improve compliance with the vaccination schedule and incentives for general practitioners to provide age-specific immunisation services for children. Since this program has been established, the overall age-specific vaccination coverage for children at one year of age increased from 74.9% in 1997 to 91.2% in 2001 and for children at two years of age increased from 63.8% in 1997 to 84.7% in 2000 (AIHW 2002).

Unfortunately, no vaccine offers 100% protection and so a small proportion of people get infected despite being vaccinated. Most vaccines that are recommended for universal use in children are known to be effective for between 80% and 95% of recipients following a primary series (Orenstein et al 2005). In addition, any vaccine may cause an adverse event, that is, 'an unwanted or unexpected event following immunisation' (NHMRC 2003 p 20). 'Such an event may be caused by the vaccine or may occur by chance after immunisation (that is, it would have occurred regardless of vaccination)' (NHMRC 2003 p 20). Most vaccines cause minor adverse events such as fever, pain or redness at the site of injection, commonly following vaccination and these should be anticipated (NHMRC 2003).

Box 10.2: Public health interventions: the case of immunisation

One of the major priorities set by the federal government has been to make an impact on the low rates of childhood immunisation in Australia. Many deaths in children are vaccine preventable. Immunisation against childhood diseases is one of the well-documented public health strategies to address this problem. A range of initiatives has been implemented nationally to improve the rates of childhood immunisation against such diseases as measles, mumps, rubella (German measles), diphtheria and pertussis (whooping cough). Although Australia instituted a childhood vaccination program in the 1920s, information on coverage was less than satisfactory until the establishment of the *National Notifiable Diseases Surveillance Scheme* (NNDSS) in 1991, and the *Australian Childhood Immunisation Register* (ACIR) in 1996 (AIHW 2002). The importance of this public health issue is demonstrated by the data that show that vaccine-preventable diseases killed 87 children between 1986 and 2004 (NCIRS 2007).

ACTIVITY

- What do you believe are the barriers for parents in immunising their children?
- As a population health strategy how effective is childhood immunisation?
- As an emerging health professional, what are your views on compulsory immunisation for children prior to entry to day care and school? Why have you taken that position?
- Why is this issue a public health concern?
- What other factors need to be considered to increase and maintain high rates of childhood immunisation?

REFLECTION

Immunisation is the cornerstone of the control of infectious diseases in our society, yet there remain significant scientific, ethical, social and economic issues that impact on the level of immunisation. In many poor countries, people simply cannot afford the vaccines. The scientific data supporting the required vaccination schedules are not clear. The schedules are often based on the achievement of 100% effectiveness in all people, whereas fewer and/or less frequent doses may be equally effective in most people. We need more scientific data on how to tailor vaccination schedules to individual needs. Some people object to vaccines as a form of mass medication and others believe that vaccines have serious adverse side effects in some people and do not wish to take the risk. How much of a responsibility do we all share for maintaining the 'herd immunity'?

Vector control

A 'vector' is defined as 'a carrier, especially one that transmits disease' (Glanze 1990 p1227). Earlier in this chapter we introduced the *Chain Model of Infection* and in this model a critical link in the chain is the mode of transmission. We identified that 'transmission' is where the infectious agent needs to be transmitted, directly or indirectly, from one place to another, and there are four routes of transmission: contact, common vehicles, airborne, and vector-borne. Vector-borne transmission of an infectious agent is undertaken by an arthropod and this may be by simple mechanical transfer of microorganisms on the external appendages of the vector, or the vector may internalise the agent requiring subsequent regurgitation, defecation or penetration of the skin or mucosal surface of the susceptible host (Weber & Rutala 2001).

There is a large range of arthropods associated with transmitting disease. These include cockroaches, ants, flies, biting midges, mosquitoes, fleas, bedbugs, lice, ticks, scabies, fabric pests, stored product pests and rodents. Throughout the world, vectors such as these are responsible for a substantial level of disease, disability and illness, with vector-borne disease accounting for about 17% of the estimated global burden of infectious diseases (WHO 2004). The most deadly vector-borne disease, malaria, kills over 1.2 million people annually, mostly African children under the age of five. In addition, dengue fever, together with its associated dengue haemorrhagic fever (DHF), is the world's fastest growing vector-borne disease. The environmental health links with vector-borne diseases are extremely strong, with poorly designed irrigation and water systems, inadequate housing, poor waste disposal and water storage, deforestation and loss of biodiversity, all being contributing factors to the most common vector-borne diseases.

Given such a substantial disease burden associated with vector-borne diseases, vector control activities are, therefore, an important disease control and prevention measure. Unfortunately, even though well-planned vector control measures can significantly contribute to reducing this disease burden, the preventative power of vector control is grossly under-utilised in public health (Townson et al 2005). Rather than relying on a single method of vector control, WHO recommends implementing integrated vector management (IVM), which stresses the importance of first understanding the local vector ecology and local patterns of disease transmission, and then choosing the appropriate vector control tools from the range of options available. Characteristic features of IVM include (WHO 2004):

- methods based on knowledge of factors influencing local vector biology, disease transmission and morbidity
- using a range of interventions, often in combination and synergistically
- collaboration within the health sector and with other public and private sectors that impact on vectors
- engaging with local communities and other stakeholders
- a public health regulatory and legislative framework.

The primary purpose of IVM strategies is therefore to achieve the greatest disease control benefit in the most cost-effective manner, while minimising negative impacts on ecosystems (e.g. depletion of biodiversity) and adverse side effects on public health from the excessive use of chemicals in vector control.

Personal protection

Our societies take actions that seek to protect the individual personally. We have initiated such measures as:

- encouraging behaviours that ensure safe practices
- encouraging 'safe sex' to reduce disease transmission, particular sexually transmitted diseases, including HIV/AIDS
- encouraging the safe use of clean needles for drugs addicts to reduce risks associated with cross infection from dirty needles
- encouraging the use of personal protective barriers, for example, condoms for safe sex, and mosquito netting
- encouraging and supporting the use of prophylactic medication in circumstances where exposure is possible, for example, malaria prophylaxis for travellers to malaria-prone areas
- actively managing secondary (post-exposure) prophylaxis, for example, in the event of needle stick injuries to health workers.

Surveillance, early recognition and early intervention

We also ensure that systems and structures are in place and functioning to screen for the presence of disease and to investigate and manage outbreaks of disease. The early warning functions of surveillance are fundamental for national, regional and global health security. Recent outbreaks, such as the severe acute respiratory syndrome (SARS) and avian influenza, and potential threats from biological and chemical agents, demonstrate the importance of effective national surveillance and response systems (WHO 2006).

The main sources of routinely collected public health surveillance data are (Stroup et al 1994):

- *notifiable disease reporting*
- *vital statistics* – birth and death certificates
- *sentinel surveillance* – monitoring of key health indicators (early warning systems or systems to provide in-depth information on specific conditions)
- *registries* – case-series and hospital based registries; population-based registries; exposure registries, for example, cancer and birth defect registries
- *surveys* – health-interview surveys; provider-based surveys
- *administrative data-collection systems* – integrated health information systems; hospital-discharge data systems.

For communicable diseases, public health officials maintain a system of compulsory reporting of particular diseases to facilitate early recognition and intervention. In Australia, these notifiable diseases include:

- blood-borne diseases, such as hepatitis B
- gastrointestinal diseases, such as typhoid and salmonella
- other bacterial diseases, such as legionnaire's disease
- quarantinable diseases, such as cholera
- sexually transmitted diseases, such as syphilis
- vector-borne diseases, for example, dengue
- zoonotic diseases, for example, Q fever
- vaccine-preventable diseases, for example, polio.

In addition, some non-communicable diseases such as asbestos-related lung disease and excessive lead exposure are also reportable in some jurisdictions.

These diseases are reported either by diagnostic laboratories or by clinicians. The reports are made to public health agencies so that immediate outbreak investigation, contact tracing and public health interventions can occur. Part of this response is analysing the incoming data. The basic analytic approaches used in surveillance systems revolve around describing and analysing data in terms of:

- *time* – patterns of disease incidence, which may generate hypotheses, or may reflect patterns in reporting
- *place* – geographic distribution of disease or of its causative exposures or risk-associated behaviour (e.g. elevated blood-lead levels in children)
- *person* – characteristics of people or groups who develop disease or sustain injury, which helps to understand the risk factors for disease or injury and target interventions.

For analysing the majority of surveillance data, descriptive methods are usually appropriate. Displaying frequencies (counts) of the health problem in simple tables and graphs is the most common method of analysing data for surveillance. Rates are also useful, and frequently preferred, for comparing the occurrence of disease for different geographic areas or periods, because they take into account the size of the population from which the cases arose (CDC 2006).

Communicable disease surveillance in Australia

National surveillance of communicable disease has been undertaken in Australia since 1917, with the current *National Notifiable Diseases Surveillance System* (NNDSS) established in 1990. This system coordinates the national surveillance of more than 60 communicable diseases or disease groups. Under this scheme, notifications are made from doctors and laboratories to state or territory health authorities and electronic, de-identified unit records of notifications are then supplied to the Australian Government Department of Health and Ageing for collation, analysis and reporting in the journal *Communicable Diseases Intelligence* (CDI). Aggregated data are presented on the Communicable Diseases Australia internet site (www.health.gov.au/cda) and updated three times a week. Data are also published in CDI every quarter and in an annual report.

The NNDSS is a passive surveillance in that it is based on legislative requirements in each state for medical practitioners and laboratories to report confirmed or suspected cases of disease. As such, the NNDSS recognises that the notified cases represent only a fraction of the total incidence in the community and this is graphically described in Figure 10.5.

Surveillance systems such as the NNDSS can therefore be used for a range of purposes including describing the natural history of a disease, facilitating research and investigating trends or other interesting outcomes from the routine analysis of the data. An example

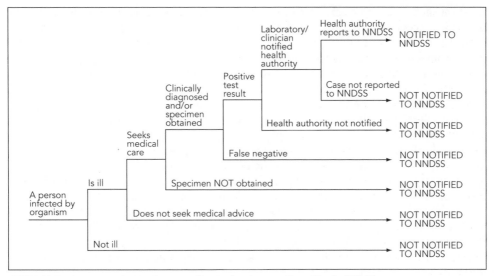

FIGURE 10.5: The communicable disease notification fraction as collected by the NNDSS

(Source: Owen et al 2007. Copyright Commonwealth of Australia, reproduced by permission)

of research conducted using routinely collected communicable disease surveillance data is a study that reviewed the incidence (notification data) of campylobacter infection in Queensland for a five-year period between 1991 and 1995 (Stafford et al 1996). As campylobacter infection consistently has one of the highest annual notification rates of all communicable diseases, and has a characteristic age distribution, an analysis of any long-term trends in incidence can be useful to more fully understanding this disease and for implementing control measures that may be able to reduce this high incidence. This study therefore analysed the following variables associated with the campylobacter notification data: incidence, age and sex distribution, seasonality, geographic distribution, and socioeconomic status. The review found that the highest notification rate was in children aged 12–23 months, and there was no distinct seasonal pattern of infection. Campylobacter infection was reported more frequently in urban areas and for persons residing in higher socioeconomic areas. The study concluded that factors which influence notification rates in the general population do not seem to have the same influence on the 0–4 years age group.

Managing a disease outbreak

The third level of management is considered to be tertiary prevention, which involves managing disease outbreaks in order to reduce the risks associated with transmitting that disease to unaffected people. This involves attention to infection control in health facilities and services, and the appropriate management of infected patients.

Infection control

The control of infectious diseases is dependent on adequate infection control procedures, particularly in environments of special risk such as health facilities or services. Infection control describes the systems, behaviours and structures that are designed to break the transmission of microorganisms from infected patients to unaffected people.

Infection control practice is an evolving discipline and prior to the 1980s, infection control systems were based on identifying at-risk patients in hospitals and applying isolation systems or special treatments. Unfortunately, this approach failed to take into account the possibility of transmitting infection from asymptomatic individuals, particularly those with blood-borne viruses or antibiotic-resistant bacteria (Commonwealth of Australia 2004).

By the mid 1980s, the AIDS epidemic created an urgent need for new strategies to protect health care workers from blood-borne infections in their working environment. Therefore, health authorities adopted a new approach in which all blood and body substances were to be considered potentially infectious and therefore introduced the principle of 'standard precautions'. This level of care was applied to all people, regardless of their perceived or confirmed infectious status, as a strategy for minimising health care associated infections from both asymptomatic and symptomatic people. The scope of this approach was later broadened by adopting a two-tier approach to infection control that consists of 'standard precautions' and 'additional precautions' (Commonwealth of Australia 2004).

Standard precautions involve a series of system and structures that should always be used in managing all patients so as to minimise the risks associated with infection. Standard precautions include hand washing between patients, appropriate clothing to reduce cross infection, wearing gloves where necessary and wearing masks to reduce respiratory transmission.

Additional precautions are recommended for patients known or suspected to be infected or colonised with disease agents that cause infections in health care settings and that may not be contained by standard precautions alone. These include situations where patients are particularly at risk (e.g. during a surgical procedure, particularly those involving implants) or in managing patients with particular infectious diseases that pose a heightened risk to other people. Additional precautions are generally targeted to the particular circumstances and may include the highest standard of respiratory protection, isolation and barrier nursing and care in a positive-pressure environment with closed-circuit air control.

Box 10.3: Tattoos and body piercing

Even though the infection control principles and practices have been developed for use in hospitals, there is a range of activities undertaken in non-medical settings that present potential to transmit infectious diseases. Such activities include hairdressing, body piercing, tattooing, hair replacements/implants and permanent make-up. Therefore appropriate infection-control practices are equally important for these activities.

Tattooing and body piercing are now a worldwide fashion craze that started in the 1990s and body piercing, in particular, is considered to be the fastest growing form of body decoration in the modern world, practised mainly by the young (Polhemus 1996, Vale et al 1989). In Australia, the most recent population survey available on this topic found that 10% of the population has had a tattoo at some point in their life and 8% have had some form of body piercing (excluding ear piercing). Men were found to be more likely to have tattoos, while women were more likely to report body or ear piercing (Makkai & McAllister 2001).

However, this 'craze' has also coincided with the emergence of blood-borne viral diseases such as hepatitis B and C, and HIV/AIDS. With the prevalence of tattooing and body piercing being considerably higher among injecting drug users, and along with a strong association with youth, these factors suggest a high potential for transmitting blood-borne viral diseases (Makkai & McAllister 2001).

Surprisingly, there appears to be a very low medical complication rate with tattoos, with only sporadic reports of viral transmission of blood-borne viruses. However, plastic surgeons report that much of the tattoo-related medical issues they encounter are concerned with treating patients who are dissatisfied with their tattoos (or permanent make-up) (Parliament of South Australia 2005).

In contrast, the medical evidence regarding complications from body piercing indicates an association with a large range of health issues. These range in severity from simple infections around the piercing site to the more serious localised and systemic infections. In addition to these infections, the other common medical issues caused by body piercing are inclusion cysts, hypertropic scars (scars that grow excessively) and metal allergies. There are also complications that occur in some specific piercings. These include genital complications, such as urethral rupture and sexual dysfunction, due to pain and scarring; and oral complications, such as chipped teeth, aspiration of the device and speech impediment. Patients often present with a severe infection at the piercing site, for example, the lips, which requires extensive treatment and may leave a scar that causes permanent problems with eating or drinking (Parliament of South Australia 2005).

ACTIVITY

- Do you or any friends have either a tattoo or a body piercing? If so, what were the motivating factors to obtain these? When deciding on getting a tattoo or piercing, did you (or your friends) consider the infection risks associated with such a procedure? If so, what sort of information was available to help with decision making, and was the tattooist or body piercer able to supply information on the risks? Finally, what sort of post-procedure care instructions were given in order to minimise infection?

REFLECTION

It is clear that the infection risks for body piercings are substantial – the procedure creates a wound and the body often rejects the foreign material. Accordingly, infection control focuses on appropriately trained and licensed operators; using sterile instruments and appropriate piercing techniques; and suitable post-procedure care.

Secondary prophylaxis

In certain circumstances, post-exposure prophylaxis is appropriate. There are two strategies used including the use of antibiotic or antiviral agents or passive immunisation with immunoglobulins. With regard to antibiotic or antiviral agents there is a massive range of such drugs and the choice of drugs is generally dependent on the known or presumed organism causing the illness. There are, however, increasing problems encountered with the development of resistant strains, thus reducing the effectiveness of antibiotics. Two important strategies for reducing this growing problem are minimising the unnecessary use of antibiotics, or using antibiotics that are targeted specifically to the organism concerned and its known sensitivities. One point to note with using antiviral agents is that as they generally act by reducing the reproduction of the virus; to be effective they have to be used (in a large number of cases) prior to the virus developing.

Secondary prophylaxis is particularly important in circumstances of known or suspected exposure to an infective agent. For example, antiviral agents are used to reduce the risks of viral agents following needle stick injury, and rabies immunoglobulin is used following exposure to a rabid animal.

Outbreak investigation and contact tracing

The public health strategies implemented to investigate a disease outbreak are an essential part of communicable disease management. These strategies involve:

- identifying the disease and the causative agent – this requires specimens from the infected patient(s) and the collection and testing of specimens of any possible or likely causes; for example, during an outbreak of a food-borne illness, specimens from food sources, food handlers and environmental contaminants may assist with tracking the cause
- investigating the circumstances of the infection – this may involve taking a detailed history of exposure and contacts
- identifying and testing others who may have been the source of the infection
- identifying others who may be at risk from similar exposure and who may knowingly or unwittingly be a source of further transmission
- timely implementation of appropriate control measures to minimise further illness.

The choice and type of control measure should be guided by the results of the epidemiological and environmental investigations. However, any delay in implementing control measures may expose the public to unacceptable risks, and so sometimes controls are implemented based on limited information. Control measures include food recalls, restaurant closures, excluding food handlers, decommissioning food-processing equipment and revising maintenance and operating procedures. The selection criteria for the most appropriate measures for the situation are based on their effectiveness for interrupting transmission, as well as their ease of implementation, expense and safety.

Case study: Outbreak investigation

The following is a case study of a food-borne illness outbreak that occurred in Queensland in 2001 that involved the following elements:

- a rare strain of a common food-borne pathogen was identified by the disease surveillance system
- the implicated food was sold by a major fast-food restaurant chain and cases were widely distributed throughout Queensland
- the implicated ingredient had traditionally been considered to present minimal risk
- the source of the outbreak was traced to the manufacturer of the ingredients.

In May 2001, 10 cases of *Salmonella bovismorbificans* (SB) were reported within seven days in south east Queensland compared with an average of three cases per month. Based on this 'spike' in incidence, enhanced surveillance was implemented and all current and new cases were interviewed. A case-control study was also conducted until 17 June 2001 and any implicated retail outlets and manufacturers were inspected. Results for this incident are summarised as:

- Up to 30 July 2001, 41 cases of SB were identified, 36 of which were SB phage type 32 (SB PT 32) (a rare type).
- Nationally, the majority of SB PT 32 cases occurred in Queensland in the first seven months of 2001.
- 63% of cases reported eating at one of 15 outlets of a fast food chain (company A) in the week preceding illness.
- 70% of these cases consumed product X.
- In the case control study, the matched odds ratio for eating at a company A outlet was found to be 17.5 (p<0.004) and p<0.001 for consuming product X. No

significant association was found for any other products or for eating at any other fast food chain.

● Inspections of the food safety standards at individual retail outlets of company A revealed no concerns.

● An audit of manufacturer M of the salad mixture for product X identified deficiencies in the cleaning procedures undertaken for the equipment used for shredding lettuce.

● A swab of food residue from the lettuce shredder was found to be positive for SB PT 32.

Based on these findings, company A changed suppliers for its salad mixtures and there were no further cases reported after this date.

Overall, this case study illustrates how a disease surveillance system can help to identify an outbreak and how the combination of epidemiological approaches (e.g. case-control studies) and environmental investigations can be used to identify the cause of, and control, an outbreak.

(Source: Stafford et al 2002)

Barriers to effectively managing communicable diseases

There are however many barriers to effective disease control. These generally relate to the failure of systems and structures, which in turn relate to general societal problems. Some examples include:

- poverty and its associated failure of infrastructure, education and awareness, and resources
- community ignorance associated with poor education standards
- ideological views – in some circumstances individuals or communities hold ideological views that are contrary to known communicable disease management strategies; for example, some individuals believe on religious or personal grounds that vaccination is 'unnatural', while others believe that vaccines sourced from Western countries are an attempt to subjugate the people of developing nations
- failure of communication either about the importance and value of prevention strategies or about the particular circumstances and risks – this failure may simply reflect poverty and associated poor educational standards or it may be due to the impediments associated with conflict whereby communities are deliberately deprived of information for the purposes of exercising political control

Case study: Legionnaire's disease

Legionnaire's disease is an atypical pneumonia caused by *Legionella* bacteria, often inhaled in contaminated aerosols. *Legionella pneumophila* serogroup 1 is the major notified cause of legionellosis in Australia. Sources linked to outbreaks worldwide include cooling towers, piped water, fountains and spas.

On 26–27 April 2000, routine follow-up by the Victorian Department of Human Services of three notifications of legionnaire's disease revealed that all three patients had visited the recently opened Melbourne Aquarium in the 10 days before illness onset. As this suggested a potential source at the aquarium, environmental

Continued

Case study: Legionnaire's disease—cont'd

investigations were begun immediately. Notifications increased rapidly, becoming Australia's largest outbreak of legionnaire's disease, with a total of 125 confirmed cases and four deaths. The epidemiological analysis identified an association between visiting the Aquarium in the risk period, and the environmental investigations found that the cooling towers were contaminated with legionella organisms. In fact, the cooling towers did not contain any detectable biocide, indicating that there was no effective disinfection of the cooling tower water. This was most likely to be due to faulty equipment and a lack of regular maintenance. Under these circumstances, it is likely that aerosols containing legionella organisms were dispersed into the environment and visitors to the aquarium inhaled the contaminated aerosols. This outbreak was the catalyst for new risk-based legislation in Victoria, which requires high-level maintenance of all water-cooled air conditioning systems.

(Source: Greig et al 2004)

- lack of infrastructure related either to poverty or to the failure of appropriate investment in necessary systems and structures required to deliver on the public health measures
- lack of resources such as equipment, personnel or consumables.

A final word

This chapter has covered a wide range of issues related to the development, prevention, management and care of chronic and communicable diseases. We have defined both chronic and communicable diseases and spent some time in the chapter discussing medical microbiology, which is the study of microbes that cause disease in humans.

We have included an extensive section on managing and preventing diseases and managing disease outbreaks as well as discussing the importance of public health throughout the continuum of care for both chronic and communicable diseases.

REVIEW QUESTIONS

1 How would you define a chronic disease?
2 What is a communicable disease? Is this definition different to the definition of an infectious disease? What then is a zoonotic disease?
3 What is medical microbiology and why do you think public health workers need to understand medical microbiology?
4 How is chronic disease managed at state/territory and federal government levels?
5 The Australian Government's *National Chronic Disease Strategy* concentrates on four key areas for improving outcomes. In a table identify the four key areas and describe the contribution of each to the prevention and management of chronic disease.
6 What is the range of ways in which microorganisms can cause disease?
7 What protective mechanisms does the body use to prevent infection?
8 How might we prevent and how might we manage infectious diseases?
9 What are the major strategies you would use to manage a disease outbreak?

USEFUL WEBSITES

Blue Book – Guidelines for the control of infectious diseases (Department of Human Services, Victoria): www.health.vic.gov.au/ideas/bluebook

Centers for Disease Control and Prevention (USA): www.cdc.gov

Centre for Healthcare Related Infection Surveillance and Prevention (CHRISP): www.health.qld.gov.au/chrisp

Communicable Diseases Australia: http://www.health.gov.au/internet/main/publishing.nsf/Content/cda-about.htm

Communicable Disease Network Australia: http://www.health.gov.au/internet/main/publishing.nsf/Content/cda-cdna-index.htm

Epidemic and Pandemic Alert and Response (World Health Organization): www.who.int/csr/en/

Epidemologic Case Studies (Centers for Disease Control and Prevention, USA): www2a.cdc.gov/epicasestudies

Global Defence Against the Infectious Disease Threat (World Health Organization): http://www.who.int/infectious-disease-news/cds2002/

Immunise Australia Program: www.immunise.health.gov.au

Medical Microbiology Book (University of Texas): http://gsbs.utmb.edu/microbook/toc.htm

REFERENCES

APIC infection control and applied epidemiology: principles and practice 1996 Association for Professionals in Infection Control and Epidemiology, Inc. Mosby, St. Louis

Australian Chronic Disease Prevention Alliance (ACDPA) 2004 Chronic Illness: Australia's Health Challenge. The Economic Case for Physical Activity and Nutrition in the Prevention of Chronic Disease. Available: http://www.goforyourlife.vic.gov.au/hav/articles.nsf/pracpages/The_Economic_Case_for_Physical_Activity_and_Nutrition?open 18 Feb 2008

Australian Institute of Health and Welfare 2002 Chronic diseases and associated risk factors in Australia, 2001. Available: www.aihw.gov.au/publications/phe/cdarfa01 18 Feb 2008

Australian Institute of Health and Welfare 2005 Chronic diseases and associated risk factors website. Available: http://www.aihw.gov.au/cdarf/index.cfm 24 April 2008

Australian Institute of Health and Welfare 2006 Australia's health 2006. AIHW cat. no. AUS 73. AIHW, Canberra

Australian Institute of Health and Welfare 2006 Chronic diseases and associated risk factors in Australia, 2006. Available: http://www.aihw.gov.au/publications/phe/cdarfa06/cdarfa06.pdf 12 Feb 2008

Australian Institute of Health and Welfare 2008 Chronic Disease and Associated Risk Factors. Available: http://www.aihw.gov.au/cdarf/index.cfm 7 Feb 2008

Begg S, Vos T, Barker B et al 2007 The Burden of Disease and Injury in Australia 2003, PHE 82, AIHW, Canberra

Brownson R C, Bright F S 2004 Chronic disease control in public health practice: Looking back and moving forward. Public Health Reports 119:230–238

Centers for Disease Control and Prevention 2003 Promising Practices in Chronic Disease Prevention and Control: A Public Health Framework for Action. Department of Health and Human Services, Atlanta. Available: http://www.cdc.gov/nccdphp/publications/PromisingPractices/pdfs/PromisingPractices.pdf 18 Feb 2008

Centers for Disease Control and Prevention 2004 Indicators for chronic disease surveillance. Morbidity and Mortality Weekly Report 53(No. RR-11). Available: http://www.cdc.gov/mmwr/preview/mmwrhtml/rr5311a1.htm 18 Feb 2008

Centers for Disease Control and Prevention (CDC) 2006 Principles of Epidemiology in Public Health Practice, 3rd edn, Self-Study Course SS1000, Centers for Disease Control and Prevention, Atlanta

Coligiuri R 2004 Diabetes as a health promotion focus: a disease for all reasons. Health Promotion Journal of Australia 15:95–99

Commonwealth of Australia 2004 Infection Control Guidelines for the prevention of transmission of infectious diseases in the health care setting. Department of Health and Ageing, Canberra

Department of Education and the Arts 2005 Activate website. Available: http://education.qld.gov.au/schools/healthy/active-ate/index.html 18 Feb 2008

Australian Government Department of Health and Ageing 2004 Building Healthy Communities. A Guide for Community Projects. Australian Government Department of Health and Ageing, Canberra

Department of Health and Ageing 2005 Sharing Health Care Initiative. Available: http://www.health.gov.au/internet/main/Publishing.nsf/Content/chronicdisease-sharing.htm 18 Feb 2008

Department of Health and Ageing 2006 Chronic Disease Management. Available: http://www.health.gov.au/internet/main/publishing.nsf/Content/pcd-programs-epc-chronicdisease 18 Feb 2008

Department of Human Services 2006 'Go For Your Life' website. State Government of Victoria. Available: http://www.goforyourlife.vic.gov.au/hav/articles.nsf?open 17 Feb 2008

Flinders Human Behaviour and Health Research Unit 2005 The 'Flinders Model' of Chronic Condition Self-Management. Flinders University, Adelaide. Available: http://som.flinders.edu.au/FUSA/CCTU/Self-Management.htm 17 Feb 2008

Frohlich K, Potvin L 1999 Health promotion through the lens of population health: toward a salutogenic setting. Critical Public Health 9:211–221

Glanze W D (ed) 1990 Mosby's Medical, Nursing and Allied Health Dictionary. The C V Mosby Company, St Louis

Glasgow R, Wagner E, Kaplan R et al 1999 If diabetes is a public health problem, why not treat it as one? A population-based approach to chronic illness. Annals of Behavioral Medicine 21:159–170

Greig J E, Carnie J A, Tallis G F et al 2004 An outbreak of Legionnaires' disease at the Melbourne Aquarium, April 2000: investigation and case–control studies. Medical Journal of Australia 180:566–572

Holman H, Lorig K 2000 Patients as partners in managing chronic disease. BMJ 320:526–527

Hurster M M 1997 Communicable and Non-Communicable Disease Basics: A Primer. Bergin & Garvey, Westport

Irving W L, Ala'Aldeen D, Boswell T 2005 Medical Microbiology. Taylor & Francis, New York

Kesteloot K 1999 Disease Management: a new technology in need of critical assessment. International Journal of Technology Assessment in Health Care, 15:3:506–519

Kindhauser M K 2003 Communicable Diseases 2002: Global Defence Against the Infectious Disease Threat, WHO, Geneva. Available: http://www.who.int/infectious-disease-news/cds2002/ 8 Feb 2008

Le Gales-Camus C 2005 Fighting Chronic Disease. Bulletin of the World Health Organization 83(6):407–8

Lopez A D, Mathers C D, Ezzati M et al 2006 Global Burden of Disease and Risk Factors. The World Bank and Oxford University Press, New York

Lorig K, Sobel D, Ritter P et al 2001 Effect of a Self-Management Program on Patients with Chronic Disease. Effective Clinical Practice November/December. Available: http://www.acponline.org/journals/ecp/novdec01/lorig.htm 18 Feb 2008

Makkai T, McAllister I 2001 Prevalence of tattooing and body piercing in the Australian community. Communicable Diseases Intelligence 25(2):67–72

Mathers C, Vos T, Stevenson C 1999 The burden of disease and injury in Australia. AIHW cat. no. PHE 17. AIHW, Canberra

National Centre for Immunisation Research and Surveillance of Vaccine Preventable Diseases (NCIRS) 2007 Vaccine preventable diseases and vaccination coverage in Australia 2003 to 2005, Communicable Diseases Intelligence, Volume 31, June, Supplement, pp S1–S152

National Health and Medical Research Council 2001 Tackling Chronic Disease: Exploration of Key Research Dimensions, Synopsis of Workshop, 5–6 July, 2001. NHMRC and Commonwealth Department of Health and Aged Care, Canberra

National Health and Medical Research Council 2003 The Australian Immunisation Handbook, 8th edn. NHMRC, Canberra

National Health Priority Action Council. National Chronic Disease Strategy 2006 Australian Government Department of Health and Ageing, Canberra. Available: http://www.health.gov. au/internet/main/publishing.nsf/Content/7E7E9140A3D3A3BCCA257140007AB32B/$File/ stratal3.pdf 17 Feb 2008

National Public Health Partnerships 2001 Preventing Chronic Disease: A Strategic Framework Background Paper. Available: http://www.nphp.gov.au/publications/strategies/ chrondis-bgpaper.pdf 17 Feb 2008

Orenstein W A, Wharton M, Bart K J et al 2005 Immunization. In: Mandell G L, Bennett J E, Dolin R (eds) Principles and Practice of Infectious Diseases, 6th edn. Elsevier Churchill Livingstone, Philadelphia, pp 3557–3589

Owen R, Roche P W, Hope K et al 2007 Australia's notifiable disease status, 2005: Annual report of the National Notifiable Diseases Surveillance System. Communicable Diseases Intelligence 31(1):1–70

Parliament of South Australia 2005 Report of the Select Committee on the Tattooing & Body Piercing Industries PP228, Parliament of South Australia, Adelaide

Polhemus T 1996 The Customised Body. The Serpant's Tail, New York

Pruitt S, Epping-Jordan J 2005 Preparing the 21st century global healthcare workforce. BMJ 330:637–639

Salisbury D, Ramsay M, Noakes K 2006 Immunisation against infectious disease. The Stationery Office, London

Sierra Club – Oklahoma Chapter website 1999 Bringing Urban Sprawl Into Focus. Available: http://oklahoma.sierraclub.org/sprawl/sprfocus.html 9 May 2008

Stafford R J, McCall B J, Neill A S et al 2002 A statewide outbreak of Salmonella Bovismorbificans phage type 32 infection in Queensland. Communicable Diseases Intelligence 26(4):568–573

Stafford R, Tenkate T, McCall B 1996 A five year review of Campylobacter infection in Queensland. Communicable Diseases Intelligence 20(22):478–482

Stroup N E, Zack M M, Wharton M 1994 Sources of routinely collected data for surveillance. In: Teutsch S M, Churchill R E (eds) Principles and Practice of Public Health Surveillance. Oxford University Press, New York pp 31–85

Townson H, Nathan M B, Zaim M et al 2005 Exploiting the potential of vector control for disease prevention. Bulletin of the World Health Organization 83(12):942–947

Vale V, Juno A (eds) Modern Primitives: an investigation of contemporary adornment, Research Publications, San Francisco

Velasco-Garrido M, Busse R, Hisashige A 2003 Are disease management programmes (DMPs) effective in improving quality of care for people with chronic conditions? WHO Regional Office for Europe (Health Evidence Network report), Copenhagen. Available: http://www. euro.who.int/document/e82974.pdf 17 Feb 2008

Weber D J, Rutala W A 2001 Biological basis of infectious disease epidemiology. In: Thomas J C, Weber D J (eds) Epidemiologic Methods for the Study of Infectious Diseases. Oxford University Press, New York, pp 3–27

Weeramanthri T, Hendy S, Connors C et al 2003 The Northern Territory Preventable Chronic Disease Strategy – promoting an integrated and life course approach to chronic disease in Australia. Australian Health Review 26:31–42

World Health Organization 1999 Removing Obstacles to Healthy Development, WHO, Geneva

World Health Organization 2000 Global Strategy for the Prevention and Control of Non-communicable Diseases, Report by the Director General WHA 53/14, Fifty-third World Health Assembly, Geneva. Provisional agenda item 12.11

World Health Organization 2002 Health Care for Chronic Conditions Team: Innovative Care for Chronic Conditions: Building Blocks for Action: Global Report. Geneva, Noncommunicable Diseases and Mental Health, WHO, Geneva

World Health Organization 2003a Global Strategy on Diet, Physical Activity and Health. Available: http://www.who.int/hpr/NPH/docs/gs_global_strategy_general.pdf 17 Feb 2008

World Health Organization 2003b Global Strategy on Diet, Physical Activity and Health – Chronic Disease. Available: http://www.who.int/hpr/NPH/docs/gs_chronic_disease.pdf 17 Feb 2008

World Health Organization 2004 Global Strategic Framework for Integrated Vector Management. WHO, Geneva

World Health Organization 2005a Preventing chronic diseases: a vital investment: WHO global report. Available: http://www.who.int/chp/chronic_disease_report/full_report.pdf 17 Feb 2008

World Health Organization 2005b Noncommunicable Diseases and Mental Health Cluster (NMH). Available: http://www.who.int/noncommunicable_diseases/en/ 17 Feb 2008

World Health Organization 2005c Preparing a workforce for the 21st century: the challenge of chronic conditions. WHO, Geneva

World Health Organization 2006 Communicable disease surveillance and response systems: Guide to monitoring and evaluating WHO/CDS/EPR/LYO/2006.2, WHO, Geneva

Yach D, Hawkes C, Linn Gould C et al 2004 The Global Burden of Chronic Diseases Overcoming Impediments to Prevention and Control. JAMA 291:2616–2622

CHAPTER 11

Health protection

Thomas Tenkate

Learning objectives

After reading this chapter, you should be able to:

- describe environmental health, and how human health can be protected from environmental hazards
- recognise the general tools used to manage environmental health issues
- identify key environmental health issues and how they are managed
- understand the importance of managing our environment in a sustainable manner so as to protect human health.

Introduction

Our understanding of how the environment can impact on human health has evolved and expanded over the centuries, with concern and interest dating back to ancient times. For example, over 4000 years ago, a civilisation in northern India tried to protect the health of its citizens by constructing and positioning buildings according to strict building laws, by having bathrooms and drains, and by having paved streets with a sewerage system (Rosen 1993).

In more recent times, the 'industrial revolution' played a dominant role in shaping the modern world, and with it the modern public health system. This era was signified by rapid progress in technology, the growth of transportation and the expansion of the market economy, which led to the organisation of industry into a factory system. This meant that labour had to be brought to the factories and by the 1820s, poverty and social distress (e.g. overcrowding and infrequent sewage and garbage disposal) was more widespread than ever. These circumstances, therefore, led to the rise of the 'sanitary revolution' and the birth of modern public health (Rosen 1993).

The sanitary revolution has also been described as constituting the beginning of the first wave of environmental concern, which continued until after the Second World War when major advances in engineering and chemistry substantially changed the face of industry, particularly the chemical sector. The second wave of environmental concern came in the mid to late 20th century and was dominated by the environmental or ecology movement. A landmark in this era was the 1962 publication of the book *Silent Spring* by Rachel Carson. This book, for the first time, identified the dramatic effects of the organochlorine pesticide DDT on the ecosystem. The third wave of environmental concern commenced in the 1980s and continues today. The accelerated rate of economic development, the substantial increase in the world population and the globalisation of trade have dramatically changed the production methods and demand for goods in both developed and developing countries. This has led to the rise of 'sustainable development' as a key driver in environmental planning and economic development (Yassi et al 2001).

The protection of health has, therefore, been a hallmark of human history and is the cornerstone of public health practice. This chapter introduces environmental health and how it is managed in Australia, including a discussion of the key generic management tools. A number of significant environmental health issues and how they are specifically managed are then discussed, and the chapter concludes by discussing sustainable development and its links with environmental health.

What is environmental health?

Many people think that environmental health refers to the health of the environment. This view conjures images of wilderness, rivers and oceans and is a term that is synonymous with environmental protection. For others, environmental health is recognised as human health issues associated with poor living conditions, contaminated water and vermin infestation: all old battles that were fought – and generally won – over the past century. Unfortunately, both views are wrong (however, the second view could be considered the 'old' view of environmental health). The easiest way to describe environmental health is to say that it is 'concerned with creating and maintaining environments which promote good public health' (enHealth Council 1999 p 1). There is a large range of definitions of 'environmental health' and a few of these that provide differing perspectives are:

> Those aspects of human health including quality of life, that are determined by physical, chemical, biological and social factors in the environment.
>
> (enHealth Council 1999 p 3)
>
> Refers to the protection against environmental factors that may adversely impact human health or the ecological balances essential to long-term human health and environmental quality, whether in the natural or man-made environment.
>
> (National Environmental Health Association 1996)
>
> Focuses on the health inter-relationships between people and their environment, promotes human health and wellbeing, and fosters a safe and healthful environment.
>
> (Milne 1998)

It is clear from these definitions that environmental health is an integral component of the broad field of 'public health' but also has some overlap with the field of 'environmental protection'. The relationship between these areas is shown in Figure 11.1.

Environmental health management

Environmental health practice has been defined as:

> the assessment, correction, control and prevention of environmental factors that can adversely affect health, as well as the enhancement of those aspects of the environment that can improve human health.
>
> (enHealth Council 1999 p 3)

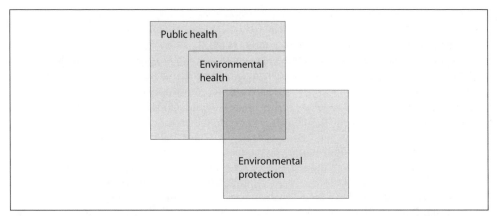

FIGURE 11.1: Relationships between the related fields

(Adapted from: enHealth Council 1999. Copyright Commonwealth of Australia, reproduced by permission)

Due to the nature of environmental health, most environmental health practice is conducted within the government context and is backed up by specific legislation and policy. The three levels of government in Australia each have a specified (and sometimes overlapping) role in providing environmental health services. Examples of the role of each level of government are:

- *federal* – development of national policy (e.g. *National Environmental Health Strategy, National Strategy for Ecologically Sustainable Development,* national food safety standards) and quarantine services
- *state* – enforcement of state legislation (e.g. public health Acts, food Acts, environmental protection Acts), surveillance and monitoring of environmental health issues, and investigation and control of disease outbreaks
- *local* – direct service delivery role; provide infrastructure and policy for environmental health issues at a local level. This includes waste management services, licensing and auditing of food premises, enforcement of environmental protection regulations (e.g. for nuisances), health promotion programs, and planning and development assessment.

Case study: Food safety management in Australia

The complexity of roles played by the various levels of government is highlighted in the following examples that relate to managing food safety in Australia.

Federal: Food Standards Australia New Zealand (FSANZ) is a bi-national independent statutory authority that develops food standards for composition, labelling and contaminants, including microbiological limits, that apply to all foods produced or imported for sale in Australia and New Zealand. The policy guidelines under which FSANZ works are set by the Australia New Zealand Food Regulation Ministerial Council, with the Food Regulation Secretariat within the Australian Department of Health and Ageing responsible for managing the implementation of the regulatory arrangements. The key policy/guideline produced by FSANZ is the *Australia New Zealand Food Standards Code* (FSC). This does not have any legal power itself, but gains legal authority by adoption through state legislation. The Australian Department of Health and Ageing also coordinate *OzFoodNet*, which is a national surveillance system for food-borne illness.

Continued

> ## Case study: Food safety management in Australia—cont'd
>
> *State*: In each state, the FSC is adopted through the state food Act, which is generally administered by the state health department. In Queensland, the *Food Act 2006* is the responsibility of Queensland Health which undertakes the following food safety activities: monitoring and enforcing food standards and food labelling (specified by the FSC), food safety in government premises, food-borne illness surveillance and investigation, and compliant investigation. In addition, Safe Food Queensland is a statutory authority under the Department of Primary Industries and is responsible for food safety in primary production.
>
> *Local*: Local governments are responsible for enforcement of food safety standards in local businesses and licensing and registration of local food businesses. This includes enforcement of the *Food Safety Standards* (Chapter 3 of the FSC; adopted under the Queensland Food Act).

The following generic tools are generally used to manage environmental health at each level of government (Stoneham et al 2004):

- *legislation* – enforcing particular behaviours and standards
- *funding* – encouraging appropriate health-supporting activities and discouraging other activities that are harmful
- *education* – using education, research and communication strategies to provide information and to form the basis for community involvement.

The extent to which each of these tools is used will depend on the environmental health issue being addressed and will be based on appropriate policy development (Stoneham et al 2004). These tools are described diagrammatically in Figure 11.2.

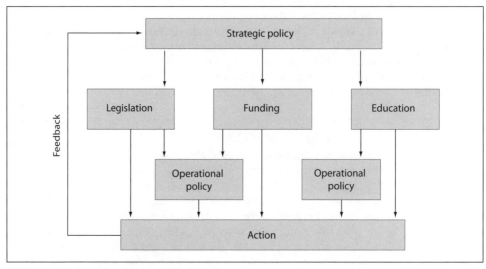

FIGURE 11.2: Tools of the environmental health trade

(Adapted from Stoneham, Dodds & Buckett 2004)

As can be seen from Figure 11.2, each of the tools can be used in response to an overall policy directive (this is usually determined through political processes); however, policies can also be developed to assist in implementing the tools to enable specific actions to be achieved.

Because of the large range of stakeholders (e.g. a multitude of government agencies) involved in environmental health, the *National Environmental Health Strategy* highlighted the need for collaboration between government, community, industry and academia to progress the effective management of environmental health issues. This national strategy stated that 'a major impediment to better environmental health management is the fragmentation of responsibility across a large range of groups'. It goes on to state that 'no single organisation has the capacity to manage environmental health in isolation' and 'improving environmental health in Australia requires all stakeholders and affected groups to recognise their common aspirations, develop common goals, work to strengthen their communication and links, and to forge partnerships on common actions' (enHealth Council 1999 p 12).

Management tools

In addition to the generic tools described above, there are a number of tools that are frequently used to assist environmental health managers in the decision-making process. These specific management tools include risk assessment (and its closely aligned tool, the *Health Impact Assessment*), economic evaluation and environmental/public health indicators. Environmental health risk assessment is the principal tool for providing scientific information into the risk management decision-making process, and is one element of the health impact assessment process, which is predominantly used to assess health impacts related to major development projects. Economic evaluation (particularly cost–benefit and cost–effectiveness analysis) and environmental/public health indicators are relatively new tools for use in environmental health and are gaining wider acceptance in environmental health management.

Legislation

Legislation continues to be the most widely used tool to improve environmental/public health conditions. Under the Australian Constitution the federal government has no direct public health power apart from the power to make laws with respect to quarantine. However, the High Court has broadly interpreted the Commonwealth's powers relating to trade and commerce and as such has enabled federal 'public health' legislation in areas such as: food, therapeutics, tobacco, occupational health and safety, consumer protection and safety, environment and conservation.

The various state and territory constitutions, therefore, provide powers for enacting public health laws, of which environmental health laws are a significant component. Local governments also share responsibility with the state governments for the enforcement and administration of environmental/public health legislation, and they also enjoy the power to make local laws on any matter of good governance for their areas as long as they are consistent with state and federal laws. With such a broad range of legislation and with so many levels of government involved, the opportunity for over-regulation and inconsistent enforcement has led to a number of arrangements being put in place to ensure uniformity and consistency across the states in regard to public health laws and their application.

The use of legislation as a management tool has a long history, with the first dedicated public health Act being the English *Public Health Act 1848*. This was developed in response to high rates of death and illness in the rapidly expanding urban areas of the major cities in the UK. In Australia, Victoria was the first colony to pass a health Act in 1854 and this was very similar to the English law. The need for this Victorian legislation was due to a large increase in migrant numbers, particularly in the goldfield's canvas towns, resulting in disease epidemics due to unsanitary conditions. The other colonies in Australia soon passed similar laws with sanitary controls to prevent the spread of disease.

A more recent development for environmental/public health law is the introduction of risk assessment and risk management as an underlying approach for managing public health issues. Risk management is the process through which risk, once identified and assessed, is dealt with, minimised, monitored and taken account of in decision making. It involves evaluating alternative options and selecting an appropriate action in response to the information derived in the assessment (NPHP 2000). From a legislative perspective, risk can be incorporated in two main ways:

1 *Standard setting* – this is where acceptable exposure or emission standards are developed through a risk assessment process and then incorporated into legislation. In general, public health legislation does not rely on standard setting to any great extent, whereas it is a common element of environmental protection legislation. Examples of public health-related standards are the *National Environmental Protection Measures* (NEPMs) (e.g. for ambient air pollution) and the *Australian Drinking Water Guidelines.*

2 *Administrative controls/decision making* – the power to 'abate' a 'nuisance' and to require action to be taken in cases where a risk to health exists is a traditional public health response and dates back to the earliest public health laws. The modern approach for managing these 'public health risks' is for the legislation to include a proactive framework that identifies the way in which the 'public health risk' is to be identified and assessed prior to the issuing of an 'abatement notice'. The Australian Capital Territory's *Public Health Act 1997* is a good example of this sort of approach, as is the Queensland *Public Health Act 2005.*

The use of risk management within environmental/public health legislation is now well established, with Reynolds (2004 p 168) stating that 'good public health practice must be aware of risk and its management, and it is therefore crucial that laws, which are "friendly to dealing with risk", are developed as the core body of public health laws for the 21st century'.

Risk assessment

There are many approaches for assessing risk; however, risk assessment that focuses on environmental/public health risks has been defined as 'the process of estimating the potential impact of a chemical, physical, microbiological or psychosocial hazard on a specified human population system under a specific set of conditions and for a certain timeframe' (enHealth Council 2004 p xxv). The purpose of undertaking risk assessment has been described as 'to provide pertinent information to risk managers, specifically policymakers and regulators, so that the best possible decisions are made' (Paustenbach 2002 p 4).

In Australia, the Australian Standard *AS/NZS4360:2004 Risk Management* provides a generic framework for risk assessment and risk management. However, this framework takes more of a 'corporate' or 'organisational' approach to risk assessment and risk management, and therefore informs the risk management approaches used in public health, but is not generally used to assess public/environmental health risk. Therefore, the principal framework that we use for assessing and managing environmental/public health risks is the *Australian Framework for Environmental Health Risk Assessment* that was developed by the enHealth Council (2004).

Environmental health risk assessment (EHRA) is a process or a way of thinking for assessing human health risks from exposure to environmental hazards. It is used to help set health-based standards and guidelines (e.g. air pollution, drinking water), and when defined standards are non-existent to assess the health risks from exposure to a particular chemical, product or activity. The EHRA process can also be applied to an existing or proposed scenario or as part of the health impact assessment process. The EHRA process is described diagrammatically in Figure 11.3 and consists of the following steps:

1 *Issue identification* – this step identifies issues relevant to the risk assessment and assists in establishing the context within which the risk assessment will be

undertaken. Issues to be identified include what is the concern (e.g. what are the health effects); what is causing the identified concern (e.g. what is the environmental exposure perceived to be associated with the health effects); why is the concern an issue; is risk assessment appropriate for this issue and in this situation; and what are the public perceptions about the hazard and what is the expected response.

2 *Hazard assessment* – this consists of two parts: hazard identification and dose–response assessment. Hazard identification involves determining what types of adverse health effects might be caused by the implicated agent, and how quickly the adverse health effects might be experienced. Data for hazard identification generally come from human studies (observational and clinical epidemiological studies) and animal studies (toxicological studies on animals where they are exposed to a range of doses and various end points/effects observed). For dose–response assessment, information on the toxicity of the hazardous agent is considered to determine the relationship between various exposure levels and their effects, particularly adverse effects.

3 *Exposure assessment* – this involves determining the magnitude, frequency, extent, character and duration of exposures in the past, at present and in the future. It also includes identifying the exposed populations and potential exposure pathways (e.g. exposure through the air, food, water or soil). A key requirement for conducting exposure assessment is an understanding of the presence (or absence) of the agent and its concentrations and distribution.

4 *Risk characterisation* – this final step in the process seeks to integrate the information from the hazard assessment and exposure assessment steps and describe the risks to individuals and populations in terms of the nature, extent and severity of potential adverse health effects.

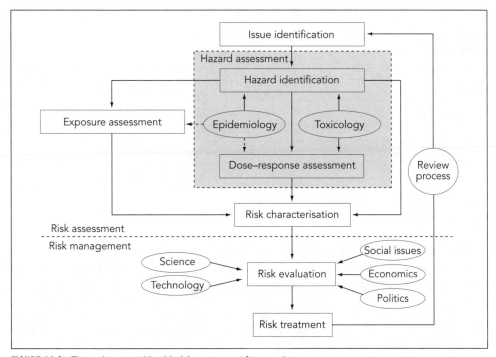

FIGURE 11.3: The environmental health risk assessment framework

(Adapted from enHealth Council 2004. Copyright Commonwealth of Australia, reproduced by permission)

The risk assessment process therefore provides a standard approach for assessing human health risks from environmental exposures, with the outcomes of the assessment providing managers/decision makers with information to: (1) compare the level of risk against predetermined standards or other criteria to determine if the risk is acceptable or not acceptable (i.e. undertake risk evaluation); (2) make decisions about the various options available for addressing the risk and implementing appropriate options (i.e risk treatment); and (3) undertake effective risk communication.

Risk perception and risk communication

From an environmental health management perspective, technical and scientific approaches form the basis of risk assessment. However, much of the social science literature argues that risk is inherently subjective and based on the perceptions held by the individuals involved or affected (Slovic 1997). Therefore, a key issue for risk perception is definition – how each of us defines risk and establishes our own risk priorities. It is widely acknowledged that in addition to the scientific elements that underpin the definition of risk, there are many qualitative aspects of risk that include values, emotions, power relations and the need for action (Sandman 1987). These qualitative aspects of risk have been described in terms of 'outrage factors'. These factors influence a person's perception of the level of risk and include whether the risk is imposed or voluntary, whether the person feels they have some level of control of the risk, and whether the risk is familiar or unfamiliar. Ten of the outrage factors that most often arise in environmental health are listed in Table 11.1.

FACTORS THAT DECREASE RISK	FACTORS THAT INCREASE RISK
Voluntary	Imposed
Control	Lack of control
Fair	Unfair
Ordinary	Memorable
Not dreaded	Dreaded
Natural	Technological, artificial
Certain	Uncertain
Familiar	Unfamiliar
Morally acceptable	Morally unacceptable
Trustworthy source	Untrustworthy source

TABLE 11.1: Outrage factors for individual risk perception
(Source: Blake 1995)

The influence of the outrage factors generally results in very different definitions of risk being held by scientific/technical experts versus that held by the public (Fischhoff et al 1984, Slovic 1987). In particular, the 'technical' models of risk are relatively narrow and quantitatively precise, whereas the 'public' model of risk includes a broad set of qualitative factors relating to the potential seriousness of the issue/mishap, the nature of exposure and their beliefs about the level of knowledge and credibility of science, industry and government (Slovic 1987).

Appropriate risk communication provides a way of bridging the gap between the 'experts' and the public's definitions of risk, particularly in light of the outrage factors

> ### Example: Risk perception of 'experts' versus the 'public'
> In a study by Kraus et al (1992), members of the public and a group of toxicologists were asked to express their attitude and beliefs about chemicals and chemical risk assessment. Examples of the differences in views can be seen in the responses to the following statements: *'If you are exposed to a toxic chemical substance, then you are likely to suffer adverse health effects'* – 32.3% of toxicologists agreed with this statement, whereas 85.5% of the public respondents agreed with the statement: *'There is no safe level of exposure to a cancer-causing agent'* – 25.3% of toxicologists agreed with this statement, whereas 53.9% of lay respondents agreed.

described in the preceding section. Risk communication is more than just disseminating risk information, but involves elements of conflict resolution, public participation and two-way messages. Aakko (2004) states that in the 'traditional' communication model, the risk messages flow in one direction – from regulator to public – but risk communication has to be a two-way process with active participation from both the sender and the audience. In addition, building and maintaining trust between the spokesperson and the audience is a key factor in effective risk communication. Four characteristics that effective spokespeople exhibit in establishing and maintaining trust are: caring and empathy, dedication and commitment, competence and expertise and honesty and openness (Peters et al 1997).

ACTIVITY
- Consider the following scenario: you work for a public health agency and a major chemical fire takes place in your area. Shortly after the fire is extinguished, the local residents start to complain of a range of adverse health effects. A health risk assessment is conducted and this indicates that the health risk posed to the residents is minimal.
- In this scenario, what are the 'perceptions' of risk likely to be held by the residents and the 'experts', and what 'outrage factors' may influence this perception of the risk?

REFLECTION

Scenarios like the one described above are regularly faced by public health agencies. For example, in Sydney a contaminated and disused gasworks site was being cleaned up and some of the perceptions of the risk held by various stakeholders were:
- 'There are no real emissions leaving the site, so there are no real risks to health' (environmental engineers).
- 'People are experiencing health effects, but they can be reassured that these will not cause long-term damage' (health agency).
- 'It is okay for the professionals to think that there is no health risk, because they don't have to live here' (residents).
- 'We are experiencing significant effects on our health and no-one is taking our complaints seriously' (residents).

This case highlights the challenge for public health practitioners to combine 'scientific' information from a risk assessment with qualitative approaches that recognise the differing perceptions of risk held by the various stakeholders (Rutherford 2003).

Health impact assessment

Health Impact Assessment (HIA) has been described as 'a process that systematically identifies and examines, in a balanced way, both the potential positive and negative health impacts of an activity (e.g. policy, program, project or development)' (enHealth Council 2001 p vii). The two key principles that distinguish HIA from other processes are: (1) that it takes the broad World Health Organization (WHO 1948 p 2) view of health, this being that health is 'a state of complete physical, mental and social wellbeing and not merely the absence of disease or infirmity'; and (2) that 'health impacts' can be anything that alters (either positively or negatively) one of the underlying determinants of health. Some of the factors that are normally considered in a HIA are shown in Table 11.2.

General impacts	• Increased demand and/or improvements to public infrastructure (water, sewerage, waste, health, education) • Altered risk from acute hazards (e.g. fires) • Damage to vulnerable ecosystems that impact on human health • Impacts on health or amenity – odour, noise, dust, insects, shade, vibration, etc • Encourage/discourage healthy forms of physical activity
Physical impacts	• Communicable and non-communicable diseases • Exacerbation of existing conditions • Injury, for example, from trauma
Social impacts	• Employment opportunities created or lost • Effects on government revenues • 'Spin-off' effects on local industry • Changes in social conditions • Mental and emotional wellbeing • Opportunities for recreation or socialisation • Increased/decreased isolation of individuals.
Special populations	• The elderly, people with a disability, low-income earners, children, those from a non-English speaking background, Indigenous Australians.

TABLE 11.2: Factors generally considered when undertaking an HIA
(Adapted from: enHealth Council 2001 Health Impact Assessment Guidelines, Commonwealth Department of Health and Aged Care, Canberra)
(Copyright Commonwealth of Australia, reproduced by permission)

HIA is usually undertaken in conjunction with an *Environmental Impact Assessment* (EIA) for a particular project or development. The types of projects/developments for which HIA is applied are usually ones that will have 'significant' impact on the local environment, however, the specific 'triggers' for implementing HIA vary among states. For example, the Tasmanian Government (through the *Environmental Management and Pollution Control Act 1994*) has made the link between HIA and EIA quite clear by giving the director of public health the power to require a HIA as part of an EIA. Undertaking an

HIA should however be more commonplace than is the current experience, particularly as the definition of 'environment' under most state environmental protection Acts identifies ecosystems as including people and communities. As such, any impacts being considered on the environment should include a consideration and assessment of the impacts (e.g. health impacts) on individuals and the community.

Environmental health hazards

There are a range of environmental threats that are *either* independent of human activity and can impair human health by either their presence (e.g. radon, ultraviolet radiation, disease carrying mosquitoes) or absence (e.g. iodine, iron), *or* are a result of human activity (e.g. nitrogen oxides and particulates that come from fossil fuel combustion and can result in air pollution). These threats can be divided into 'traditional hazards' and 'modern hazards'. Traditional hazards are often associated with poverty and a lack of development and include (WHO 1997):

- lack of access to safe drinking water
- inadequate basic sanitation in the household and the community
- food contamination with pathogens
- indoor air pollution from cooking and heating using coal or biomass fuel
- inadequate solid waste disposal
- occupational injury hazards in agriculture and cottage industries
- natural disasters, including floods, droughts and earthquakes
- disease vectors, mainly insects and rodents.

Modern hazards are related to any rapid development that lacks health and environment safeguards, and also to the unsustainable consumption of natural resources. These include (WHO 1997):

- water pollution from populated areas, industry and intensive agriculture
- urban air pollution from motor vehicles, coal power stations and industry
- solid and hazardous waste accumulation
- chemical and radiation hazards following the introduction of industrial and agricultural technologies
- emerging and re-emerging infectious diseases
- deforestation, land degradation and other major ecological change at local and regional levels
- climate change, stratospheric ozone depletion and trans-boundary pollution.

One of the main differences between traditional and modern hazards is that the adverse health outcomes from traditional hazards are often immediate or rather quickly expressed, whereas modern hazards often have a long latency period before the adverse health effect is realised. Differences such as this mean that a variety of management approaches are required to adequately address these issues.

An important concept associated with managing the risks posed by these hazards is risk transition. This term is used to describe the reduction in 'traditional risk' and increase in 'modern risks' that takes place with advances in economic development. However, when environmental health risks are poorly managed, the traditional risks are not adequately eliminated and remain important health threats to the poor and disadvantaged in the community, while the modern risks continue unabated. Whereas, when the environmental health risks are well managed, the traditional risks can be almost completely eliminated and the modern risks can be reduced through effective prevention programs (WHO 1997). Overall, the following are considered to be the basic requirements for a healthy environment:

- clean air
- safe and sufficient water

- adequate and safe food
- safe and peaceful settlements
- safe workplaces
- stable global environment.

Each of these environmental health issues and their current management approaches will now be discussed in the following sections.

Air pollution

Air pollution can be defined as 'the result of emission into the air of hazardous substances at a rate that exceeds the capacity of natural processes in the atmosphere (e.g. rain and wind) to convert, deposit or dilute them' (Yassi et al 2001 p 180). Air pollution can have the following effects:

- *human health effects* – acute respiratory illness, aggravation of pre-existing illnesses (e.g. cardiac or respiratory conditions, asthma), cancers (triggered by pollutants), eye or nose irritation, stress or loss of general wellbeing
- *loss of amenity* – odour, poor visibility, dust and residue deposits on surfaces (e.g. clothes, vehicles)
- *damage to property* – acidic pollutants, deposition of soot and particles
- *effect on the environment* – death or injury to sensitive species, loss of biological diversity, excess nutrient loads in waterways, loss of specific ecosystems, acid rain
- *economic impact* – reduced property values, deterrent to new industries or residents, reduced crop production, loss of tourism, loss of productivity due to illness.

From an environmental/public health perspective, we are mainly interested in the human health effects of air pollution. On a worldwide scale, WHO estimates that over 2.5 million people die each year from indoor and outdoor air pollution (WHO 2002), with many more people suffering from disabling or restrictive health conditions (e.g. asthma and other respiratory conditions). Of particular concern is the household use of biomass fuels and coal by over half of the world's population, exclusively in developing countries, which results in 1.5 million deaths a year from indoor air pollution-related respiratory diseases (Pruss-Ustun & Corvalan 2006). In contrast, developed countries are more concerned about outdoor air pollution, and for Australia the health consequences have been summarised as follows:

> Mortality due to (outdoor) air pollution in Australia is higher than the road toll. Each year on average 2400 deaths are linked to air quality and health issues – more than the 1700 people who die on our roads. That's an average of a death every four hours. This number increases if the long-term effects of air toxics on cancer are included.

> (Beer 2004)

Air quality in Australia is managed by all levels of government. At the national level, uniform air quality standards were agreed to in 1998 by the National Environment Protection Council, which comprises ministers from all states and territories as well as the Commonwealth. The *National Environment Protection Measure for Ambient Air Quality* (Air NEPM) sets maximum levels for six pollutants (carbon monoxide, nitrogen dioxide, photochemical oxidants (as ozone), sulphur dioxide, lead and particles) and goals for their long-term management. The Commonwealth Government also has other programs that directly impact on air pollution, and these include motor vehicle emissions standards and national fuel quality standards.

At a state level, air pollution is generally regulated through environmental protection legislation, which generally adopts or refers to the Air NEPM. At a local level, many councils protect air quality by banning backyard burning/incinerators and requiring developers to minimise burning of land for clearing; effective town planning to keep industry separate from residential areas, with appropriate areas of vegetation buffer zones; and improving public transport services to reduce the use of private cars. Council provision of bikeways and roads with wider verges can also encourage bicycle use.

In addition, it is widely recognised that developing air quality standards should be based on a health risk assessment approach. The NHMRC has recently released guidance on the appropriate use of risk assessment for setting ambient air quality standards. These guidelines recommend the use of the *Environmental Health Risk Assessment* approach developed by the enHealth Council which was discussed in the previous section on environmental health management.

Safe water

The importance of water quality and sanitation for public health has been summarised as follows by WHO's director-general, Dr Lee Jong-wook:

> Water and sanitation is one of the primary drivers of public health. I often refer to it as 'Health 101', which means that once we can secure access to clean water and to adequate sanitation facilities for all people, irrespective of the difference in their living conditions, a huge battle against all kinds of diseases will be won.
>
> (WHO 2004)

As a resource, water is our most important one. However, despite the large amount of water that makes up our planet, only a small amount is suitable and available for drinking. For example, only 2.5% of all the water is fresh water (97.5% is salt water), and of this freshwater, only 0.5% is accessible for drinking because the rest of it is frozen in glaciers or the polar ice caps, or is unavailable in the soil (NHMRC 2004).

For Australia, water is a particularly fragile resource. We are one of the driest continents and have about 1% of the water carried by the world's rivers, despite occupying 5% of the world's land area. In regard to water usage in Australia, agriculture is by far the biggest user,

---

Box 11.1: The global water crisis

The 2006 *Human Development Report* from the United Nations *Development Programme* focussed on the 'global water crisis'. It identified that access to water is a basic human need and a fundamental human right, however, more than 1 billion people are denied access to clean water and 2.6 billion people lack access to adequate sanitation. The human cost of the 'global water crisis' can be seen in the following statistics:

- Approximately 1.8 million children die each year as a result of diarrhoea – which is 4900 deaths a day. This is equivalent to the under-five population in London and New York combined.
- Deaths for diarrhoea in 2004 were about six times greater than the average annual deaths in armed conflict for the 1990s.
- 443 million school days each year are lost to water-related illnesses.
- Millions of women spend up to four hours each day collecting water.
- Almost 50% of all people in developing countries are suffering at any given time from a health problem caused by water and sanitation deficits.

The gulf between rich and poor countries that exacerbates the 'global water crisis' is illustrated in the following statements 'while basic needs vary, the minimum threshold is about 20 litres a day. Most of the 1.1 billion people categorised as lacking access to clean water use about five litres a day – one-tenth of the average daily amount used in rich countries to flush toilets', and 'dripping taps in rich countries lose more water than is available each day to more than 1 billion people' (UNDP 2006).

consuming more than 70% of our water supplies. Some industries are also heavy users, such as manufacturing (around 3%) and electricity and gas production (around 8%). Approximately 8% of water use is in the home. However, despite all of the water supplied to homes being of a drinkable quality, only 1% is used for drinking. The rest is used for cooking, washing clothes, showering and flushing the toilet. Most of the water supplied to households is used on the garden – on average, this is 35% of the water used, but this can reach as high as 90% during some hot and dry summers (NHMRC 2004). Clearly, sustainable water usage should be a key priority for governments, industry and consumers alike.

From a public health perspective, water can be contaminated with pathogenic microorganisms and with a range of chemical and other substances. Water provides the vehicle for spreading a range of communicable diseases and these can be classified as follows (WHO 1992):

- *waterborne diseases* – contamination of water by human/animal faeces or urine infected by pathogenic viruses or bacteria; directly transmitted when water is consumed or used in preparing food (e.g cholera, typhoid)
- *water-washed diseases* – quantity of water; a lack of access to safe water supplies leads to infrequent washing or inadequate personal hygiene that then results in disease/illness (e.g diarrhoeal diseases, eye infections)
- *water-based diseases* – water provides the habitat for intermediate host organisms where parasites can pass through their life cycle; later, these parasites can infect humans in larval forms, by boring into the skin or being injected (e.g. schistosomiasis – a worm carried by snails living in the water)
- *water-related diseases* – water provides the habitat for vectors of disease (e.g. mosquito breeding leading to malaria and dengue fever)
- *water-dispersed infections* – infections can proliferate in water and enter the body through the respiratory tract (e.g. *Legionella* spp.).

Case study: Chemical contamination of drinking water

Groundwater contamination by arsenic is a global health problem of enormous significance. Long-term exposure to arsenic in drinking water is associated with painful and debilitating skin lesions, skin cancers and cancers of the lungs and bladder. Many developing countries rely almost entirely on drinking water from bores and tube-wells; however, in many of these countries the groundwater is contaminated with naturally occurring inorganic arsenic. The country most affected by this is Bangladesh.

Historically, the surface water in Bangladesh has been highly contaminated with microorganisms that have caused a significant burden of disease and mortality. To overcome this problem, UNICEF worked with the Bangladeshi Government in the 1970s to install large numbers of tube-wells, and this endeavour was continued by the private sector during the 1980s. However, at the time when the tube-wells were installed, arsenic was not recognised as a problem in water supplies and so the water from the wells was never tested.

In 1993 arsenic contamination of water from tube-wells was confirmed and it is now estimated that up to 77 million people are at risk of drinking this contaminated water. Unfortunately, the cost of removing or capping the wells is prohibitive and the options for sourcing other safe water are limited. This is now considered to be the largest ever poisoning of an entire population (Smith et al 2000).

Water quality is managed in Australia under the framework established by the *National Water Quality Management Strategy* (NWQMS). The objective of this strategy is the sustainable use of water resources through protecting and enhancing their quality while maintaining economic and social development. Even though managing water resources is a state and territory government responsibility, the NWQMS emphasises the important role of the community in setting and achieving water quality objectives and developing management plans. A key approach of the NWQMS is the development of national guidelines to cover issues across the whole of the water cycle – ambient and drinking water quality, monitoring, groundwater, rural land uses and water quality, storm water, sewerage systems and effluent management for specific industries. Guidance on what constitutes good-quality drinking water is provided by the *Australian Drinking Water Guidelines* (ADWG). The ADWG incorporate a preventive risk management approach and apply to any water intended for drinking, irrespective of its source (municipal supplies, rainwater tanks, bores or point-of-use treatment devices) or where that water is to be used (e.g. in homes and restaurants).

Safe food

Food is a fundamental human need, a basic right and a prerequisite to good health. From an environmental/public health perspective, the supply of both nutritious and safe food to the consumer is vitally important. The following statistics provide a summary of why food safety is important for both public health professionals and the wider community:

- The Australian food industry is a large and integral part of the Australian economy. In 2001–02, consumer spending on food was nearly $75 billion, and exports were over $26 billion (DAFFA 2003).
- There are over 131,500 food businesses in Australia (KPMG 1998).
- It is estimated that there are 4–7 million cases of gastroenteritis each year in Australia caused by contaminated food (Hall et al 2005).
- Food-borne illness results in significant impacts on the health system: 18,000 hospitalisations and 400,000 GP visits in Australia (Food Science Australia & Minter Ellison 2002).
- The cost of food-borne illness in Australia each year is estimated to be more than $1.67 billion (Food Science Australia & Minter Ellison 2002).

There are a number of current factors that are influencing food safety to an increasing extent. These factors include:

- *Centralisation and globalisation* – food is increasingly being produced by larger and larger firms, is being processed by more industrial and mechanical means and is being sold in supermarkets by multinational companies. These factors result in decreased cost per item, an increased variety of food items, and present an increased opportunity to impact large numbers of people if the food is contaminated. This is highlighted in the following example.

Example: The cost of supplying prawns to Scots

A total of 19,000 km is the round-trip journey planned for prawns caught in Scottish waters before they reach British stores. The seafood firm that catches the prawns calculates that hand peeling in Thailand will be cheaper than machine peeling in Scotland with 50c being the hourly wage paid to Thai prawn peelers. The move will mean the loss of 120 jobs in Scotland where workers are paid $11 per hour (Time Magazine 2006).

- *National and trans-national FBI outbreaks* – there is an increasing trend for food-borne illness outbreaks to have national and international impacts, particularly due to the centralisation and globalisation of the food supply process.

- *A widening gap between first and third world countries* – this impacts on food supply, nutrition and safety.
- *An increasing number of emerging pathogens being identified* – some of these have drug-resistant strains that present difficulties for control and treatment.
- *New production technologies are being developed* – these technologies (e.g. genetic modification, antibiotics) help improve efficiencies in the centralisation and globalisation of the food supply, and help to increase production, but the long-term impacts of these technologies are not well understood.
- *Increasing pressures on food supply* – with the world's population predicted to double over the next 50 years, this will require food production to be undertaken in a more sustainable manner.

In Australia, food safety is managed by all levels of government. At a national level, Food Standards Australia New Zealand (FSANZ) is a statutory body tasked to develop food standards, which are generally consistent with international standards. The key document that provides food standards is the *Australia New Zealand Food Standards Code*. This code consists of the following four chapters:

1 *General food standards* – this lists general food standards on issues such as labelling, contaminants and residues, substances allowed to be added to food, and microbial requirements.
2 *Food product standards* – specific standards are provided for a range of food products, including cereals, meat, eggs, fish, dairy products, beverages and special purpose foods (e.g. infant formula).
3 *Food safety standards* – there are four food safety standards and these are adopted through the food Acts of each state. These form the basis of food safety regulation in Australia. The standards cover food safety practices and general requirements, food premises and equipment and food safety programs, and are generally administered by local governments.
4 *Primary production standards* – these are national primary production and processing standards that focus on food safety. Standards are proposed for seafood, meat, dairy, horticulture, honey, eggs and grains.

The built environment

The built environment is 'part of the overall ecosystem of our earth. It encompasses all of the buildings, spaces and products that are created, or at least significantly modified by people. It includes our homes, schools and workplaces, parks, business area and roads. It extends overhead in the form of electric transmission lines, underground in the form of waste disposal sites and subway trains and the country in the form of highways' (Health Canada 1997 p 141).

The built environment is arguably our main environment and, thus, the most important environmental health setting. This is because developed countries (e.g. Australia, the United States and European countries) are 80% urbanised and people spend nearly 90% of their time indoors (plus 5% in cars). Therefore, modifying the built environment will have significant impacts on the health of the public. For example, some of the direct health effects are the availability of shelter, water and food (positive effects), whereas direct negative impacts include indoor and outdoor air pollution, as well as traffic accidents. Indirect health effects result from changes in the natural environment that are due to human modification of or by the built environment. For example, various communicable diseases are predicted to increase due to global warming, which is due to an increase in greenhouse gas emissions that are a result of human activity.

WHO has summarised the impacts of the built environment on health in the following statement:

> The health of a city's people is strongly determined by physical, social, economic, political and cultural factors in the urban environment, including the process of social aggregation, migration, modernisation and industrialisation, and the circumstances of urban living ... the impact of urban processes on health is not just the sum of the effects of the various factors taken individually, since they interact synergistically with each other.

(WHO 1991 p 11)

Urbanisation and urban systems

Urbanisation is the process by which an increasing proportion of the population comes to live in urban areas. In 1999 the world's population reached six billion – three times the population in 1900. It is predicted that there will be a 30% rise in population by 2010, with most of this occurring in developing countries. For example, the urban populations of developing countries are expected to double between 1990 and 2010, so that by 2010 over half of the world's population (four billion people) will live in urban centres. In Australia, over 80% of the population live in major cities and towns, with this population concentrated along the coast.

It is important to view a city or town as consisting of a network of interdependent human systems to meet our needs for raw materials, finished goods and services, and also to dispose of the waste we generate. Some of these systems are:

1 *transportation system* – roads, highways, petrol stations, cars, buses, trucks, airports
2 *energy system* – gas stations, power plants, underground pipes, power lines
3 *water supply* – wells, dams, reservoirs, water treatment plants, pipe network, users
4 *waste management system* – collection services, recycling centres, landfills, sewage treatment plants, hazardous waste facilities.

Unfortunately, it is generally acknowledged that our current urban systems are unsustainable because they produce waste and pollution in excess of the earth's capacity to absorb them, thereby poisoning humans and other species, resulting in climate change, and depleting resources (both renewable and non-renewable). The challenge, therefore, is to revamp the existing infrastructures and build new sustainable infrastructures.

Land use planning

Land use planning establishes the locations of various structures and activities and keeps incompatible uses apart; sustainable land use planning attempts to achieve a more efficient use of land, thereby creating patterns of land use that minimise 'urban sprawl'. Urban sprawl has been described as:

> Haphazard growth or extension outward, especially that resulting from real estate development on the outskirts of a city; or low density, haphazard, car-dependent urban development at or beyond the edges of existing urban service areas.

(Sierra Club – Oklahoma Chapter website)

It is clear that the type of development philosophy that underpins the way development occurs in a region has a significant influence on the sustainability of the area. There are four main types of development; they are described briefly below and are listed in decreasing order of their sustainability:

1 *Compact* – this is a dense type of development and requires the least amount of land to accommodate people and provide services. It helps preserve open space, farmland and nature reserves. Some of the design principles/measures include smaller lots, more efficient placement of house in subdivisions, inner city redevelopment, increase

in multifamily dwellings and a more compact placement of services. Some negatives of this type of development include crowding and potentially unpleasant living conditions.

2 *Satellite* – development is undertaken in outlying communities that are connected to a metropolitan area. A key positive of this type of development is an improved quality of life, but negative aspects include conversion of open space and farmland to housing and increases in commuting time, energy consumption and air pollution.

3 *Corridor* – this involves concentrating housing and business growth along a major transportation corridor. The major negative aspect of this type of development is increased vehicle usage.

4 *Dispersed* – this is the main type of development that is undertaken in most developed countries and typifies 'urban sprawl'. In this case, urban areas indiscriminately take over farmland, forest and grassland. This results in a decreased capacity to produce food, a loss of habitat, an increase in the potential for flooding, poor aesthetic appeal, and increases in travel time, energy consumption and air pollution. In addition, more costly and widespread infrastructure is needed to service this type of development.

One response to urban sprawl is 'smart growth'. This is a set of land use and transportation principles that are the opposite of sprawl. Smart growth recognises connections between development and quality of life and invests time, attention and resources into restoring community and vitality to the centre of cities and in older suburbs. New development under smart growth is more town centred, is transit and pedestrian oriented and has a greater mix of housing, commercial and retail uses. It also preserves open space and many other environmental amenities. However, smart growth recognises that there is no 'one-size-fits-all' solution. Successful communities tend to have one thing in common – a vision of where they want to go and of what things they value in their community – and their plans for development reflect these values (Frumkin et al 2004).

Case study: Urban design, transport and health

Cities are largely shaped by their transport systems and this is primarily due to the 'Marchetti constant' – people do not want to travel more than one hour each day to and from work. As such, for Australian cities, the current urban design and land use patterns mean that many people have no choice but to use a car, with the more sustainable options (e.g. efficient public transport, walking or cycling) often being too difficult to access. In 2006 it was estimated that there were 14.4 million motor vehicles in Australia, with an estimated 209,405 million kilometres each year travelled in these vehicles. This heavy dependency on the car has a range of public health impacts:

- *Road accidents* – there are around 1600 deaths and 22,000 serious injuries associated with motor vehicles each year in Australia. Even though there is a decreasing trend in Australia, the current patterns of industrialisation throughout the world suggests that road accidents will become more prominent as a cause of death and injury.
- *Air pollution* – there is increasing evidence of an association between fine particulate matter and mortality, and so it is considered that the burden of disease from traffic emissions is at least as great as that caused by road accidents.
- *Physical inactivity* – car dependency encourages sedentary lifestyles, with the proportion of trips made by walking, cycling or public transport dropping substantially

in recent times. For example, less than 5% of Australian workers travel to work by bicycle compared with 15% to 20% in European cities. Consequences of this decline in physical activity include increasing bodyweight and cardiovascular disease risk, an increase in diabetes and an association with certain cancers (e.g. colon and breast cancer).

● *Social networks and community connectedness* – the link between strong social networks and health is well established, but busy roads can disrupt and sever communities and heavy use of the car results in fewer people interacting on the streets in the ways that pedestrians and cyclists are able to.

Therefore, from both an environmental and health perspective, significant changes are required in the way we travel within our cities. There are a large number of options for this and these include: more fuel-efficient vehicles; a better public transport system (particularly a substantial increase in light-rail infrastructure); active transport strategies; workplace incentives to reduce car travel such as public transport vouchers instead of company cars, and changing rooms and showers for cyclists; removing economic subsidies that hide the true costs of roads and parking facilities; and of most importance, creative and sustainable approaches to land use planning that help people to access public transport and to live closer to their work, shopping and recreational activities.

(Sources: ABS 2006, ATSB 2005, Davis et al 2005, Newman 2004, Woodward et al 2002)

The occupational environment

The workplace can be thought of as a localised subset of the larger environment, a setting in which people become exposed to environmental hazards while they earn their living. The occupational environment is particularly complex and important because (Perry & Hu 2005):

- Work remains the central activity in which most people throughout the world spend most of their time outside of the home.
- Many hazardous substances are experienced at their highest level in the workplace.
- The workplace represents a broad range of exposures, from acute chemical poisoning to catastrophic injuries, from long-term chemical effects to psychological stress.
- Occupational health is not only a subset of public health, it is also a subset of industrial relations, which consists of complex inter-relationships between politics, power, history, justice and law.
- The workplace setting provides many opportunities for health interventions, from health education to medical screening.

To clarify some of the key links between environmental health and occupational health, Yassi et al (2001) describe the following aspects of the occupational environment:

- The workforce of a country is the backbone of its development. Therefore, a healthy workforce increases productivity and generates wealth that is necessary for the good health of the community at large.
- Health concerns in the occupational and general environments often have the same or similar source of hazard. As such, a coordinated approach to addressing particular issues may be needed and may also be the most effective way of dealing with the issue.
- As workplace exposures are generally significantly higher than similar exposures in the general community, the workplace provides the role of a sentinel for environmental health hazards. As such, many studies that have investigated workplace exposures have had wide ranging implications for protecting the health of the general public.

- To adequately assess health impacts and dose–response relationships, the sum of all exposures needs to be measured. As people spend a significant amount of their life at work, exposures in the workplace, at their home and in the community need to be considered when investigating health impacts. These impacts may not only be on the worker themselves, but may include exposures to other family members that result from secondary exposure at home following exposure at work.

On a global scale, it has been estimated that occupational injuries and illnesses kill between 1.9 and 2.2 million people each year, which is a number that exceeds the death toll from traffic crashes and war combined (International Labour Organization 2004). Unfortunately, a disturbing development of globalisation is that there is a continuing transfer of hazards from developed countries to developing countries who have inadequate safeguards for workers (Perry & Hu 2006).

Occupational health and safety issues are primarily managed through state-based legislation with this being similar throughout Australia and also having a number of similarities with legislation in other developed countries. This includes legislative requirements that impose 'duties of care' or 'obligations' on both employers and employees in regard to safe work places and safe work practices. In addition, risk assessment and risk management principles provide the basis for this legislation as well as for many of the key prevention and protection approaches that are adopted in this setting.

Case study: Sun exposure and outdoor workers

With Australia having the highest incidence of skin cancers in the world and with an estimated 1.2 million outdoor workers, occupational exposure to solar ultraviolet (UV) radiation is a significant public health issue. This issue gains more significance when it is considered that it is estimated that around 200 melanomas and 34,000 skin cancers per year are caused by occupational UV exposure, and that outdoor workers are often inadequately protected and exposed to extremely high UV levels.

The legal obligations and risk management approaches discussed in this section mean that workplaces should have a comprehensive sun protection program that includes:

- having a written sun protection policy
- reducing the amount of time outdoor workers spend in the sun
- providing and maintaining equipment needed to protect workers from the sun
- information, training and supervision to reduce UV exposure
- evaluation of the effectiveness of the sun protection program to identify if any changes are needed to further reduce UV exposure.

(Source: Cancer Council Australia 2007)

The global environment

Throughout this chapter, the dependency of human life and wellbeing on the environment in which we live has been continuously discussed. Unfortunately, we are currently experiencing the start of a global ecological crisis, the outcomes of which are predicted to have a significant impact on our way of life in the coming century. The factors for this crisis should hopefully be obvious by now, but some of the fundamental reasons are (Yassi et al 2001):

- rapid technological development in the developed world has and is introducing new potential hazards

- rapid population growth and industrial development, based largely on obsolete technologies in the developing world, is accelerating existing environmental degradation
- environmental degradation is being aggravated by poverty, urbanisation without adequate infrastructure, rural development policies that do not strengthen local economies and a limited economic base that is dependent on commodity prices.

The global nature of this environmental degradation is a new phenomenon for humans to deal with. Previously localised environmental problems (e.g. air pollution) are now becoming widespread, regional and global, and are affecting areas that are not the sources of the pollution. In addition, the economic and political systems that create and sustain these problems are now influenced by the global marketplace, which is beyond the capacity of individual governments to regulate effectively.

In the past, the ecological systems of the planet (particularly local systems) have been capable of adapting to the changes forced onto them by human development. However, these changes are now producing an imbalance in global systems (e.g. climate), and the actual long-term outcomes of these changes are hard to comprehend.

Global environmental change is being observed in a range of systems, with the main systems affected being climate, stratospheric ozone, land, freshwater, biodiversity and general functioning of the world's ecosystems. Unfortunately for humans, we are at the centre of all of these systems and so the adverse impacts on each of these systems will affect us directly and synergistically. The inter-relationships between the major types of environmental change are shown in Figure 11.4.

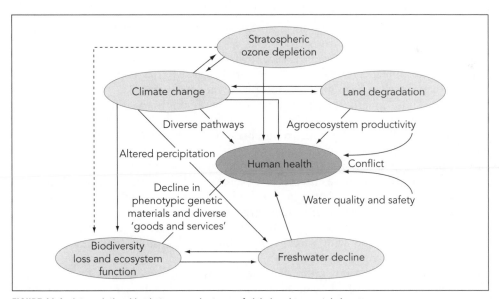

FIGURE 11.4: Inter-relationships between major types of global environmental change

(Source: McMichael et al 2003)

Given the magnitude of this issue, it is too broad and complex to cover in great detail in this component of the chapter. As such, we will therefore focus on climate change as it is the issue that attracts most of the political and public attention.

Global climate change

Global climate change has been defined as 'a change of climate which is attributed directly or indirectly to human activity that alters the composition of the global atmosphere and which is in addition to natural climate variability observed over comparable time periods' (United Nations 1992 p 3).

This definition highlights that it is human activity that is altering the world's climate, primarily through the production of 'greenhouse' gases that amplify the natural 'greenhouse effect' that makes Earth habitable. Greenhouse gases (e.g. carbon dioxide, methane and nitrous oxide) are naturally present at low concentrations in the lower atmosphere and keep Earth's mean surface temperature at around 15°C. Without this trapping of heat, the mean air temperature would be –18°C. However, greenhouse gas concentrations have been increasing rapidly due to increased combustion of fossil fuels, increased deforestation, irrigated agriculture, animal husbandry, coal mining, cement manufacture and a range of other human activities. Unfortunately, the warming effects of these gases are much larger than atmospheric cooling caused by aerosols. This has resulted in Earth's climate now being warmer than at any time since records were kept, with the 1990s the warmest decade in the past 1000 years.

The Intergovernmental Panel on Climate Change has concluded that the global average surface temperature is projected to rise by 1.1 to 6.4°C between 1990 and 2100, with this being a two to 15 times greater increase than in the previous 100 years (IPCC 2007a). Carbon dioxide is responsible for more than 60% of this enhanced 'greenhouse effect', with current annual emissions at more than 23 billion metric tonnes and carbon dioxide levels having risen more than 30% since 1800 (IPCC 2001).

Currently observed changes in climate

Carbon dioxide is the most important anthropogenic greenhouse gas and its atmospheric concentration has increased from a pre-industrial value of about 280 ppm to 379 ppm in 2005 (see Fig 11.5). This 2005 value exceeds by far the natural range over the past 650,000 years, with the annual carbon dioxide concentration growth rate being larger in the past 10 years than since the beginning of atmospheric measurements. The primary source of the increased atmospheric concentration of carbon dioxide is fossil fuel use, with land-use change providing another significant but smaller contribution.

The IPCC (2007a) have compiled a number of key facts in relation to climate change including:

- The atmospheric concentrations of the other significant greenhouse gases, methane and nitrous oxide, have also increased substantially since pre-industrial values.
- Eleven of the 12 years between 1995 and 2006 rank among the 12 warmest years since surface temperatures were first recorded in 1850.
- There has been a linear upward trend for global surface temperatures of around 0.13°C per decade, with a total temperature increase from 1850–1899 to 2001–2005 of 0.76°C.
- Average surface temperatures of the oceans have increased, with the oceans absorbing more than 80% of the heat added to the climate system. Such warming causes the seawater to expand, contributing to sea level rise.
- Mountain glaciers and snow cover have declined on average in both hemispheres.
- Losses from the ice sheets of Greenland and Antarctica have very likely contributed to sea level rise between 1993 and 2003.
- Global average sea level rose at an average rate of 1.8 mm per year between 1961 and 2003, with a faster rate of 3.1 mm per year between 1993 and 2003.

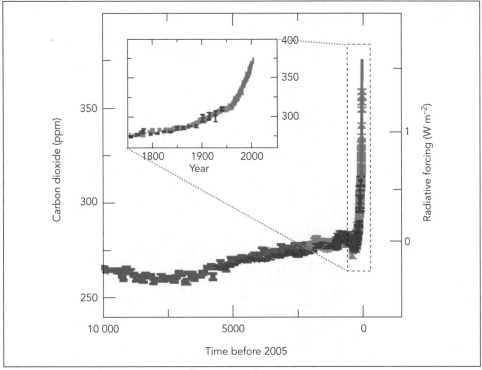

FIGURE 11.5: Changes in atmospheric concentrations of carbon dioxide over the past 10,000 years

(Source: IPCC 2007a Climate Change 2007, Figure SPM1, p 3)

- Average arctic temperatures have increased at almost twice the global average rate in the past 100 years.
- More intense and longer droughts have been observed over wider areas since the 1970s, particularly in the tropics and subtropics.
- The frequency of heavy precipitation events has increased over most land areas.
- Widespread changes in extreme temperatures have been observed in the past 50 years. Cold days, cold nights and frost have become less frequent, while hot days, hot nights and heat waves have become more frequent.

Some of the projected impacts of the observed and predicted climate changes are described in Table 11.3 for a range of sectors, including for human health.

Managing climate change

The principal organisation responsible for monitoring and assessing climate change is the Intergovernmental Panel on Climate Change (IPCC). This was established in 1988 by the World Meteorological Organization (WMO) and the United Nations Environment Program (UNEP) to assess scientific, technical and socioeconomic information relevant for the understanding of climate change, its potential impacts and options for adaptation and mitigation. The IPCC is an intergovernmental body that is open to all member countries of the UNEP and of WMO.

The main IPCC products are assessment reports, special reports, methodology reports and technical papers. Each IPCC report includes a 'summary for policymakers' published in all official UN languages. These summaries reflect the state-of-the-art understanding of the subject matter and are written so that they are comprehensible to the non-specialist. The most current assessment report is the fourth assessment report, *Climate Change 2007*.

PHENOMENON	LIKELIHOOD OF FUTURE TRENDS	EXAMPLES OF MAJOR PROJECTED IMPACTS			
		AGRICULTURE	WATER RESOURCES	HUMAN HEALTH	INDUSTRY, SETTLEMENT AND SOCIETY
Over most land areas, warmer and fewer cold days and nights, warmer and more frequent hot days and nights	Virtually certain	Increased yields in colder environments; decreased yields in warmer environments; increased insect outbreaks	Effects on water resources relying on snow melt; effects on some water supply	Reduced human mortality from decreased cold exposure	Reduced energy demand for heating; increased energy demand for cooling; declining air quality in cities; reduced disruption to transport due to snow, ice; effects on winter tourism
Warm spells/heat waves; frequency increases over most land areas	Very likely	Reduced yields in warmer regions due to heat stress; wild fire danger increase	Increased water demand; water quality problems (e.g. algal blooms)	Increased risk of heat-related mortality, especially for the elderly, chronically sick, very young and socially isolated	Reduction in quality of life for people in warm areas without appropriate housing; impacts on elderly, very young and poor
Heavy precipitation events; frequency increases over most areas	Very likely	Damage to crops; soil erosion, inability to cultivate land due to water logging of soils	Adverse effects on quality of surface and groundwater; contamination of water supply; water scarcity may be relieved	Increased risk of deaths, injuries, infectious, respiratory and skin diseases	Disruption of settlements, commerce, transport and societies due to flooding; pressures on urban and rural infrastructures; loss of property

Area affected by drought increases	Likely	Land degradation, lower yields/crop damage and failure; increased livestock deaths; increased risk of wildfire	More widespread water stress	Increased risk of food and water shortage; increased risk of malnutrition; increased risk of water- and food-borne diseases	Water shortages for settlements, industry and societies; reduced hydropower generation potentials; potential for population migration
Intense tropical cyclone activity increases	Likely	Damage to crops; uprooting of trees; damage to coral reefs	Power outages cause disruption of public water supply	Increased risk of deaths, injuries, water- and food-borne diseases; post-traumatic stress disorders	Disruption by flood and high winds; withdrawal of risk coverage in vulnerable areas by private insurers, potential for population migrations, loss of property
Increased incidence of extreme high sea level (excludes tsunamis)	Likely	Salinisation of irrigation water, estuaries and freshwater systems	Decreased freshwater availability due to saltwater intrusion	Increased risk of deaths and injuries by drowning in floods; migration-related health effects	Costs of coastal protection versus costs of land-use relocation; potential for movement of populations and infrastructure; also see tropical cyclones above

TABLE 11.3: Example of the possible impacts of climate change due to projected extreme weather and climate events

(Source: IPCC 2007b Climate Change 2007, Figure SPM1, p 18)

Further details on all reports and the activities of the IPCC can be found on their website, which is listed at the end of this chapter.

As climate change is a global issue, international agreement is necessary to appropriately manage such an enormous issue. In 1992 the world's governments came together and developed the UN *Framework Convention on Climate Change*. The objective of this convention was 'stabilisation of atmospheric concentrations of greenhouse gases at levels that would prevent "dangerous" human interference with the climate system' (UN 1992 p 4). These levels (which were not quantified at the time) were to be achieved within a timeframe to allow ecosystems to adapt naturally to climate change to ensure that food production was not threatened and to enable economic development to proceed in a sustainable manner. Industrialised countries that have contributed the most to climate change (that is, the United States, Australia, the United Kingdom and European Union nations) agreed to a non-legally binding aim of reducing greenhouse gas emissions to 1990 levels by 2000. These countries were known as 'Annex 1 countries'.

By 1997, it was apparent that these targets were not close to being achieved. The international community once again came together and developed the *Kyoto Protocol*. Under this protocol, the Annex 1 countries agreed to individual emissions targets, with these adding up to a total reduction in greenhouse emissions of at least 5% (of 1990 levels) by 2008 to 2012. For most countries this meant a reduction in emissions, but a few countries (e.g. Norway, Iceland and Australia) were allowed increases in their emissions.

Unfortunately, the conditions that were set under which the *Kyoto Protocol* would become law meant that it took a long time for the protocol to come into force. The *Kyoto Protocol* finally became legally binding on its parties from 16 February 2005. At that time, 150 states and regional economic integration organisations had ratified/approved the protocol. Currently, only three industrialised countries have not ratified the protocol: Liechtenstein, Monaco and the United States, with the United States accounting for around one-third of all the greenhouse gas emissions.

Under the *Kyoto Protocol*, a large number of industrialised countries have legally binding targets for reducing/limiting their greenhouse gas emissions. An international carbon trading market has been formalised, a 'clean development mechanism' is now operating to provide investment in developing-country projects, and an 'adaptation fund' has also commenced that will assist developing countries to cope with the negative effects on industry of the reduction in emissions.

Given the nature of the issue, it is understandable that the politics of climate change is constantly changing because of new scientific information and changing public sentiment. For Australia, this was most clearly seen in 2007 when there was a change in federal government and the new prime minister ratified the *Kyoto Protocol* as the first official act of the new Australian Government. Even though the previous federal government did not ratify the *Kyoto Protocol*, it did develop a national greenhouse strategy that described how Australia would still meet the Kyoto targets. At the time of writing, a new national strategy for climate change has not been developed, but the government has indicated that the strategy will consist of the following key elements (Wong 2008):

- *reducing greenhouse gas emissions* – the government has committed to a longer term target of a 60% reduction in greenhouse gases by 2050 (based on 2000 levels), with a medium term target currently being determined
- *climate change adaption* – implementing strategies to adapt to the inevitable changes in climate that will occur and which will impact on the economy, human amenity and the environment
- *global solution* – recognising that climate change is a global problem that requires global cooperation and global solutions. With ratifying the *Kyoto Protocol*, Australia

is now able to fully engage in international negotiations, and the government has committed to working towards a post-Kyoto agreement for addressing climate change.

The key strategy to reduce greenhouse emissions is an 'emissions trading scheme' that is planned to commence in 2010. The proposed scheme will be a 'cap and trade' scheme in which an overall cap on emissions will be set by issuing a set number of permits, and allowing industry to trade these permits, thereby putting a price on carbon. A key input into this process is the *Garnaut Review*, which is to examine the impacts of climate change on the Australian economy and to recommend medium and long-term policies to improve the prospects for sustainable prosperity. In addition to these national approaches to climate change, each state in Australia also has its own greenhouse strategy, with the federal and state governments also working cooperatively to implement a national 20% renewable energy target.

It should be noted that due to the politics surrounding this issue, it took eight years to get the required number of countries to ratify the *Kyoto Protocol* and thus bring it into force. As the conditions of the *Kyoto Protocol* expire in 2012, concerted efforts are needed to ensure that new targets are in place by this date. Encouragingly, with the increasing public and political pressures that are evident worldwide, most countries have identified the critical need to cooperate to ensure a smooth transition to new global climate change regulations. Further details on the rapidly changing landscape of climate change politics can be found at the websites listed at the end of this chapter.

Environmental health and sustainable development

It is clear from the preceding sections that human activity has had a significant impact on biodiversity and on most of the world's ecosystems. It is also clear that the current level of human impact on the environment is unsustainable for both the environment and people. The concept of 'sustainability' therefore assists us to manage and measure the human impacts on the environment. As with most terminology, there are a range of definitions to describe sustainability, but a good definition is:

> It is a balance that integrates: protection of the ecological processes and natural
> systems at local, regional, state and national levels; and, economic development;
> and maintenance of the cultural, economic, physical, and social wellbeing of
> people and communities.
>
> (Queensland Integrated Planning Act 1997 p 36)

The term 'sustainable development' was originally conceived by the 1987 World Commission on Environment and Development (the 'Brundtland Commission'), and was defined as 'development that meets the needs of the present without compromising the ability of future generations to meet their own needs' (WCED 1987 p 54).

This definition was initially developed to bring 'environmental' issues into the mainstream of development, recognising that in order to address the escalating problems related to the environment, the root causes that lay in the broader development process and the global economic system needed to be addressed. This concept has since been broadened, in recognition of the non-environmental aspects of sustainability, and the non-economic aspects of development.

Even though people often think of sustainable development as an 'environmental protection' approach, an underlying concept of sustainable development is that the goals of sustainable development cannot be achieved when there is a high prevalence of debilitating illnesses (e.g. diseases of poverty), and the health of the population cannot be maintained without 'ecologically' sustainable development. In this respect 'ecological' has both social (as in social capital) as well as physical (as in natural capital) dimensions.

Therefore, if development occurs in unsustainable ways, population health gains may accompany improving economic conditions in the short term, but the health gains might not be sustainable in the long term. Thus, time scales matter with sustainable development and health.

Measuring ecosystem sustainability

There are a number of measures that are used to describe how 'sustainable' a country or nation might be, however, there is much debate about which measure is the most appropriate. As always, each measure has its strengths as well as its limitations. A key consideration in measuring sustainability is that it is a characteristic of dynamic systems and so it will always be difficult to measure at a fixed point in time.

The ecological footprint is one of the earliest attempts to measure sustainability and is based on the concept of 'carrying capacity'. This is defined as 'the maximum rate of resource consumption and waste discharge that can be sustained indefinitely in a given region without progressively impairing the functional integrity and productivity of relevant ecosystems' (Rees 1992 p 125). As many regions and nations require land areas that exceed their natural boundaries and depend on trade to supply their needs, they therefore are impacting on the resources and carrying capacity of other countries.

To account for this, a measure described as an 'appropriated carrying capacity', or ecological footprint, was developed. This is considered to be a measure of how much land area is required by an individual/city/region/nation both to produce all the natural resources they consume and to absorb all the waste generated using existing technology (Wackernagel et al 1993). The ecological footprint approach therefore provides a link between consumption patterns of a population, the environmental impact and sustainability.

The ecological footprint is described in terms of hectares/person for each nation. For example, a five-hectare footprint would mean that five hectares of biologically productive space (with world average productivity) are in constant production to support the average individual of that country. If the footprint exceeds the available biologically productive area of the country, it runs an ecological deficit. In this case, the country's area alone cannot provide sufficient ecological services to satisfy its population's current patterns of consumption. A selection of ecological footprints for countries is shown in Table 11.4.

COUNTRY	FOOTPRINT (HA/CAP)	BIOCAPACITY (HA/CAP)	ECOLOGICAL DEFICIT (-) OR RESERVE (+) (HA/CAP)
Australia	6.6	12.4	5.9
China	1.6	0.8	−0.9
Germany	4.5	1.7	−2.8
Bolivia	1.3	15.0	13.7
Republic of Korea	4.1	0.5	−3.5
United States	9.6	4.7	−4.8
World	2.2	1.8	−0.5

TABLE 11.4: Ecological footprints for selected countries – 2003 data

(Source: Global Footprint Network 2006)

This table illustrates that Australia has the second highest ecological footprint of all the nations analysed, however, due to the availability of a large amount of natural resources we do not have an ecological deficit. Unfortunately, other countries, such as the Republic of Korea and Germany, also have high resource consumption rates, but do not have any local capacity, resulting in a large deficit in ecological resources. It should also be noted that the world average is in deficit and this deficit is predicted to increase dramatically due to the rapid industrialisation/westernisation of China and India.

The ecological footprint concept can also be applied to individuals and you can calculate your own footprint by using a range of programs, including the website provided in the following activity. However, be prepared to be shocked at the results, as these will probably indicate that your resource consumption is substantially more than what can be sustained.

ACTIVITY

- Calculate your own ecological footprint by answering the questions provided on the following website:
  www.earthday.net/footprint
- Once you have calculated your own footprint, make up some data for someone who you feel has an 'environmentally friendly' lifestyle (e.g. someone living on a commune dedicated to the environment) and compare the outcome.

Arguably, the most comprehensive assessment of sustainability is the *Environmental Sustainability Index* (ESI). The ESI benchmarks the ability of nations to protect the environment over the next several decades. It does so by integrating 76 data sets – tracking natural resource endowments, past and present pollution levels, environmental management efforts and the capacity of a society to improve its environmental performance – into 21 indicators of environmental sustainability. These indicators permit comparison across a range of issues that fall into the following five broad categories:

1 environmental systems
2 reducing environmental stresses
3 reducing human vulnerability to environmental stresses
4 societal and institutional capacity to respond to environmental challenges
5 global stewardship.

The higher a country's ESI score, the better positioned it is to maintain favourable environmental conditions into the future. Currently, the five highest-ranking countries are Finland, Norway, Uruguay, Sweden and Iceland – all countries that have substantial natural resource endowments and low population density. The lowest ranking countries are North Korea, Iraq, Taiwan, Turkmenistan and Uzbekistan. These countries face numerous issues, both natural and manmade, and have not managed their policy choices well (Esty et al 2005). More detail on the ESI is available from their website that is listed at the end of this chapter.

A final word

This chapter has provided an introduction to what environmental health is, some of the key environmental health issues faced in Australia and in other countries, and the various tools and approaches used to manage these issues. In Australia, environmental health activities are primarily undertaken by all levels of government, with legislation and policy being the main tools through which environmental health conditions are improved, and with risk assessment underpinning many of the regulatory approaches now used.

Hopefully this chapter has reinforced how dependent human life and wellbeing is on the environment in which we live. Despite a slow start, we are starting to accept and realise the potential implications of the global ecological crisis we are facing and that it is arguably the greatest challenge faced by the world today. However, the history of environmental health has shown that we have been able to develop effective strategies to address issues of the time and so we should be optimistic that solutions to the enormous and complex challenges that we now face are within our reach, as long as there is enhanced community and political support that emphasises the motto 'think globally, act locally'. Overall, the importance of environmental health is nicely summarised in the following quotation:

> Human health ultimately depends on society's capacity to manage the interaction between human activities and the physical and biological environment in ways that safeguard and promote health but do not threaten the integrity of the natural systems on which the physical and biological environment depends.

(WHO 1992)

REVIEW QUESTIONS

1 If someone said to you that environmental health related only to the health of the environment, are they correct and what would you say to them in response?
2 What is the role of government in managing environmental health and what are the general management tools they use?
3 How is the process of risk assessment incorporated into legislation and can you provide an example of an environmental health issue in which this approach is used?
4 Can you describe the concept of risk transition as it relates to environmental health hazards?
5 What are the adverse effects of air pollution?
6 How is water quality and quantity related to human health?
7 For the city you live in, can you identify the various human systems that have been established, and are there any examples of 'urban sprawl'?
8 What impacts do you think global climate change will have on your lifestyle during your lifetime and what actions can you take to promote sustainability?

USEFUL WEBSITES

Australian Business Roundtable on Climate Change: www.businessroundtable.com.au
Australian Drinking Water Guidelines: http://www.nhmrc.gov.au/publications/synopses/eh19syn.htm
Australian Institute of Environmental Health (professional association): www.aieh.org.au
Department of Climate Change: www.greenhouse.gov.au
Department of the Environment, Water, Heritage and the Arts (Australia): www.environment.gov.au
enHealth Council: http://enhealth.nphp.gov.au
Environment Protection and Heritage Council: www.ephc.gov.au
Environmental Health (free access journal): www.ehjournal.net
Environmental Health Perspectives (journal): www.ehponline.org
Environmental Protection Agency (United States): www.epa.gov
Environmental Sustainability Index: http://sedac.ciesin.columbia.edu/es/esi/
Food Standards Australia New Zealand: www.foodstandards.gov.au
Garnaut Climate Change Review: www.garnautreview.org.au
Global Footprint Network: www.footprintnetwork.org
Human Development Reports: http://hdr.undp.org/en/
Inter-Governmental Panel on Climate Change: www.ipcc.ch
National Center for Environmental Health (US Centers for Disease Control and Prevention): www.cdc.gov/nceh
National Institute of Environmental Health Sciences (USA): www.niehs.nih.gov
OzFoodNet: www.ozfoodnet.org.au

Smart Growth Online: www.smartgrowth.org

Sustainable Development Gateway (Australian Broadcasting Commission): www.abc.net.au/
science/sustainable

United Nations Division for Sustainable Development: www.un.org/esa/sustdev

World Health Organization, Public Health and Environment homepage: www.who.int/phe/en/

REFERENCES

Aakko E 2004 Risk communication, risk perception, and public health. Wisconsin Medical
Journal 103(1):25–27

ABS 2006 2006 Survey of motor vehicle use. Australian Bureau of Statistics, Canberra

ATSB 2005 Road crash casualties and rates, Australia, 1925 to latest year. Australian Transport
Safety Bureau, Canberra

Australian Greenhouse Office (AGO) 1998 The National Greenhouse Strategy: Strategic
Framework for Advancing Australia's Greenhouse Response. Australian Greenhouse Office,
Canberra

Beer T 2004 Air Pollution Death Toll Needs Solutions, CSIRO Atmospheric Research, 2 March.
Available: http://www.csiro.au/files/mediaRelease/mr2004/PrAirPollution2.htm 10 Jan 2006

Blake E R 1995 Understanding outrage: How scientists can help bridge the risk perception gap.
Environmental Health Perspectives supps 103(supp. 6):123–125

Cancer Council Australia 2007 Media release: Sun is a deadly risk for outdoor workers
says Cancer Council, 20 November. Available: http://www.cancer.org.au/Newsmedia/
mediareleases/mediareleases2007/20November2007.htm 9 Feb 2008

Davis A, Cavill N, Rytler H et al 2005 Making the case: improving health through transport.
Health Development Agency, London

Department of Agriculture, Fisheries and Forestry 2003 Australian Food Statistics 2003.
Department of Agriculture, Fisheries and Forestry, Canberra

enHealth Council 1999 National Environmental Health Strategy. enHealth Council,
Canberra. Available: http://www.health.gov.au/internet/wcms/Publishing.nsf/Content/
C642C824473E84D3CA256F190004250C/$File/envstrat.pdf

enHealth Council 2001 Health Impact Assessment Guidelines, Commonwealth Department of
Health and Aged Care, Canberra. Available: http://enhealth.nphp.gov.au/council/pubs/pdf/
hia_guidelines.pdf

enHealth Council 2004 Environmental Health Risk Assessment: Guidelines for Assessing
Human Health Risks from Environmental Hazards. Commonwealth Department of Health
and Ageing, Canberra. Available: http://enhealth.nphp.gov.au/council/pubs/pdf/envhazards.
pdf

Esty D C, Levy M, Srebotnjak T et al 2005 2005 Environmental Sustainability Index:
Benchmarking National Environmental Stewardship. Yale Center for Environmental Law &
Policy, New Haven

Fischhoff B, Watson S, Hope C 1984 Defining risk. Policy Sciences 17:123–139

Food Science Australia & Minter Ellison 2002 National Risk Validation Project: Final Report.
Department of Health and Ageing, Canberra

Frumkin H, Frank L, Jackson R 2004 From urban sprawl to health for all, Urban Sprawl and
Public Health: Designing, Planning and Building for Healthy Communities. Island Press,
Washington DC, pp 201–222

Global Footprint Network 2006 Ecological Footprint and Biocapacity. Available: http://www.
footprintnetwork.org/download.php?id=305 14 Feb 2008

Hall G, Kirk M D, Becker N et al 2005 Estimating foodborne gastroenteritis. Emerging
Infectious Diseases 11(8):1257–1264. Available: http://www.cdc.gov/ncidod/EID/vol11no08/
pdfs/04-1367.pdf

Health Canada 1997 Health and Environment: Partners for Life. Health Canada, Ottawa

International Labour Organization 2004 Global Estimates of Fatalities Caused by Work-Related Diseases and Occupational Accidents, 2002. Available: http://www.ilo.org/public/english/protection/safework/accidis/globest_2002/dis_world.htm

IPCC 2001 Climate Change 2001: Synthesis report – a contribution of working groups I, II, and II to the Third Assessment Report of the Intergovernmental Panel on Climate Change. Cambridge University Press, Cambridge

IPCC 2007a Climate Change 2007: The physical science basis. Contribution of Working I to the Fourth Assessment Report of the Intergovernmental Panel on Climate Change. Cambridge University Press, Cambridge

IPCC 2007b Climate Change 2007: Impacts, Adaptation and Vulnerability. Contribution of Working II to the Fourth Assessment Report of the Intergovernmental Panel on Climate Change. Cambridge University Press, Cambridge

KPMG 1998 Food Regulation: Current Costs to State and Local Governments, KPMG Management Consulting Pty Ltd report to the Australia New Zealand Food Authority, October

Kraus N, Malmfors T, Slovic P 1992 Intuitive toxicology: Expert and lay judgements of chemical risks. Risk Analysis 12:215–232

McMichael A J, Campbell-Lendrum D H, Corvalan C F (eds) 2003 Climate Change and Human Health: Risks and Responses. World Health Organization, Geneva

Milne TL 1998 National Association of County and City Health Officials (personal communication). In: An Ensemble of Definitions of Environmental Health, US Department of Health and Human Services. Available: http://web.health.gov/environment/DefinitionsofEnvHealth/ehdef2.htm

National Environmental Health Association 1996 Definition of environmental health. Adopted April 1996. Available: http://www.neda.org/position_papers/def_env_health.html

National Health and Medical Research Council 2004 Water Made Clear: A Consumer Guide to Accompany the Australian Drinking Water Guidelines 2004. Australian Government, Canberra

National Public Health Partnership 2000 The Application of Risk Management Principles in Public Health Legislation. NPHP, Melbourne. Available: http://www.nphp.gov.au/publications/legislation/riskmgtrep.pdf

Newman P 2004 Sustainable transport for sustainable cities, United Nations Asia-Pacific Leadership Forum: Sustainable Development for Cities, Hong Kong. Available: http://www.susdev.gov.hk/html/en/leadership_forum/

Paustenbach D J 2002 Primer on human and environmental risk assessment. In: Paustenbach D J (ed). Human and Ecological Risk Assessment: Theory and Practice. John Wiley, New York, p 1–83

Perry M, Hu H 2005 Workplace health and safety. In: Frumkin H (ed) Environmental Health: From Global to Local. Jossey-Bass, San Francisco, pp 648–682

Peters R G, Covello V T, McCallum D B 1997 The determinants of trust and credibility in environmental risk communication. Risk Analysis 17:43–54

Pruss-Ustun A, Corvalan C 2006 Preventing Disease Through Healthy Environments: Towards an estimate of the environmental burden of disease. World Health Organization, Geneva

Queensland Government 1997 Integrated Planning Act 1997. GoPrint, Brisbane

Rees W E 1992 Ecological footprints and appropriated carrying capacity: What urban economics leaves out. Environment and Urbanization 4:121–130

Reynolds C 2004 Public Health Law & Regulation. The Federation Press, Sydney

Rosen G 1993 A History of Public Health (Expanded Edition). Johns Hopkins, Baltimore

Rutherford A 2003 But you don't have to live here! Risk assessment and contaminated sites: a case study. NSW Public Health Bulletin 14(8):171–173

Sandman P 1987 Risk communication: Facing public outrage. EPA Journal 13(9):21–22. Available: http://www.psandman.com/articles/facing.htm

Slovic P 1987 Perceptions of risk. Science 236:280–285

Slovic P 1997 Public perception of risk. Journal of Environmental Health 59(9):22–24

Smith A H, Lingas E O, Rahman M 2000 Contamination of drinking-water by arsenic in Bangladesh: A public health emergency. Bulletin of the World Health Organization 78(9):1093–1103

Stoneham M, Dodds J, Buckett K 2004 Policy in the government context. In: Cromar N, Cameron S, Fallowfield H (eds). Environmental Health in Australia and New Zealand. Oxford University Press, Melbourne, pp 127–141

Time Magazine 2006 'Numbers', 27 November 2006, p. 32

The World Commission on Environment and Development 1987 Our Common Future. Oxford University Press, Oxford. Available: http://www.undocuments.net/wced-ocf.htm

United Nations 1992 United Nations Framework Convention on Climate Change. United Nations, New York

United Nations Development Programme 2006 Human Development Report 2006. UNDP, New York

Wackernagel M, McIntosh J, Rees W E et al 1993 How Big is Our Ecological Footprint? A Handbook for Estimating a Community's Appropriated Carrying Capacity. Task Force on Planning Healthy and Sustainable Communities. Vancouver

Wong P 2008 Climate change: a responsibility agenda. Speech to the Australian Industry Group Luncheon, 6 February 2008. Available: http://www.environment.gov.au/minister/wong/2008/pubs/tr20080206.pdf 9 Feb 2008

Woodward A J, Hales S, Hill S E 2002 The motor car and public health: are we exhausting the environment? Medical Journal of Australia 177:592–593

World Health Organization 1948 Constitution. WHO. Available: http://www.searo.who.int/LinkFiles/About_SEARO_const.pdf 14 Feb 2008

World Health Organization 1991 Environmental Health in Urban Development. Technical Report Series no. 807, World Health Organization, Geneva

World Health Organization 1992 Our Planet Our Health. World Health Organization, Geneva. Available: http://www.ciesin.org/docs/001-232/chpt1.html

World Health Organization 1997 Health and Environment in Sustainable Development: Five Years after the Earth Summit. World Health Organization, Geneva

World Health Organization 2002 World Health Report 2002: Reducing Risks, Promoting Healthy Life. World Health Organization, Geneva

World Health Organization 2004 Water, Sanitation and Hygiene Links to Health: Facts and Figures Updated November 2004, World Health Organization, Geneva. Available: http://www.who.int/water_sanitation_health/publications/facts2004/en/print.html 2 Feb 2006

Yassi A, Kjellstrom T, deKok T et al 2001 Basic Environmental Health. Oxford University Press, New York

CHAPTER 12

Health promotion

Elizabeth Parker

Learning objectives

After reading this chapter you should be able to:

- define health education and health promotion, and understand their conceptual definitions, histories and place in public health
- discuss health promotion actions and strategies, and their applications for practice in various settings and population groups
- identify levels of prevention and how health promotion works across these levels
- discuss different practices in health promotion for health professionals and the 'new health education'.

Introduction

The 'promotion of health' has become everybody's business including the marketers of 'healthy' products/lifestyles and gym memberships; government media campaigns such as 'Go for 2&5®' (fruit and vegetables every day); special 'extra' benefits for joining a private health insurance fund; and workplace 'wellness' programs that include yoga and pilates. For consumers, the list is endless. Health professionals need to understand the background to this growth in promoting 'health' and the place health promotion plays in public health. We begin this chapter with a discussion on health education, we then trace the evolution of health promotion from health education, to the strategies and settings for health promotion, and conclude with challenges for health promotion. Case studies, activities and reflections on the material are presented to assist you.

History of health education

Health education has had a long history in public health. Education concerning prevailing health problems and the methods of preventing and controlling them is the first of the eight basic elements of primary health care (WHO 1978). Health education is about providing information and education to individuals about specific illnesses and disease, so that they can make informed decisions to prevent the onset of these conditions, or maintain and restore good health, usually by changing their behaviour.

Ritchie (1991) described four phases of health education activity and experience in Australia. The first stage was education through health information provision. Health professionals were 'perceived as being invested with all pertinent knowledge, and health practitioners were seen as the prime source responsible for the health of individuals' (Ritchie 1991 p 157). Even though there were great efforts made by health professionals in providing information to patients/clients, information alone was not producing the desired effects. In Stage 2 (the early 1970s), health information and education programs were delivered through audio-visual channels, such as films, leaflets, posters, booklets and teaching kits. Ritchie (1991) claimed that even with all these additions, health professionals were still 'talking heads' and some of the printed brochures were in scientific language that was not easily understood. In Stage 3, health educators used adult education principles. First espoused by Malcolm Knowles (1913–1998), adult education principles include empathy, experiential learning, participation and authenticity. He coined the term 'androgogy' (the study of adult learning) and education was through 'guided interaction' (Boshier 1998). Adults learned by building on their own experiences, particularly in groups with other adults. For health professionals, group work that used these principles was energetically pursued, with the assumption that behaviour change to improve health was a voluntary choice. The premise was that receiving the correct information would automatically lead to behaviour change. When people did not change, despite the best efforts of health professionals, patients/clients tended to be 'blamed'. This led to the term 'victim-blaming' (Ritchie 1991 p 160). Stage 4 in health education development in Australia was the combination of improving individuals' knowledge, skills and understanding, but within the context of their social and environmental milieu.

Mass health education campaigns were broadened from a focus on educating individuals about their health, to health education campaigns aimed at changing the behaviour of populations in the 1970s and 1980s. These campaigns were extensive and vigorously pursued in the United States and in Finland. The two earliest of these large community-wide programs were the *Stanford Three-Community Study* in California, and the *North Karelia Project* in Finland, both initiated in 1972. The study in North Karelia (with a population of 180,000) showed that Finnish men had the world's highest mortality rate from ischaemic heart disease in 1972. A health education program was started to see whether the main risk factors of high blood pressure, high cholesterol and smoking could be reduced in the population and whether this would reduce mortality from cardiovascular diseases (Vartianen et al 2000).

The *Stanford Three-Community Study* in California (1972–1975) 'targeted cardiovascular disease (CVD) risk factors through a health promotion program that used mass media supplemented by individual and group education for high-risk persons in one town and mass media alone in a second town; a third town served as a control' (Fortmann & Varady 2000 p 316). This program promoted a reduction in cholesterol levels through dietary changes, a reduction in blood pressure with regular blood pressure monitoring, an increase in physical activity and a reduction in cigarette smoking, salt intake and obesity. These behaviours are known risk factors for heart disease, and it was for this purpose that major investments were made in these campaigns. However, the campaigns had limited effects in these trial communities so the outcomes of these community education approaches were limited in the short term (Fortmann & Varady 2000). In North Karelia, however, there have been documented declines in coronary heart disease since 1972; surveys are conducted every fifth year and there is some evidence that these declines are attributable to the focussed health education program (Vartianen et al 2000).

Despite its limitations as a population health strategy, health education still has a significant role to play in providing health information to raise awareness of health issues in the community, to assist patients in exploring their attitudes and values about health problems and to educate policymakers about important health issues. Knowledge of effective health education strategies, in particular the application of theories about individual behaviour change, is essential for those health professionals who work with individual patients/clients. This knowledge takes on a special significance as the health profile of the population changes, with the consequent rise in chronic diseases, such as diabetes, mental health problems (e.g. depression) and arthritis. Health education definitely has a place in the individual counselling of patients about self-management, and all health professionals play some role in educating the public through patient education. For example, nurses educate patients/clients, environmental health officers are health educators in ensuring that restaurant staff apply safe food handling practices and physicians educate their patients/clients about vaccinations. Patients have the right to know about their care, but as a whole-of-population approach, health education alone is limited.

The concept of wellness

Wellness is a term that has evolved through health interests in the United States. Unsatisfied with the term 'health' and its origins in the 'absence of disease', some American health professionals claimed this definition of 'health' was limited. Health education should be about improving 'wellness'; that is, people's sense of wellbeing. Wellness programs have sprung up in organisations as employee wellness programs. They focus not only on keeping employees physically active and healthy, but also on the spiritual, emotional and social aspects of health. Navarro et al (2007), in an article about new strategic directions for public health, assert that there is a need to examine new approaches for health and wellness. They note that 'fragmentation and overemphasis on the physical aspects of health exclude mental health, spirituality and complementary and alternative medicine (CAM) as integral parts of wellness' (Navaro et al 2007 p 4), and call for funding of research to investigate further these influences on community health outcomes.

Emergence of health promotion in the 'new public health'

After the World Health Organization (WHO) *Declaration of Alma-Ata* in 1978 (WHO 1978), and its *Health for All* strategy, the concept of health promotion emerged. Catford (2004) argued that 'health promotion' was becoming increasingly used by a new wave of public health activists who were dissatisfied with the traditional and top-down approaches of 'health education' and 'disease prevention'. Health promotion, as a public health strategy, was a more radical approach, because it assumed that people's health was determined not only by their own behaviour but by the contexts in which they lived and worked. Therefore, health opportunities were mediated through people's social, emotional and physical environments. For example, it is difficult to purchase healthy food if you have little money or access to stores where fruit and vegetables are available at a reasonable cost. To improve health within a population, a 'new public health' was needed to tackle these socio-environmental determinants of health. Health promotion became an integral part of the new public health, particularly as research revealed that multiple strategies across many sectors – government, non-government and industry – were needed to create and provide health opportunities for all. Health education provided by health professionals to individuals, and mass media campaigns exhorting people to practice 'healthy lifestyles', had a limited impact on improving population health. The analysis of promoting and improving population health became more sophisticated.

Catford (2004) claimed that there have been three stages in the development of health promotion since the 1970s. The first dimension was 'tackling preventable diseases and risk behaviours' (e.g. heart disease, cancer, tobacco and nutrition), through education

(Catford 2004 p 3), commonly termed 'health education'. The Stanford and North Karelia programs could be included here. The second dimension of health promotion was the 'complementary intervention approaches' (Catford 2004 p 3), with a range of action areas such as the development of healthy public policy, personal skills, supportive environments, community action and health services. These were the pivotal actions in the *Ottawa Charter for Health Promotion*, promulgated in 1986 at a seminal WHO conference in Ottawa, Canada (WHO 1986). The third dimension was recognising 'the value of reaching people through the settings and sectors in which they live and meet (e.g. schools, cities, health care settings, workplaces)' (Catford 2004 p 3). This became known as the 'settings' approach for health promotion. The fourth dimension for the 2000s is the need to examine, even more, the social determinants of health in a changing global world. Although Catford (2004) did not expand specifically on the dimensions of this changing world, some issues come to mind. The migration and movement of people in Europe, since the establishment of the European Union; and the pressure on the world's cities as increasing numbers of people move from agrarian-based economies to market-based economies – for example, the mass migration to cities in South Asia and South-East Asia to work in clothing and textiles and technology industries. In addition, there are the increasing disparities in the standard of living between developed countries and less developed countries; changing weather patterns that impact on water supplies, and hence agriculture; and never-ending war and the displacement of millions of people to refugee camps, especially in Africa. All these factors create challenges for public health. Therefore, health promoters need the skills to unravel and analyse the impact of such social determinants on health and to advocate for public health policies that create health opportunities for all.

ACTIVITY

Discuss the following questions with other students and write down your answers.

- Why do you think the early community health education programs that focussed on educating the public about multiple risk factors for cardiovascular disease through behaviour change were not as successful as planned?
- Are there lessons to be learned from Ritchie's (1991) analysis of health education?
- Define 'wellness', and comment on whether you believe there is a lot of attention in the community for wellness, including complementary medicines.
- Where does wellness fit in your understanding of health?

REFLECTION

Did you consider that it is difficult for people to change their behaviour and that education alone may not be enough motivation? As you will learn in this chapter, health education is only one aspect of health promotion, and community change requires numerous strategies in a variety of settings. If your group thought there were more people interested in alternative paths to wellness, what does this mean for the education of health professionals or health science students?

Aboriginal and Torres Strait Islander concepts of health promotion

In Chapter 2, you were introduced to the Aboriginal and Torres Strait Islander definition of health. For Aboriginal and Torres Strait Islander peoples, 'health' is interlinked with families, communities and land. Aboriginal and Torres Strait Islander health promotion needs to consider the individual, family and community. Health professionals need to understand the dynamics of Aboriginal and Torres Strait Islander culture and be culturally competent.[1] Health promotion uses a primary health care approach to improve health in communities. A primary health care approach integrates 'both an individual and the population' as its hallmark (Couzos & Murray 2003 p xxxi). 'Primary health care', according to the National Aboriginal Community Controlled Health Organisation (NACCHO), is designed as 'essential, integrated care based upon scientifically sound and socially acceptable procedures and technology made accessible to communities (as close as possible to where they live) through their full participation, in the spirit of self-reliance and self-determination' (Couzos & Murray 2000 p xxxii). Through the more than 130 Aboriginal community-controlled health services (ACCHSs) that are managed by boards of elected Aboriginal members, integrated care for the community is offered through individual treatment and promotion programs, as well as extensive community health screening and health promotion programs. For a full account of the development and structure of these Aboriginal medical services, and for a wide-ranging profile of Indigenous health, policies and services, see the NACCHO website listed at the end of this chapter.

Principles of health promotion

In 1986, WHO declared a set of principles that underpinned health promotion. 'These principles were developed as "health" was the extent to which individuals and groups are able to realise their aspirations and satisfy needs and to change or cope with the environment' (Health Promotion International 1986 p 73). The principles underpinning health promotion are:

- Health promotion involves the population as a whole in the context of their everyday life, rather than focussing on people at risk for specific diseases.
- Health promotion is directed towards action on the determinants or causes of health.
- Health promotion combines diverse, but complementary, methods of approaches, including communication, education, legislation, fiscal measures, organisational change, community development and spontaneous local activities against health hazards.
- Health promotion aims particularly at effective and concrete public participation.
- Health professionals, particularly in primary health care, have an important role in nurturing and enabling health promotion (WHO 1984 p 20).

The *Ottawa Charter for Health Promotion* (WHO 1986) articulated a way forward for the new public health. While not explicit, it posed the question, 'What really creates health?' (Kickbusch 2007). The charter used the WHO (1984) health promotion principles as a foundation for five action areas. It outlined a decisive platform for health promotion action. Significantly, there were specific prerequisites for health. These were 'peace, shelter, education, food, income, a stable ecosystem, sustainable resources, social justice and equity' (WHO 1986 p 1). More than 20 years on, these prerequisites remain the cornerstone for health actions. Health was seen as a 'resource for everyday life, not the object of living' (WHO 1986 p 1). This represents a positive concept of health instead of explaining 'health' as merely the absence of disease. The definition of health promotion was to 'enable people to take control over their health'. Implicit in this platform for health promotion was the concept of empowerment. In health promotion, empowerment is described as 'a process through which people gain greater control over decisions and actions affecting their health' (WHO 1998). '*Health promotion* not only encompasses actions directed at strengthening the basic life skills and capacities of individuals, but also at influencing underlying social and economic conditions and physical environments which impact upon *health*' (WHO 1998). The role of health professionals in health promotion is to practice 'with' people not 'on' them.

The *Ottawa Charter for Health Promotion* became a 'focal point in the work of the World Health Organization (WHO) in advocating a comprehensive approach to public health and health promotion practice' (Fleming & Parker 2007 p 6). It was based on the social democratic principles of justice, equity and access. This translates to a public health practice that addresses the determinants of ill health in societies. Health actions are expanded. The charter builds on the *Health for All* declaration (WHO 1978), and is therefore universal in its belief that health should indeed, be for all! The charter emphasises the role of healthy public policy, education in health advocacy and action, and the development of individual skills in advocacy. It reinforces the need to reorient community services towards prevention. There are five essential actions, outlined in Figure 12.1.

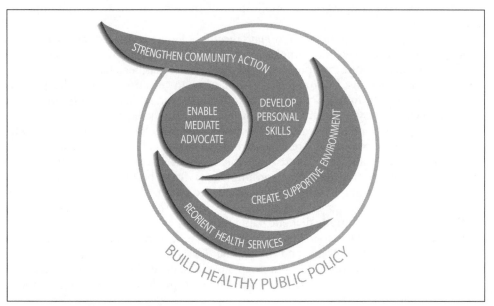

FIGURE 12.1 The Ottawa Charter emblem for health promotion

(Source: WHO 1986)

1 *Build public policies that support health* – Health promotion goes beyond health care (e.g. hospitals that treat the sick) and makes health an agenda item for policymakers in all areas of governmental and organisational action. Health promotion requires that the obstacles to adopting health-promoting policies be identified in non-medical sectors together with ways of removing them. The aim must be to make healthier choices easier.

2 *Create supportive environments* – Health promotion recognises that at both the global and local level, human health is tied to nature and the environment. Societies that exploit their environments without attention to ecology reap the effects of that exploitation in ill health and social problems. Health cannot be separated from other goals and changing patterns of life. Work and leisure have a definite impact on health. Health promotion therefore must create living and working conditions that are safe, stimulating, satisfying and enjoyable.

3   *Strengthen community action* – Health promotion works through effective community action. Communities need to have control of their own initiatives and activities. Health professionals must learn new ways of working with individuals and communities – working *for* and *with,* rather than *on* them.

4   *Develop personal skills* – Health promotion supports personal and social development through providing information and education for health and by helping people to develop the skills they need to make healthy choices. By doing so, it enables people to exercise more control over their own health and over their environments, making it possible for people to learn through life, to prepare themselves for all of its stages and to cope with chronic illness and injuries. This process has to be assisted in the school, at home, at work and in community settings.

5   *Reorient health services* – The responsibility for health promotion in health services is shared among individuals, community groups, health professionals, medical care workers, bureaucracies and governments (WHO 1986).

Here are some examples of the application of these action areas to contemporary health problems.

- *Building public policies that support health* – Government policies have been developed to make non-smoking an easier choice. For example, smoking in workplaces, public transport, hospitals and schools has been banned.

- *Create supportive environments* – Actions to ensure sustainable physical environments, for example, not building housing on toxic landfills or ensuring a safe working environment through workplace health programs.

- *Strengthen community action* – Examples include health professionals who work with newly arrived refugee communities and advocate on their behalf to ensure that health services are accessible and that interpreters are available; and nutritionists who work with a community service to build a community kitchen and provide cooking classes for disadvantaged youth.

- *Develop personal skills* – Health professionals (e.g. nurses, podiatrists and dieticians) who educate diabetic patients about managing their diabetes.

- *Reorienting health services* – For example, healthy messages are displayed in hospital waiting rooms and individual lifestyle assessments are conducted during the intake procedures in many hospitals; general practitioners undertake individual lifestyle counselling; and some hospitals have 'health promoting hospital' committees.

ACTIVITY

● Apply the five actions steps of the *Ottawa Charter* (WHO 1986) to reducing road accidents in Australia.

● Write a short paragraph about how the concept of health and health promotion in Indigenous communities differs from that of non-Indigenous communities?

REFLECTION

In the road accident exercise, you can notice how extensive the application of the five action steps can be. These action steps have been used extensively to design health promotion programs. There are differences in the Indigenous and non-Indigenous concepts of health promotion because of the significance of ties to the land and community for Aboriginal and Torres Strait Islander peoples and, therefore, a particular focus on local community-based services.

Health promotion strategies

One of the principles of health promotion is that the strategies need to be intersectoral and engage participants, as the focus of health promotion is to 'enable all people to achieve their fullest potential' (WHO 1986). WHO articulated a broad range of approaches to health promotion, summarised below.

- The focus of promotion is access to health, to reduce inequalities and to increase opportunities to improve health. This involves changing public and corporate policies to make them conducive to health, and involves reorienting health services towards the maintenance and development of health in the population, regardless of current health status.
- Improving health depends upon the development of an environment conducive to health, especially in conditions at work and in the home. Since this environment is dynamic, health promotion involves the monitoring and assessment of technological, cultural and economic influences on health.
- Health promotion involves the strengthening of social networks and social supports. This is based on the recognition of the importance of social forces and social relationships as determinants of values and behaviour relevant to health, and as significant resources for coping with stress and maintaining health.
- Promoting lifestyles conducive to health involves consideration of personal coping strategies and dispositions, as well as beliefs and values relevant to health, all shaped by lifelong experiences and living conditions. Promoting positive health behaviour and appropriate coping strategies is a key aim in health promotion.
- Information and education provide an informed base for making choices. They are necessary and core components of health promotion that aim at increasing knowledge and disseminating information related to health. Addressing information and education needs should include consideration of the public's perceptions and experiences of health; knowledge from epidemiology, social and other sciences; patterns of health and disease, and factors affecting them; and descriptions of the 'total' environment in which health and health choices are shaped. The mass media and new information technologies are particularly important (Health Promotion International 1986).

You can see that the main theme of health promotion strategies is improving the health of the population as a whole, not solely that of individuals.

Since 1986, WHO assemblies focussing on health promotion have been held regularly. The *Second International Conference on Health Promotion* was held in Adelaide, in 1988. It explored in greater depth the concept of 'healthy public policy'. Remember in Australia, healthy public policies, particularly about sales of cigarettes and advertising of cigarettes, had not been enacted at that time. Healthy public policy occupies a unique position: it provides a framework within which strategic advances can be made in relation to personal development, public participation and healthy environments. Public policies in all sectors have some bearing on health and are an important agency for decreasing social and economic injustice, for example, facilitating equal access to resources, in addition to health services (WHO 1988). The focus at the *Third International Conference on Health Promotion*, held in Sundsvall, Sweden, in 1991 brought the world's attention to 'creating supportive environments for health'. The conference identified war, fast population growth, insufficient food, being deprived of the instruments of self-determination and the destruction of natural resources as some of the factors detrimental to wellbeing (WHO 1991). The *Fourth International Conference on Health Promotion* was held in Jakarta, Indonesia in 1997 (WHO 1997a). Its dominant themes were partnerships and settings. The *Fifth International Conference on Health Promotion* was held in Mexico City in 2000 (WHO 2000). Its theme was bridging the equity gap with a focus on the determinants of health. The *Bangkok Charter for Health Promotion in a Globalized World* (WHO 2005) stressed that 'progress towards a healthier world requires strong political action, broad participation and sustained advocacy' (WHO 2005). These subsequent documents are frameworks for action. They continue to embed the principles of health promotion as a sustaining and integral part of public health.

How would the *Ottawa Charter* appear if written now? Nutbeam provides some commentary, claiming that 'health promotion will certainly involve partnerships with the private sector in ways that were inconceivable in 1986' (2005 p 2). A range of businesses and organisations promote fundraising for breast cancer research through selling pink ribbons. Several years ago, such a promotion would have received scant attention in the media, and would certainly not have the profile through the private sector that it has now.

If we use 'supportive environments for health' to focus on the physical environment, much has changed since the *Ottawa Charter* in 1986. Climate change and the degradation of the world's rainforests, and other environmental damage, has primarily been the domain of environmentalists. Now, health professionals and environmentalists have common ground because degradation of rainforests increases mosquito-borne disease and climate change alters ocean flows, with the consequential depletion of fish stocks and, therefore, food resources.

Has the *Ottawa Charter for Health Promotion* and its action areas been effective? Jackson et al (2006) analysed eight reviews of the health action areas, published between 1999 and 2004, which assessed the efficacy and cost-effectiveness of health promotion interventions. Significant lessons are:

- *Investment in building healthy public policy is a key strategy* – Successful actions include 'investment in government and social policy, creation of legislation and regulations and intersectoral and inter-organisational partnerships and collaboration' (Jackson et al 2006 p 76). Road safety legislation is an example.
- *Supportive environments need to be created at all levels* – Supportive conditions and environments require a variety of actions. Successful youth health promotion programs require psychosocial and emotional supports such as counselling, outreach and life skills training, and also joint programs with parents/professionals and community leaders (Warren 1999, in Jackson et al 2006).
- *Interventions employing multiple strategies and actions at multiple levels and sectors are most effective* – Multiple strategies and actions at multiple levels were most evident in successful programs (Hoffman & Jackson 2003, in Jackson et al 2006). Those interventions shown to be effective for 'reducing tobacco use, increasing physical activity, preventing cardiovascular disease and increasing food security involved a combination of health promotion strategies occurring at the personal, community and structural (policy) levels' (Jackson et al 2006 p 79).

Successful health promotion actions featured the following elements:

- *Intersectoral collaboration and inter-organisational partnerships at all levels* – Developing alliances and partnerships to pool resources and personnel and to work collaboratively on priority areas has become an increasingly important role for health promoters and allied health professionals doing health promotion work.
- *Community participation and engagement in planning and decision making* – A health promotion approach engages clients in the design, implementation and evaluation of programs. Clients/community members are active decision-makers and 'owners' of planned programs, as opposed to being passive recipients of programs.
- *Creating healthy settings, particularly focussing on the settings of schools, workplaces and cities and communities/municipalities (councils)* – Settings such as these

provide opportunities to reach large numbers of people with sustained programs. For example, in Australia, local councils are influential in designing walking paths and promoting shade cloths over swimming pools.

Strategies for health promotion

Multiple strategies are used to promote population health including individual counselling and group work; development of print and web-based materials; social marketing campaigns; advocacy, policy and legislative changes; and the development of networks.[2] We will introduce social marketing and then discuss how the combination of social marketing, advocacy, policy and legislative changes and the development of networks have had an impact on the rates of tobacco smoking in Australia.

Social marketing is 'the application of commercial marketing techniques to the achievement of socially desirable goals' (Egger et al 2005 p 96). Social marketing campaigns are used in Australia to raise awareness of specific health issues, particularly through short television commercials. *Slip, Slop, Slap and Wrap* is one of Australia's best-known health slogans, *Every Cigarette is Doing You Damage* and *Every K over is a Killer* signal prompts to consumers to reflect on their smoking and driving behaviour. More recently, Donovan and Henley (2003, in Egger et al 2005) propose that target audiences (usually consumers) be expanded to include those who influence consumers, for example, while campaigns can target families as 'consumers' of junk food, campaigns should simultaneously be targeting the manufacturers of such food to reduce fat and sugar, and broadcasting authorities to ban the advertising of such products during children's television programs. So how do social marketing and other strategies make a difference? To answer that question, we examine tobacco control.

The most successful nations at controlling smoking prevalence (indicated by total population smoking rates) are Sweden (16%), Canada (19%), Australia (20.6%) and the US (20.9%) (Chapman 2007). Tobacco control is one of the most successful public health efforts in Australia. Australia has used an integrated and dedicated approach to tobacco reduction. The strategies used are broad-based, and through their consistent application over 30 years, tobacco smoking within Australia has declined.

Case study: Tobacco control

In Australia, the consumption of cigarettes has been steadily declining. The report by the Australian Institute of Health and Welfare (2005) demonstrates this steady decline. In 2004 Australians aged 20–29 years were more likely to be daily or occasional smokers than those in any other age group, with 24% smoking daily. People aged 60 years and over were least likely to be daily smokers (9%) and most likely to be ex-smokers (39%). Males were more likely to smoke than females in every age group, except at ages 14–19 years. Some 10% of males aged 14–19 years were daily smokers, compared with 12% of females aged 14–19 years (AIHW 2005 p 5).

The achievements in tobacco control over 30 years are the result of a variety of factors, including both health education and health promotion strategies, such as:

- *Harm reduction* – Australian advocates were among the first to arrange for the tar and nicotine content of cigarettes to be tested.
- *Advertising bans* – Australia was one of the first democracies to ban all tobacco advertising and sponsorship.

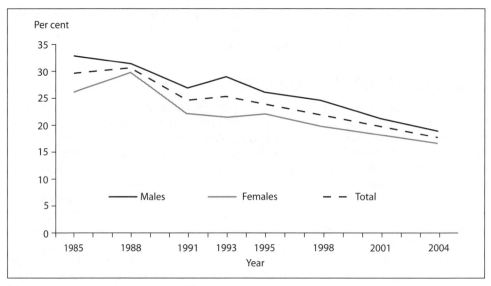

FIGURE 12.2: Smoking rates in Australia, 1985–2004

(Source: AIHW 2006)

- *Pack warnings* – We have one of the world's largest pack warnings, with pioneering research that ensures maximum impact on youth.
- *Mass-reach campaigns* – Mass community antismoking campaigns were one of the first, and were countered forcefully by the tobacco industry.
- *Civil disobedience* – Health and community activists 'graffitied' tobacco billboards, focussing on the harm the tobacco industry was causing.
- *Smokeless tobacco* – South Australia banned smokeless tobacco in 1986. This was a world first. All states followed. Similarly, South Australia banned small 'kiddie' packs (less than 20 cigarettes).
- *Tax* – Australia has a relatively high tobacco tax, with intense lobbying against this by the tobacco industry.
- *Replacement of tobacco sponsorship* – Victoria paved the way by establishing the Victorian Health Promotion Foundation (VicHealth), which was funded by a tax on tobacco.
- *Clean indoor air* – Australia has one of the highest rates of smoke-free workplaces and environments, such as restaurants, bars and clubs, and all public transport (Chapman & Wakefield 2001 pp 275–276).

Multiple strategies to promote better health for Aboriginal and Torres Strait Islander mothers and babies is illustrated by the following case study, which took place in Townsville, Queensland.

The *Strong Women, Strong Babies, Strong Culture Program* (d'Espaignet et al 2003) and the *Living with Alcohol* program (Chikritzhs et al 2005) are more examples of successful health promotion programs in Aboriginal and Torres Strait Islander communities in the Northern Territory.

ACTIVITY

● Write a short paragraph on the decline in tobacco smoking in Australia. Would this decline have been achieved without the identified actions? Could some of these strategies be applied to another health issue? And how would they be implemented? What strategies worked in the *Mums and Babies Program* in Townsville?

Case study: Aboriginal and Torres Strait Islander health promotion

Aboriginal and Torres Strait Islander health promotion is integrated in a primary health care approach, through the Aboriginal community-controlled health organisations, of which there are 130 in Australia. The Townsville Aboriginal and Islander Health Services' *Mums and Babies Program* illustrates 'developing personal skills', 'reorienting health services' and 'creating supportive environments' in their goal of improving the health of young mothers and children in Townsville.

The Townsville Mums and Babies Program

The Townsville Aboriginal and Islander Health Services established the *Mums and Babies Program* in 2000 – a morning clinic for pregnant women and young mothers with limited staff (two doctors, two health workers, a child-care worker and a driver). The service responded to 'long waiting times and a historically unwelcoming hospital environment that had kept many Indigenous women from using mainstream health services' (Panaretto 2007 p 8). In the first month, the service saw 40 clients; in 2001 there were 500 clients a month, and now there is a purpose-built family-friendly centre with a growing number of clients from outside Townsville. There has been a reduction in low-birth-weight babies (<2500 grams, Panaretto et al 2007) from 16% to 11.7%; and mean birth weights have increased by 170 grams; perinatal deaths have fallen from 58 per thousand to 22 per thousand. 'We wanted to create an environment where women felt comfortable, treated as people and where they could bring children along' (Panaretto 2007 p 8). Other ancillary programs are now offered, encouraging breastfeeding, nutrition support, increasing immunisation rates and monitoring healthy child development. This program demonstrates health promotion in action, in a supportive health service where the majority of staff are Indigenous.

REFLECTION

Did you note that the decline in tobacco smoking has taken many years and it has taken concerted effort, as the tobacco-smoking case study points out? Often in health promotion, there are expectations that population health change is simple, and can be done quickly. Did you find that the strategies that worked in Townsville utilised a unified approach across services?

We extend our discussions on health promotion by seeing how it is linked across various levels of prevention.

Levels of prevention in public health and health promotion

Health promotion is about prevention, and your work in health promotion, irrespective of your health profession, will fall within this paradigm. There are three levels of prevention: primary, secondary and tertiary. Primary prevention 'refers to strategies to reduce incidence and prevent occurrence of poor health' (Oldenburg et al 2004 p 218). This includes vaccinations to prevent disease, tobacco control measures such as workplace policies that prevent people smoking, banning of cigarette advertising in all media and changing legislation or public policies that assist people to make 'healthy choices'. Strategies such as these are sometimes called 'upstream' strategies as they work on creating healthy public policy. Secondary prevention aims at detecting and curing the disease before it causes symptoms – examples include cervical cancer screening, and tertiary prevention aims at minimising the consequences for a patient who already has a disease, such as the implementation of cardiac rehabilitation programs for patients with heart disease (Couzos & Murray 2003 p xxxv).

The relationship between primary, secondary and tertiary levels of prevention is well illustrated through Figure 12.3.

	Primary prevention	Secondary prevention	Tertiary prevention
Target group	Healthy individuals Whole populations	Individuals at risk The early stages of a condition	Individuals with the condition Conditions that have already occurred
Aim	Prevent occurrence Reduce incidence	Prevent progression Slow progression Minimise duration Risk reduction	Minimise complications Optimise functioning Limit recurrence
Strategies	Promote health-enhancing and preventive practices Create supportive environments Develop healthy public policy	Screening Early detection Early intervention Risk assessment and reduction	Treatment or rehabilitation Reduce psychological, social, physical distress Enhance support networks Enhance self-management

FIGURE 12.3: The relationship between primary, secondary and tertiary levels of prevention.

(Reproduced by permission of Oxford University Press Australia from Environmental Health in Australia and New Zealand by Croman, Cameron & Fallowfield © Oxford University Press)

Health promotion works across a number of settings and these are introduced to give you an idea of the extent of health promotion in action.

Health promotion in practice

Settings for health promotion

'A setting refers to a socially and culturally defined geographical and physical area of factual social interaction, and a socially and culturally defined set of patterns of interaction to be performed while in the setting' (Wenzel 1997). Health promotion strategies can encompass a total population and can be an effective public health strategy. For example, one of the action steps in the *Ottawa Charter* (1986) is 'reorienting health services'. So, a health service could be the focal point for health promotion programs. Similarly, schools are now used extensively for promoting healthy messages to children; workplaces are ideal sites for offering employees physical activity programs, nutrition advice and even yoga. And communities, in their various forms, such as neighbourhood centres and shopping centres, are places where health information and education can be distributed.

In addition, it is not uncommon to see blood glucose testing booths promoting diabetes prevention, healthy heart information programs and other information on specific health issues available at cultural and art centres.

Why a settings approach?

The strength of a settings approach is that it aligns with several of the health promotion principles we discussed earlier. For example, health is promoted where people live, work, love and play. It also aligns with a population health approach rather than merely a focus on individuals. In your role as a health promotion worker, nurse, medical practitioner or allied health professional (e.g. nutritionist, environmental health officer, physiotherapist, audiologist), investments in strategies that reach large groups of the population can be a more effective use of your time in 'promoting health'. Some of the initial thinking about a settings approach stemmed from the work of Hancock and Duhl (1988) who began working on the concept of the 'healthy city'. The city was a setting where health opportunities or lack of them occurred. This work was extended to include other 'places' where opportunities to promote health could be exploited (outside the health system or health services, be that a hospital, a doctor's office or a medical centre).

The concept that 'health' is separate from 'health services' and that a wider set of strategies was needed to promote health in the community was first canvassed at an influential conference, *Beyond Health Care*, held in Toronto in 1984. International experts in housing, the environment, agriculture, urban planning and workplaces discussed how policies from their sectors influenced the community's health. For example, if there is limited food, inadequate housing that causes housing stress, polluted cities or unsafe workplaces, the health of the community is compromised. WHO was represented at this conference. The Toronto conference was one of the forerunners of the settings approach to health promotion and stimulated thinking for developing the *Ottawa Charter* in 1986.

Schools

For children, schools play a pivotal role in health education, because of the vast array of health initiatives now being implemented in schools. Health messages are increasingly part of the curriculum. An emphasis on healthy food has seen tuckshops change their food selections, fruit and vegetables are grown in schoolyards and sun protection programs are enacted through 'no hat, no play' policies. Visiting dental staff promote tooth brushing and provide regular check-ups. Positive emotional health programs are integrated into teacher training and anti-bullying policies are common. Sustainable environments are encouraged through initiatives such as planting trees, learning to be 'water wise' and recycling. The place of schools for health education has been documented in the literature (Maes & Lievens 2003, St Leger 2001, WHO 1997b). Kolbe (2005) claimed that schools have the potential to do more than any other single agency in society to help young people live healthier, longer and more satisfying and productive lives.

The *Health Promoting Schools* framework integrates the school health curriculum, the school ethos (or philosophy), school health policies and practices, the community in which the school resides, and the school environment (physical, social and emotional) as components to create health thinking and opportunities. A 'health promoting school (HPS) is a school that is constantly strengthening its capacity as a healthy setting for living, learning, and working' (WHO School and Youth Health website). So what does a health promoting school look like? A health promoting school focuses on: caring for oneself and others; making healthy decisions and taking control over life's circumstances; and creating conditions that are conductive to health (through policies, services, and physical/social conditions) (WHO School and Youth Health website). Is there evidence that a health promoting schools approach works to promote health of children?

In a systematic review of over 111 studies, Lister-Sharp et al (1999) evaluated the effectiveness of school-based health promoting schools programs and health promotion in schools. Health promotion in schools showed 'that school health promotion initiatives can have a positive impact on children's health and behaviour but do not do so consistently' (Lister-Sharp et al 1999 p 5). There was evidence that there can be an impact on the 'social and physical environment of the school in terms of staff development, school lunch provision, exercise programmes and social atmosphere' (Lister-Sharp et al 1999 p 5).

Schools are a vital resource in the community where children's attitudes and values about health can be formed, where there are opportunities for engagement with health in the classroom and playground. If we recall that health promotion is about 'enabling people to take control over their health' (WHO 1986), what better place to begin than in school?

Communities

The concept of 'community' in health promotion is interpreted in a number of ways. First, our discussion on community health education programs previously focussed on 'community' as a 'place'. Such programs as the *Stanford Five City Project* and the *Minnesota Heart Health* program in the United States, and the *North Karelia Project* in Finland are examples of 'place'. Second, groups of people who share common bonds, such as age, gender, cultural identity or are linked to common cause, such as groups championing the environment. Third, communities of people who are coping with the same health condition, such as 'survivor' groups of cancer patients, represent another type of community where health promotion is practised (O'Connor & Parker 1995).

Health promotion practice varies in different communities. Community health nurses confront an array of health education and promotion opportunities in their work in community health centres that are run by state governments or, in the case of the Aboriginal and Islander Health services, the federal government. Individual patient/client education occurs in the home through assisting patients with the self-management of their chronic disease; and young mothers and babies' programs that provide opportunities for education about healthy child development and child rearing. Community nutritionists work with physicians in general practice, and other allied health professionals, including exercise physiologists, who work to plan healthy walking and weight control programs. The settings for this work can be sporting clubs, for example, working with tuckshop convenors to offer healthy snacks and with service clubs, to promote reminders of cancer prevention screening (e.g. bowel, cervical and breast cancer screening).

The focus is on the need for communities to identify their own health problems and direct attention to their solutions, thereby gaining control over the initiatives and solutions. The health professional is a facilitator of actions and solutions, and thus works as an advocate for communities. This is in line with the 'enabling' approach to health promotion. Strengthening community action justified a new direction in community health promotion.

This broadens the role of the community health promotion worker from solely providing health education and health information to a practice that is founded in encouraging collaborative partnerships with communities in the development, implementation and evaluation of programs.

Community development in health promotion is central to community health promotion work. 'A developmental approach involves working in ways that facilitate people and communities developing their strength and confidence while at the same time, addressing immediate problems' (Butler & Cass 1993 p 8 in Fleming & Parker

2007 p 196), with different approaches to community health identified in the literature (Labonte 1989). Figure 12.4 can assist you to conceptualise your practice. It is impossible for one health professional to reduce cardiovascular disease in a community alone or to advocate for changes to the placement of traffic lights on congested roads so that older residents in a retirement 'village' may safely cross the road. Recalling that health promotion has, at its roots, the fundamental concept of empowerment, and that practice is 'with' people not 'on' them, then the empowerment continuum is helpful in thinking about the strategies to put in place to make a difference (see Fig 12.4).

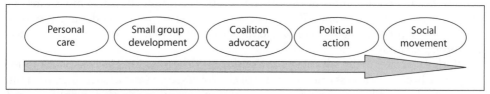

FIGURE 12.4: The Empowerment Continuum

(Source: Jackson et al 1989, Labonte 1992, Baum 1998 in Fleming ML, Parker E 2007 Health Promotion: Principles and practice in the Australian context. 3rd edn. Allen & Unwin, Melbourne, p 201)

Personal care is individual care or an education/information program with individuals. This is the 'care' that, for example, nurses and allied health professionals engage in with patients/clients. **Small group development** is where the group identifies issues of concern that need action. A small group education program could be the catalyst for broader discussions about issues that are impacting on health; for example, a group of women in a smoking cessation program discuss the lack of day-care facilities in their neighbourhood. Through mutual support, the group is strengthened, and friendships extended through other networks. **Coalition advocacy** is about issue identification, and joining together with other networks to build strong coalitions to bring about change. **Political action** is about working 'upstream' and engaging political support for policy change, resource allocation, research funding, networking and advocacy. For example, without the grass-roots activism, sound research, advocacy and lobbying, the policy changes for altering the tobacco smoking culture, and the subsequent reduction in tobacco-smoking rates and smoking-related illnesses, would not have occurred. Another example is the strong coalition advocacy and political action that are required to enhance the health of Aboriginal and Torres Strait Islander peoples. **Social movement** refers to the swell in activity and the changing community consciousness of issues. Environmental issues and the concept of sustainability were quite alien terms for the majority of Australians 30 years ago – the domain of 'radicals'! Fast forward, and climate change, destruction of forests, salination of the water supply and the shortage of water are the focus of political agendas. Dedicated social activists, and scientific research and advocacy, have brought about a change in the consciousness of Australians.

Workplaces

Promoting health in the workplace is good for business. This makes sense because healthy workers are productive workers. But what kinds of health promotion workplace opportunities exist? A comprehensive approach to workplace health promotion (WHP) is desirable, according to the National Steering Committee on Health Promotion in the Workplace (NSCHPW 1989). It defined WHP as 'those educational, organisational or economic activities in the workplace that are designed to improve the health of workers and therefore the community at large' (NSCHPW 1989 p 8).

Many workplace health promotion programs complement, and are integrated with, the occupational health and safety programs and actions in workplaces. These programs have traditionally focussed on controlling health and safety hazards in the workplace, and work through the industrial relations arena. But since legislative change in Australia in the 1980s, there has been a 'duty of care' imposed on employers to provide a safe and healthy working environment for their employees and the training of a few employees as occupational health and safety representatives (National Health Strategy Unit 1993); this has led to an increase in workplace health promotion programs.

Workplace health promotion programs can include providing workplace day care centres, healthy food options in the canteen, employee health checks, gymnasiums and employee assistance programs (EAP). These EAPs were traditionally designed to assist with personal problems, and alcohol and drug use, which may affect safe work practices and produce family conflicts.

Workplaces offer many advantages as a setting for risk reduction and health promotion programs, because of access to a wide range of employees from various socio-demographic backgrounds. In addition, Australians spend approximately one third of their life at work and are encouraged to extend their working lives past the traditional retirement age. A comprehensive workplace strategy contains four key strategies: having a defined direction and purpose through clearly defined policies; building organisational and individual efficacy (empowerment); eliminating unnecessary organisational stress; and committing to and working towards a healthier organisational culture (Dooner 1990–91).

Whitehead (2006) claimed that the workplace is an important setting as it is an environment that caters for the physical, mental, social and economic wellbeing of its employees. There is an evolving continuum of health-promoting programs in workplaces – from a traditional focus on occupational health and safety and the establishment of employee health and medical services, to behavioural risk reduction approaches (e.g. blood pressure and cholesterol monitoring programs, and improvements in the availability of healthy food choices), discounted gym memberships, and the addition of 'wellness' activities such as yoga, pilates and massage. Many Australian workplaces provide such programs, for example, see the *Queensland University of Technology Wellness Program* (QUT wellness website).

The internet

The internet is a setting for health promotion. New communication tools, such as blogs, wikis, Facebook, YouTube, MySpace, chat rooms, SMS messaging and telephone-assisted devices (TAD) expand upon traditional print communication strategies, and thus expand the repertoire of health promotion settings. Consumers can converse with each other and with health professionals through these mediums. The latest health information is easily accessible to health consumers via the Web. These health information pages, some of which may be of dubious quality, 'represent passive, non-intrusive attempts at promoting health online' (McFarlane et al 2005 S60). Health consumers are becoming savvy and educated about their own illnesses and this can present a challenge to health professionals, whose traditional role was always to know more than their patients. This vast new medium also presents new tools for advocacy. Interactive online outreach programs exist. In Houston, Texas, the Montrose Clinic staff conduct online outreach as part of *Project CORE* (Cyber OutReach Education) in a sexually transmitted disease program. The chat room outreach presents discussion topics, questions and statistics to chat room participants, and information about services and symptoms of sexually transmitted infections (STIs). Staff use instant messaging to accomplish their outreach, and referrals are made to other online resources and to their own website (McFarlane et al 2005 S60). The following provides an example of one of the new communication technologies.

Case study: TLC Diabetes Program

The *Telephone-Linked-Care (TLC) Diabetes Program* is a computer-based, interactive telephone system that acts as an educator, monitor and counsellor. Using sophisticated speech recognition software, it receives calls from diabetic patients using a regular phone, and provides information and feedback to these patients. This new telehealth system is designed to educate, monitor and coach patients to improve self-care behaviours essential to diabetes management. These behaviours include nutrition, physical activity, blood glucose testing and using medication as prescribed. The system is being trialled in Brisbane (Bird 2005, B Oldenburg, personal communication, 2007).

Interactive technologies can be used for advocacy purposes. For example, *GetUp* is a community-based advocacy organisation that gives Australians opportunities to get involved in the political process by sending emails on specific topics of community concern to politicians, or raising issues in the media.

ACTIVITY

● Are there other settings that you can think of for health promotion actions? What other interactive technologies can you identify that might be useful for health promotion actions? At what level of the empowerment continuum would your health promotion practice be situated? Write a sentence describing the three levels of prevention.

REFLECTION

A way of thinking about settings is to think of various groups of the population and where they may live, work or play. Sporting clubs are a setting, the streets and parks are settings for homeless people, and beaches are also a setting. There is an opportunity to think creatively about where your health promotion efforts can be situated. In designing interactive technologies, remember to ensure the match between the technology and the skill level of the population you're targeting. You could be working along all aspects of the empowerment continuum.

Emerging challenges for health promotion

In this final section, we present some challenges for health promotion and health education for the future. On the one hand, information about being healthy or maintaining wellness is more widely available than ever; yet disparities in health status within the Australian population persist, for example, there are still cases of trachoma (eye disease) in remote Aboriginal and Torres Strait Islanders. This health issue is virtually unheard of in other developed countries; so one of the challenges of health promotion within public health is to maintain a steady focus on addressing the social determinants of health (Marmot 2003, Smedley & Syme 2000). Chapter 6 contained an introduction and analysis of social and emotional determinants of health.

Another current health promotion challenge is diabetes. McKinlay and Marceau (2000) present a succinct overview of diabetes mellitus in the US as a focal point within the 'new public health'. They claim that there are three levels of public health intervention used to address the challenge of diabetes. 'Downstream or curative efforts' consume most the available resources; midstream or primary and secondary prevention are about community-based primary prevention programs such as diet and exercise, and significantly, 'upstream' or healthy public policies are required if there is to be a change in the patterns of diabetes-related mortality and morbidity.

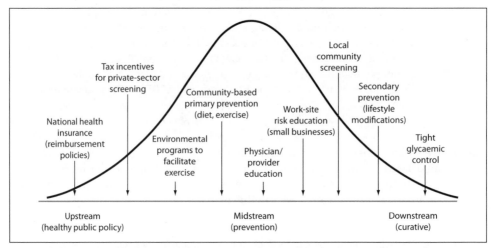

FIGURE 12.5: Some possible points of intervention for a new public health approach to diabetes given the distribution of risk

(Reprinted from The Lancet, 356, McKinlay & Marceau 2000 US public health and the 21st century: Diabetes mellitus, pp 757–761 with permission from Elsevier)

A third challenge is the changing role for health education. Nutbeam (2005) and Green (1999) argue that 'health education' has evolved into a new form. We have termed this the 'new health education'. Nutbeam is particularly interested in the role of health literacy as a means for promoting health in the population. Literacy is obviously a common term in education – the ability to read, write and comprehend; so what is health literacy? And what is its place in contemporary health promotion? There are three forms of health literacy. The first is functional literacy, which is described as 'sufficient basic skills in reading and writing to be able to function effectively in everyday situations' (Nutbeam 2000 p 263). There are two important contexts for this. First, patients/clients need to be able to read prescriptions and labels, and directions for home health care. Second, there are over 100 languages spoken in Australia, thus for many Australians English is not their first language. So functional literacy enables better access to health services and health information. The second type of literacy is communicative/interactive. This is the ability to engage in everyday activities, and to apply new information to changing circumstances (Nutbeam 2000). This has been part of health education practice for many years. The third, critical literacy, presupposes advanced cognitive and social skills and gives the ability to analyse information critically to be able to exert control over life events. It is the bedrock for personal and community empowerment, as people then have the skills, abilities and confidence to make changes to their lives and circumstances. Education and health can work together to further health literacies within the community. Internet-based technologies can aid in skills development, not only in functional literacies – reading and writing and understanding – but also communicative and critical literacies.

Self-management

Two specific developments in population health have an impact on current and future health promotion practice. These are the growth of the ageing population and an increase in chronic conditions, such as diabetes, mental health problems and depression, cancer-related illnesses, arthritis and chronic heart disease. Health professionals will need to be conversant with 'self-management' theories and practices in their work with patients. Skills in motivational interviewing will be needed (Rollnick et al 2004). The scope of practice for health promoters, nurses, podiatrists, nutritionists, dieticians and other health professionals will evolve and change to meet this changing health demographic. Expanded scopes of practice may be required through mixed general practices, community health centres, hospitals and the non-government sector in designing programs to keep people in their homes as long as possible, and for educating patients/clients about 'self-managing' their conditions. This self-management can include web-based self-management programs and the use of text messaging and email.

ACTIVITY

- Define 'upstream' and 'downstream' strategies by examining the model proposed by McKinlay and Marceau (2000). Why is health literacy important for a changing demographic in Australia? With a group of students, write your own definitions of self-management.

REFLECTION

The 'upstream' and 'downstream' strategies illustrated through the diabetes case study can be applied to other health issues, such as mental health. Such schemas provide a framework for thinking about how you can plan a number of strategies.

Did you think about the changing multicultural profile of Australians and how we make assumptions about people's ability to comprehend the health information available? With the increasing emphasis being placed on patients to understand and manage their own chronic conditions, self-management is an important term to understand.

A final word

Health promotion is part of the 'new public health'. It focuses on 'enabling' people to take control of their health. Its main focus is on addressing the determinants of health through 'upstream' policy advocacy and 'downstream' personal skills development, community empowerment and action; and it works through developing strategic partnerships across sectors to create health opportunities for all.

From its earliest roots in health education to the contemporary comprehensive approach across the prevention continuum, health professionals embrace health promotion knowledge and skills in order to make a difference to the health of individuals, communities and populations. The case studies identified the application of a variety of health promotion strategies. The internet increasingly provides a virtual reality for innovative health promotion opportunities. Self-management and health literacy were presented as new topics for health promotion research and evaluation and skilful practice. The new Australian government has indicated a commitment to a prevention agenda and health promotion will continue to be an integral and significant part of public health.

In the chapter that follows we discuss the impact of globalisation on health.

REVIEW QUESTIONS

1 What, if any, are the differences between 'health education', 'wellness' and 'health promotion'?
2 What are the strengths of using a 'settings' approach for health promotion?

3   Is there a role for health promotion for most health professionals?
4   What is meant by the 'new health education'?
5   How do the levels of prevention influence the choice of health promotion strategies in developing a health promotion program?

ENDNOTES

1   Cultural competence is defined as the 'ongoing process a health care provider continuously strives to achieve through the ability to effectively work within the cultural context of the client. This involves the integration of cultural awareness, cultural knowledge, cultural skill, cultural encounters and cultural desire' (Campinha-Bacote 2002 p 182).
2   For a comprehensive guide to health promotion strategies, see Egger et al (2005).

USEFUL WEBSITES

Australian Health Promotion Association: www.healthpromotion.org.au
NACCHO – National Aboriginal Community Controlled Health Organisation: www.naccho.org.au
Victoria Health Promotion Foundation: www.vichealth.vic.gov.au
WHO – World Health Organization: www.who.org

REFERENCES

Anonymous. Malcolm Shepherd Knowles: 1913–1997 1998 Training & Development. Alexandria 52(2):11

Australian Institute of Health and Welfare 2005 Statistics on drug use in Australia 2004. AIHW cat. no. PHE 62. AIHW, Canberra

Australian Institute of Health and Welfare 2006 Australia's health 2006. AIHW cat. no. AUS 73. AIHW, Canberra

Bird D 2005 Best of Health. Faculty of Health. Queensland University of Technology, July

Boshier R 1998 Malcolm Knowles, Archbishop of Andragogy. Adult Education Quarterly 48(2):64

Campinha-Bacote J 2002 The process of cultural competence in the delivery of healthcare services: A model of care. Journal of Transcultural Nursing 13(3):181–184

Catford J 2004 Health promotion's record card: how principled are we 20 years on? Health Promotion International 19(1):1–4

Chapman S 2007 Falling prevalence of smoking: how low can we go? Editorial. Tobacco Control 16:145–147

Chapman S, Wakefield M 2001 Tobacco control advocacy in Australia: Reflections on 30 years of progress. Health Education and Behavior 28(3):274–289

Couzos S, Murray R 2003 Aboriginal primary health care. An evidence-based approach. Oxford University Press, Melbourne

Chikritzhs T, Stockwell T, Pascal R 2005 The impact of the Northern Territory's Living With Alcohol program, 1992–2002: revisiting the evaluation. Addiction, 100(11):1625–1636

d'Espaignet E, Measay M L, Carnegie M A et al 2003 Monitoring the 'Strong Women, Strong Babies, Strong Culture program': The first eight years. Journal of Paediatrics and Child Health 39(9):668–672

Dooner B 1990–91 Achieving a healthier workplace. Health Promotion Canada 29(3):2–6

Egger G, Spark R, Donovan R 2005 Health promotion Strategies and Methods, 2nd edn. McGraw-Hill, North Ryde

Fleming M L, Parker E 2007 Health Promotion: Principles and practice in the Australian context, 3rd edn. Allen & Unwin, Melbourne

Fortmann S, Varady A 2000 Effects of a Community-wide Health Education Program on Cardiovascular Disease Morbidity and Mortality. American Journal of Epidemiology 152(4):316–323

GetUp! Action for Australia. Available: http://www.getup.org.au/ 1 Nov 2007

'Go for 2&5®' Campaign An Australian Government, State and territory Health Initiative. Available: http://www.gofor2and5.com.au/campaign.aspx?c=5&a=83&s=68&t=76&n=49 4 Nov 2007

Green L 1999 Health education's contributions to public health in the 20th century: A glimpse through health promotion's rear-view mirror. Annual Review of Public Health: Palo Alta: 1999. 20:67–99

Hancock T, Duhl L 1988 Promoting Health in the Urban Context. FADL, Copenhagen

Health Promotion International 1986 A discussion document on the concept and principles of health promotion. Health Promotion International 1(2):73–76

Jackson S, Perkin F, Khandor E et al 2006 Integrated health promotion strategies: a contribution to tackling current and future health challenges. Health Promotion International 21(S1):75–83

Kickbusch I 2007 The move towards a new public health. Promotion & Education Supplement 27:9

Kolbe L J 2005 A Framework for School Health Programs in the 21st Century. The Journal of School Health 75(6):226–228

Labonte R 1989 Commentary: Community empowerment, reflections on the Australian situation. Community Health Studies XIII(3):347–349

Lister-Sharp D, Chapman S, Stewart-Brown S et al 1999 Health promoting schools and health promotion in schools: two systematic reviews. Health Technology Assessment 3(22):1–7

McFarlane M, Kachur R, Klausner J et al 2005 Internet-Based Health Promotion and Disease Control in the 8 Cities: Successes, Barriers, and Future Plans. Sexually Transmitted Disease 32(10):S60–S64

McKinlay J, Marceau L 2000 US public health and the 21st century: Diabetes mellitus. The Lancet 356(9231):757–761

Maes L, Lievens J 2003 Can the school make a difference? A multilevel analysis of adolescent risk and health behaviour. Social Science & Medicine 56(3):517–529

Marmot M G 2003 Understanding social inequalities in health. Perspectives in Biology and Medicine 46:S9–S23

National Aboriginal Community Controlled Health Organisation (NACCHO) website. Available: www.naccho.org.au 2 Nov 2007

National Health Strategy Unit 1993 Pathways to Better Health, Issues Paper no. 7, National Health Strategy Unit, Melbourne

National Steering Committee on Health Promotion in the Workplace 1989 Health at Work Information Kit, National Heart Foundation, Western Australian Division, Nedlands

Navarro A, Voetsch K, Liburd L et al 2007 Charting the Future of Community Health Promotion: Recommendations from the National Expert Panel on Community Health Promotion. Preventing Chronic Disease 4(3). Online. Available: http://www.cdc.gov/PCD/issues/2007/jul/07_0013.htm 20 Oct 2007

Nutbeam D 2000 Health literacy as a public health goal: a challenge for contemporary health education and communication strategies into the 21st century. Health Promotion International 15(3):259–267

Nutbeam D 2005 What would the Ottawa Charter look like if it were written today? Reviews of Health Promotion and Education Online. Available: http://www.rhpeo.org/reviews/2005/19/index.htm 3 Feb 2008

O'Connor M L, Parker E 1995 Health Promotion: Principles and practice in the Australian context. Allen & Unwin, Melbourne

Oldenburg B, Burton N, Parker E 2004 Health Promotion and Environmental Health. In: Cromar N, Cameron S, Fallowfield H (eds) Environmental health in Australia and New Zealand. Oxford University Press, Melbourne

Panaretto K, Mitchell M, Anderson L et al 2007 Sustainable antenatal care services in an urban Indigenous community; the Townsville experience. Medical Journal of Australia 187(1):18–22

Panaretto K 2007 Mums and Babies Program. In: Australians for Native Title and Reconciliation. Success Stories in Indigenous Health. A showcase of successful Aboriginal and Torres Strait Islander health projects. Morprint Pty Ltd. Rydalmere, NSW, pp 8–9

Queensland University of Technology Wellness Matters Program. Available: http://www. wellness.qut.edu.au/3 Nov 2007

Ritchie J 1991 From health education to education for health in Australia: a historical perspective. Health Promotion International 6(2):157–163

Rollnick S, Mason P, Butler C 2004 Health Behavior Change: A guide for Practitioners. Churchill Livingstone. Sage Publications, London

Smedley B D, Syme S L (eds) 2000 Promotion health: Intervention strategies from social and behavioural research. National Academy Press, Washington

St Leger 2001 Schools, health literacy and public health: Possibilities and challenges. Health Promotion International 16(2):197–205

Vartianen E, Jousilahti P, Alfthan G et al 2000 Cardiovascular risk factor changes in Finland, 1972–1997. International Journal of Epidemiology 29:49–56

Wenzel E 1997 A comment on settings in health promotion. Internet Journal of Health Promotion. Available: http://www.rhpeo.org/ijhp-articles/1997/1/index.htm 6 Nov 2007

Whitehead D 2006 Workplace Health Promotion: The Role and Responsibility of Health Care Managers. Journal of Nursing Management 14:59–68

World Health Organization 1978 Declaration of Alma-Ata. International Conference on Primary Health Care, Alma-Ata, USSR, 6–12 September 1978. WHO, Geneva. Available: http://www.who.int/hpr/NPH/docs/declaration_almaata.pdf 6 Nov 2007

World Health Organization 1984 Health Promotion: Concepts and Principles. Report of a Working Group. Available: http://whqlibdoc.who.int/euro/-1993/ICP_HSR_602__m01.pdf 2 Nov 2007

World Health Organization 1986 The Ottawa Charter for Health Promotion First International Conference on Health Promotion, Ottawa, 21 November 1986. Available: http://www.who. int/healthpromotion/conferences/previous/ottawa/en/ 6 Nov 2007

World Health Organization School and youth health website. Available: http://www.who.int/ school_youth_health/gshi/hps/en/index.html 6 Nov 2007

World Health Organization 1988 Adelaide Recommendations on Healthy Public Policy Second International Conference on Health Promotion, Adelaide, South Australia, 5–9 April 1988. Available: http://www.who.int/healthpromotion/conferences/previous/adelaide/en/index1. html 6 Nov 2007

World Health Organization 1991 Sundsvall Statement on Supportive Environments for Health. Third International Conference on Health Promotion, Sundsvall, Sweden, 9–15 June 1991. Available: http://www.who.int/healthpromotion/conferences/previous/ sundsvall/en/ 6 Nov 2007

World Health Organization 1997a Jakarta Statement on Healthy Workplaces, Symposium on Healthy Workplaces at the 4th International Conference on Health Promotion (Jakarta, July 1997). Available: http://www.who.int/healthpromotion/conferences/previous/jakarta/ statements/workplaces/en/ 6 Nov 2007

World Health Organization 1997b Promoting Health through Schools. Report of a WHO Expert Committee on Comprehensive School Health Education and Promotion, Technical Report Series, No. 870

World Health Organization 1998 Health Promotion Glossary. WHO/HPR/HEP/98.1 Geneva, WHO. Available: http://whqlibdoc.who.int/hq/1998/WHO_HPR_HEP_98.1.pdf 26 Oct 2007

World Health Organization 2000 The Fifth Global Conference on Health Promotion Health Promotion: Bridging the Equity Gap 5–9th June 2000, Mexico City. Available: http://www.who.int/healthpromotion/conferences/previous/mexico/en/hpr_mexico_report_en.pdf 6 Nov 2007

World Health Organization 2005 The Bangkok Charter for Health Promotion in a Globalized World. Available: http://www.who.int/helathpromotion/conferences/6gchp/bankok_charter/en/ 26 Oct 2007

Section 5

Contemporary issues

Introduction

An understanding of the impact of globalisation on population health is essential for a public health practitioner in the 21st century. How is globalisation defined and what public health strategies might we put in place to deal with the impact of globalisation on health? Chapter 13 addresses this question as well as comparing the global burden of disease in developing and developed countries. The chapter is divided into four major sections: an introduction to globalisation; globalisation and its impact on population health; global burden of disease; and the global response from the public health community. Increasingly the way in which the planet has become relatively easy to traverse in short periods of time poses real challenges for public health into the future. Globalisation is here to stay and this chapter provides us with an opportunity to see how it impacts on the population's health and how public health might respond.

We also explore the notion of the 'new epidemics' in Chapter 14. This chapter outlines the nature and extent of current and emerging epidemics. Infectious diseases were supposed to be health conditions of the past that were rapidly being conquered by modern medicine. The unfortunate re-emergence of infectious diseases has made the public health community suddenly very aware of the consequences of these illnesses and the potential mortality that may accompany such diseases.

Chapter 14 examines what we have termed the 'old epidemics'. In countries like Australia, infectious diseases once had a much greater impact on health than they now have. However, this is not the case in developing countries where infectious diseases continue to be a major cause of death and disability. This chapter explores the reasons for this disparity but it also discusses the notion that new challenges are also emerging with many of the old infectious diseases. Emerging infectious diseases are also the subject of this chapter, this is where new diseases are recognised but there is currently no effective response. SARS, HIV and avian influenza are but three examples of novel viruses that are of significant threat to population health. The impact of new pandemics is discussed, as is the range of strategies that should be put in place to manage epidemics. The chapter concludes with a discussion about the range of management strategies that may protect the community against potential epidemics.

The final chapter in Section 5 focuses on the future of public health. Chapter 15 looks at identifying the major challenges facing public health in the 21st century and, in particular, it focuses on issues such as globalisation and health impacts, sustainable ecological public health, the re-emergence of infectious diseases, genetics, biotechnology and information technology and their impact on public health.

The chapter emphasises the importance of politics in decision making about public health resources, infrastructure and strategies. It discusses the varying roles of the public health worker in light of the re-emergence of infectious diseases and the development of a range of chronic illnesses. It also tackles the important issue of an ageing population and public health implications. Chapter 15 concludes with a discussion of the importance of a well-structured and comprehensive research agenda for public health.

CHAPTER 13

The impact of globalisation on health

Xiang-Yu (Janet) Hou

Learning objectives

After reading this chapter, you should be able to:

- understand the concept of globalisation and appreciate its complexity
- identify the significant impacts of globalisation on population health, particularly the incidence of communicable and non-communicable diseases
- understand the distribution of the global burden of disease in high-, middle- and low-income countries
- critically evaluate the factors contributing to the major causes of death in low-income countries
- understand some of the achievements of the global public health community and appreciate the challenges it faces.

Introduction to globalisation

Globalisation affects what we eat, what we drink, what we use for transport, home entertainment and professional/medical equipment. An understanding of the impact of globalisation on population health is vital for any 21st century health professional. This chapter is organised into four sections: an introduction to globalisation; globalisation in population health; the global burden of disease; and the global public health community.

Globalisation is a relatively new term used to describe a very old process, and has only been in use for around 25 years. According to Stanley Fischer, the former deputy director of the International Monetary Fund, the word 'globalisation' was never mentioned in the pages of *The New York Times* during the 1970s, and appeared less than once a week in the 1980s (Fischer 2003). Using the Google search engine, the key word 'globalisation' yielded 18.9 million links in January 2008, compared with 1.6 million links in 2002. The term is becoming more widely used every day.

Globalisation is a historical process that began with our ancestors moving out of Africa to spread all over the globe (Chanda 2002). It is likely that the first group of 'migrants' (there were no national borders then) left their homes and villages in central Africa and moved to the Mediterranean about 100,000 years ago, and the second migration was to Asia about 50,000 years ago (Chanda 2002). In the historical era (in general, the period for which we have written records), most of those people moving from country to country were traders, preachers, adventurers and soldiers.

ACTIVITY

- See if you can define globalisation in your own words.
- Can you think of the ways in which 'globalisation' might impact on your life?
- Ask three to five friends how they might define globalisation.
- Why do you think the word 'globalisation' might mean different things to different people?

REFLECTION

As you consider this activity try to think of the factors contributing to the differences among people in a society, such as the political, social, economic, ethical, educational, cultural and other factors. How are people's views of globalisation formed? You may get some idea of the different perspectives when you look at the different ways your friends have defined the term.

If you search for 'globalisation' on Google you will find more than 20 definitions, provided by governments, universities, multinational corporations and a range of other sources. For those involved in international trade, globalisation is a term describing the process of designing, developing and adapting a product for distribution in multiple countries. For those involved in public sector activities, including education, globalisation is the increased flow of goods, services, people, ideas and money across national borders resulting in a more integrated and interdependent world.

Globalisation is defined in Box 13.1. In the process of globalisation, what would bring societies and citizens closer together? According to the International Labour Office, 'trade, investment, technology, cross-border production systems, flows of information' and ease of communications are all factors that facilitate the process of globalisation (Kawachi & Wamala 2007b p 5). National and international policies are necessary to support globalisation. These policies include 'trade and capital market liberalization, and international standards for labour, the environment, corporate behaviour, and agreements on intellectual property rights' (Kawachi & Wamala 2007b p 5).

Box 13.1: Defining globalisation

Globalisation is the movement across national boundaries of people, ideas, money, goods and services, which results in the world becoming politically, economically and culturally interconnected and interdependent.

Global communication

The recent increase in globalisation is associated with technological developments, mainly in transportation and communication that have significantly reduced the 'size' of the world. The speed of communication is now faster than we could ever have imagined. For example, in the late 19th century, it took the Queen of England, Queen Victoria, 16.5 hours to send a greeting message to the American President James Buchanan across a transatlantic cable (Chanda 2002). Today we can communicate with each other through telephone, fax, email and videoconferencing almost instantaneously.

The increased speed of communication, accompanied by a decrease in cost, has made communication such an effective way of connecting the world. In 1930, a three-minute telephone call from New York to London cost US$300, now it can cost less than 10 cents (Chanda 2002). The decreasing cost of telecommunications and the advent of mobile phone technology have greatly increased accessibility for the majority of people in most countries and facilitated communications. Mobile phones were introduced into Australia in February 1987. Australia, with a population of just over 21 million people in June 2007 (Australian Bureau of Statistics 2007) and 6.5 million households, had more than 3.2 million mobile phone users in 2007 (Allen 2007).

Internet usage is another sign of globalisation in communication. A report by a marketing group in November 2007 indicated that 19.1% of the world's population (6.6 billion) use the internet (Miniwatts Marketing Group 2007). Among the 1.3 billion internet users in the world, about 37% are from Asia, 27% from Europe, 19% from North America, 10% from Latin America, 3.5% from Africa, 2.7% from the Middle East and 1.5% from Australia/Oceania (Miniwatts Marketing Group 2007). Globally, internet usage increased by an average of 250% over the period 2000 to 2007. In the Middle East the increase was 920%, in Africa – 880%, in Asia – 304% and in Europe – 227%. China, with the world's largest population, had 22.5 million internet users in 2000 (about 1.7% of the country's population); by 2007 the number had increased to 162 million (12.3% of the population) (Miniwatts Marketing Group 2007). Australia had 6.6 million internet users in 2000, and 14.7 million in 2007 (respectively, about 34 and 70% of the population) (Miniwatts Marketing Group 2007). No other communication technology has seen an increase in uptake in such a short time frame.

National and international air travel

The affordability of air travel has also dropped dramatically. In Canada, for example, there were 54 million air passengers in 2002, and 64 million in 2005 (Cherniavsky & Dachis 2007). In Australia in 1997, there were about 70,000 passengers (domestic and international) flying through Australian airports (Sydney, Melbourne, Brisbane, Adelaide and Perth). By 2006 this figure had increased to 110,000 passengers (see Fig 13.1). Air

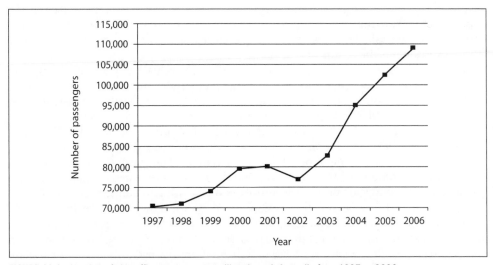

FIGURE 13.1: Number of air traffic passengers travelling through Australia from 1997 to 2006

(Source: Australian-Transport 2007 Aviation Statistics 2008)

travel contributes to local economic development itself, but in combination with related services such as hotels, local transport and food, it is an important contributor to the overall economy. The most significant impact of this increased air travel is that it has made the world a face-to-face meeting place, thus greatly enhancing global interconnectedness and interdependence. It has also meant that illness and disease spreads rapidly across the globe as people move from country to country in a relatively short amount of time.

Globalisation has positive as well as negative impacts; supporters claim it increases economic prosperity and development opportunities. The process of globalisation can also support the development of civil liberties. Another aspect of globalisation – the movement of money, goods and services – can initiate a more efficient distribution of resources, which can then enhance employment prospects, reduce the cost of goods and services, and thus increase the standard of living for the world's population.

Research has shown that poverty rates have dropped significantly in countries such as China where globalisation has taken a strong foothold, compared with regions less affected by globalisation, such as Sub-Saharan Africa, where poverty rates continue to be high (Sachs 2005). This argument was supported by the *International Monetary Fund Policy Discussion Paper* of 2001, which reported that 'countries that have embraced openness to the rest of the world' have done better in their economic development than those that have not (Masson 2001 p 1).

Critics of globalisation believe that the rapid flow of capital and consumer goods has caused damage to the planet and increased poverty, socioeconomic inequality, injustice and the erosion of traditional cultures. Many organisations in developed countries involved in globalisation have failed to consider the welfare of underprivileged countries and people of low socioeconomic status, or the interests of the natural world (Bakan 2004). To reduce the negative impact of globalisation on poorer countries, the Secretary General Mr Ban Ki-moon told the *United Nations Conference on Trade and Development* (UNCTAD) on 4 March 2008 in New York that '2008 must be devoted to helping the bottom billion of the world's poorest to tap into global economic growth … In a globalizing world, we require an international economic environment that fosters development; … today's UN cannot simply champion development, it must deliver every day on its promises' (UN 2008a).

How many people around the world do you think might be supporters of globalisation? How many people around the world do you think might be opponents? A survey on people's perceptions of globalisation was conducted in 2006 in a range of countries representing 56% of the world's population territories (University of Maryland 2007). The respondents were asked a series of questions concerning their ideas about globalisation. Table 13.1 presents the results of that study.

The survey showed that support for globalisation is remarkably strong throughout the world. The survey question, 'Globalisation, especially increasing connections of our economy with others around the world, is mostly good or mostly bad' was asked in 17 countries and the Palestinian territories. In every country positive responses outweighed negative ones. It is possible that the level of support is related to the extent of the countries' export economies. For example, respondents in China, South Korea and Israel expressed strong support for globalisation. The greatest scepticism about globalisation was found in Mexico, Russia and the Philippines, with less than 50% of the population regarding globalisation as 'mostly good' (University of Maryland 2007).

In Australia, the same survey was conducted by the Lowy Institute in July 2006 (University of Maryland 2007); it showed that most Australians viewed globalisation favourably. About 65% of Australians considered globalisation to be 'mostly good' for the country, while only a quarter (27%) said that it is 'mostly bad'. Almost all Australians interviewed (98% of respondents) believed that protecting Australian jobs should be a foreign policy goal, and 83% considered that it is 'very important'. There are links between

COUNTRY	MOSTLY GOOD (%)	MOSTLY BAD (%)
Australia	65	27
China	87	6
France	51	42
Iran	63	31
India	54	30
Israel	83	10
Mexico	41	22
Philippines	49	32
Russia	41	24
South Korea	86	12
United States	60	35

TABLE 13.1: The view of globalisation by country

(Source: WorldPublicOpinion.org 2007)

having a job and socioeconomic status, that is, people who are employed generally enjoy a higher status; moreover, socioeconomic status and health are clearly linked (see Chapter 6 for more information regarding the social determinants of health).

ACTIVITY

- If you were asked the question: *Is globalisation, especially increasing the connections of our economy with others around the world, mostly good or mostly bad?* How would you have responded?
- What information would you use to answer the question?
- Think about the positive and negative outcomes of globalisation. Make a table, with one column for the positive aspects, and the other column for the negative aspects.

REFLECTION

It is likely that your answer reflects your personal circumstances, including your educational level, financial status, country of birth, cultural background and personal beliefs. What do you consider to be some of the positive aspects of globalisation? Would you include easier access to information, a broader range of opportunities and an understanding of different cultures and the issues they face? What about the negative consequences of globalisation? Could they include unwanted economic influences or cultural changes, which some people may hold responsible for the destruction of their cultures?

Globalisation in population health

Globalisation affects population health by changing the ways in which people interact across boundaries, including 'spatial (territorial), temporal (time) and cognitive (thought processes)' boundaries (Lee 1999 p 249). For example, global trade has led to increased spatial and temporal exposure to infectious disease through the rapid cross-border transmission of communicable diseases (notable examples include SARS and avian influenza). Similarly, global trade also increases the risk of chronic diseases, through the marketing of unhealthy products, and risk behaviours, such as tobacco smoking and the consumption of fast food (Smith 2006). In addition, the global distribution of health-related goods (e.g. pharmaceutical products, medical equipment) and people (both patients and health professionals) is another example of how the health of the population might be impacted.

In this section of the chapter, we will discuss two of the main aspects of the effects of globalisation on population health. First, we will consider the impact of globalisation with regard to the increased exposure to infectious diseases, and second, the increased risk of chronic diseases. The background to infectious diseases and the individual strategies directed towards control and management are outlined in Chapter 11. The impact that infectious diseases have on population health and the strategies to manage outbreaks are covered in Chapter 14.

Globalisation of infectious diseases

Arguably, infectious diseases cause the greatest threat to population health because of the potential for such diseases to rapidly spread to large numbers of people across the world. People's travel can facilitate the movement of infectious pathogens. The potential for geographical spread is particularly apparent if you consider that most infectious diseases have an incubation period exceeding 36 hours, and that any part of the world can now be reached within 36 hours (Kawachi & Wamala 2007a). For example, SARS (severe acute respiratory syndrome) demonstrates the rapid movement of infectious pathogens from country to country.

SARS is a viral respiratory illness caused by a corona virus. In general, SARS patients have a raised body temperature (greater than 38°C), headache, diarrhoea, mild respiratory symptoms and pneumonia (US Centers for Disease Control and Prevention (CDC) 2008). The main way that SARS spreads is by close person-to-person contact. The virus is transmitted most readily by respiratory droplets (via sneezing and coughing), which can spread up to one metre in the air (CDC 2008).

SARS was first reported in China in February 2003. Within 11 weeks it had spread to 27 countries in North America, South America, Europe, and Asia (Cherry 2004). The rapid spread of SARS and the high case fatality rate prompted significant reactions around the world. Some have compared the SARS outbreak to that of the 'Spanish flu' of 1918–1919, which killed over 20 million people (Yale 2003). Spanish flu was spread by people travelling on trains and by troops on ships, while SARS was spread by people travelling by air, which facilitated the movement of SARS from Asia to North America and Europe in a matter of days (Yale 2003). While SARS has caused comparatively fewer deaths than the Spanish flu, it spread far more rapidly due to the intensification of global travel over the past several decades. The rapid spread of SARS caused fear and considerable disturbance to people's lives across the world. As we saw earlier in Figure 13.1, the reported number of domestic and international passengers flying through Australia showed a significant decrease in 2002, which is attributable, at least in part, to the SARS outbreak.

Merson (2003) claimed that 'SARS proved health is a global public good: And the need to boost domestic public health and international cooperation' (the full article can be found on the YaleGlobal website). As the economic consequences of SARS became apparent (already about US$150 billion worldwide by September 2003), countries scrambled for effective solutions. However, individual nation-states were ill equipped to manage an illness like SARS by themselves for a number of reasons, including limited medical expertise and a lack of understanding about the disease (Kickbusch 2003). This example demonstrates the need for a worldwide collaborative approach.

It was through a global public health approach and inter-country cooperation in developing and implementing 'effective control strategies, including early isolation of suspected cases, strict infection control measures' in health settings and 'meticulous contact tracing and quarantine' (Zhong & Wong 2004 p 270), that the global SARS outbreak was contained by July 2003.

The success in fighting SARS has demonstrated the importance of the global public health community working together. However, research has shown that global resources to counter emerging infectious diseases (EID) are 'poorly allocated, with the majority of the scientific and surveillance effort focussed on countries from where the next important EID is least likely to originate' (Jones et al 2008 p 990). The 'greater surveillance and infectious disease research effort' are allocated 'in richer, developed countries of Europe, North America, Australia and some parts of Asia, than in developing regions' (Jones et al 2008 p 992); while the 'predicted emerging disease hotspots due to zoonotic pathogens from wildlife and vector-borne pathogens are more concentrated in lower-latitude developing countries' (Jones et al 2008 p 992). Therefore, in the era of globalisation, the international investment needs to be targeted at lower-latitude developing countries for capacity building to detect, identify and monitor infectious diseases. As shown in SARS, emerging infectious diseases are every country's problem.

ACTIVITY

- List your ideas about how globalisation impacts on the spread of infectious diseases such as SARS.
- Now group the ideas into different categories such as political, economic, educational, research, tourism, cultural, policy and other factors.

REFLECTION

Did you think about the links between this activity and the content of Chapters 5 and 6, to clarify some of the potential factors that could either promote or impede the spread of SARS? Did you consider the contribution of research to understanding the nature of the disease, policies related to travel, social gathering or social distancing, and the possible cultural differences in managing the media and public panic?

Globalisation and chronic diseases

The main global chronic diseases today include heart disease, stroke, cancer, chronic respiratory diseases and diabetes (WHO 2008). These are generally the consequences of intermediate risk factors, such as raised blood pressure, raised glucose levels, abnormal blood lipids (particularly low-density lipoprotein and cholesterol) and overweight (Body Mass Index (BMI) ≥ 25) and obesity (BMI ≥ 30). The most important modifiable risk factors are unhealthy diet, physical inactivity and tobacco use. These risk factors, in conjunction with the non-modifiable risk factors of age and heredity, explain the majority of new cases of heart disease, stroke, chronic respiratory diseases and some cancers (WHO 2006). To explore the effects of globalisation on the modifiable risk factors, the next section discusses tobacco use and unhealthy diets.

Tobacco use

Globalisation processes including trade liberalisation, foreign direct investment and marketing have shifted the focus of the tobacco-using population in the world. Tobacco was introduced to Asia and Africa around 400 years ago.

Contemporary statistics suggest that 75% of the world's cigarette market is controlled by just four companies. They are China National Tobacco Corporation, Japan Tobacco, British American Tobacco and Philip Morris. While cigarette consumption in most high-income countries has declined, it has increased more than threefold, from 1.1 billion to 3.3 billion cigarettes in total per year in low- and middle-income countries between 1997 and 2000 (Kawachi & Wamala 2007b).

Tobacco-related diseases were responsible for nearly 4.8 million premature deaths in 2000 (Ezzati & Lopez 2003), and about 5.4 million in 2005, 6.4 million in 2015 and 8.3 million in 2030 (Mathers & Loncar 2006b). By 2015, tobacco is projected to be responsible for 10% of all deaths globally (see Table 13.2) (Mathers & Loncar 2006b). Globalisation has led to this increase in cigarette consumption in the middle- and low-income countries. Let us consider tobacco consumption in China as an example.

	CAUSE	NUMBER OF TOBACCO-CAUSED DEATHS (MILLION)
All causes		6.43
	Tuberculosis	0.09
	Lower respiratory infections	0.15
Malignant neoplasms		2.12
	Trachea, bronchus, lung cancers	1.18
	Mouth and oropharynx cancers	0.18
	Oesophagus cancer	0.17
	Stomach cancer	0.12
	Liver cancer	0.10
	Other malignant neoplasms	0.34
Diabetes mellitus		0.13
Cardiovascular disease		1.86
	Ischaemic heart disease	0.93
	Cerebrovascular disease	0.52
	Other cardiovascular disease	0.24
Respiratory disease		1.87
	Chronic obstructive pulmonary disease (COPD)	1.76
Digestive disease		0.20

TABLE 13.2: Projected global tobacco-caused deaths by 2015 – adapted from baseline scenario
(Source: Mathers & Loncar 2006a)

In China, chronic diseases account for an estimated 80% of deaths and 70% of disability-adjusted life years (DALYs) lost (Wang et al 2005). Cardiovascular diseases and cancer are the leading causes of both death and the burden of disease. The exposure to risk factors is high. For example, more than 300 million men smoke cigarettes, and if current smoking patterns persist, two million out of the seven million deaths related to smoking worldwide will occur in China (Wang et al 2005). This estimation does not include passive smokers.

The *China Guangzhou Biobank Cohort Study* (Yin et al 2007) investigated a sample size of over 20,000 and demonstrated that exposure to passive smoking is associated with an increased prevalence of COPD and respiratory symptoms. It was estimated that 1.9 million excess deaths from COPD among those who had never smoked could be attributed to passive smoking in the current population in China (Yin et al 2007).

In addition to the direct health effects of smoking, indirect consequences include the financial cost, especially for a developing country like China. It was found that in some Chinese rural areas expenditure on tobacco occurs at the expense of education, medical care, insurance and investment in farming (Wang et al 2006). The excessive medical spending attributable to smoking and consumption spending on cigarettes combined are estimated to be responsible for impoverishing 30.5 million urban residents and 23.7 million rural residents in China (Liu et al 2006). In China, smoking-related expenses push a significant proportion of low-income families into poverty, making vulnerable people more susceptible to health problems.

China's membership in the World Trade Organization (WTO) has presented unprecedented opportunities for the multinational tobacco companies to penetrate the world's largest cigarette market (Kawachi & Wamala 2007a). Since the late 1990s, these companies have signed numerous cooperation agreements with China to modernise manufacturing facilities, improve crop yields and build crop-processing plants (Kawachi & Wamala 2007a). China now grows cash crops of tobacco and produces the largest amount of tobacco in the world, whereas previously it was an agrarian, subsistence economy. It is critical that the Chinese central government, including the ministries of health, finance and foreign affairs, work together to tackle this serious tobacco problem.

ACTIVITY

- Assign the following roles to a group of seven fellow students: a representative from a global tobacco company, a Department of Health and Ageing (DoHA) spokesperson, an economist, a spokesperson for the Department of Foreign Affairs, a sports commentator, a media representative and a tobacco consumer.
- Multinational tobacco companies are approaching populations in developing countries using tactics that include mass media campaigns and generous sponsorship of large-scale popular sports. Are these tactics going to produce a large proportion of people who smoke, which then requires that these countries develop interventions to reduce the number of smokers? Or could a developing country effectively develop national strategies to promote non-smoking? What challenges would a country face in taking this approach?
- Then give each group 10–20 minutes to think about the strategies for and against tobacco importation. Each group should do their role-play for the class and then everyone can discuss the issues.

REFLECTION

This role-play will help you to understand some of the challenges health professionals face in trying to protect the health of the population during the process of globalisation. Did the 'DoHA representative' develop and implement a non-tobacco import/use policy for the population? Did the 'Department of Foreign Affairs representative' try to justify a free trade policy (e.g. tobacco) between countries? Did the 'economist' focus on the income brought into the country by exporting tobacco?

Did the sports commentator and media representatives, who may owe their jobs to tobacco company sponsorship of sports events, support the tobacco companies? Lastly, did the group representing tobacco consumers argue that they have the right to decide whether or not they use tobacco? The final outcome of this role-play should help you to understand the process of globalisation, and its potential negative impacts on population health.

Overweight and obesity

Globalisation has contributed to a worldwide epidemic of overweight and obesity. Obesity is a significant risk factor for a range of chronic diseases, and is associated with at least as much morbidity as poverty, smoking and problem drinking collectively (Sturm & Wells 2001). Prevalence rates for overweight and obesity are very different in each region, with the Middle East, central and eastern Europe and North America having higher prevalence than Asia and northern Europe (James 2004). Examine Table 13.3 below – what does the data suggest to you? This table displays evidence about the prevalence of overweight and obesity in the US, and the WHO European regions. It suggests that in the WHO European regions, depending on country, a high percentage of both men and women are pre-obese (i.e. overweight) or obese.

COUNTRY	PREVALENCE RATE OF OVERWEIGHT AND OBESE
United States in 2000 (Sturm & Wells 2001)	About 36% of adults were overweight but not obese (25<=BMI<30) Another 23% were obese (BMI>=30)
WHO European region – percentage of pre-obese or obese men, 2007	
Bulgaria (urban), Ireland, Malta and Slovenia	70%
Cyprus, the Czech Republic and Germany	75%
Albania (urban), Croatia and Slovakia (urban)	80%
WHO European region – percentage of pre-obese or obese women, 2007	
Croatia, Hungary, Ireland, Latvia and Spain	50%
Czech Republic, Cyprus, Scotland and Turkey	60%
Malta	70%
Slovakia (rural) and Albania (rural)	80%

TABLE 13.3: Prevalence of pre-obese (overweight) and obese in the world

(Adapted from Knai et al 2007, Sturm & Wells 2001)

If the prevalence of obesity continues to increase at the same rate as in the 1990s, approximately 150 million adults in the European region may be obese by 2010 (WHO 2006). Some nations, such as the US, are almost completely globalised in their food and activity patterns for all social strata. Other countries, for example China, are currently less than fully globalised, with primarily higher socioeconomic status individuals becoming incorporated into global systems, and consequently, members of this group are more likely to become obese (Sobal 2001). As developing countries 'catch up' with developed countries in the prevalence rates of overweight and obesity, the number of obese people (currently more than 315 million people in the world) could double by the year 2025 (Formiguera & Canton 2004).

Children and adolescents tend to assimilate global culture more quickly than their parents. Therefore, their eating and activity levels, and consequently their body weight, are more rapidly modified (Sobal 2001). In China, the prevalence of childhood overweight/obesity in 2000 was similar to that of Great Britain and the US in the 1980s (Liu et al 2007). While China is 'catching up' with the West, studies show that within China, rural areas are fast approaching the prevalence of overweight and obesity of urban areas (see Table 13.4) (Wang et al 2005). A study in Shenzhen (Hui & Bell 2003), a relatively wealthy city in China, found that 19% of boys and 11% of girls were overweight or obese.

	PREVALENCE OF OVERWEIGHT (%)	PREVALENCE OF OBESITY (%)
Large city	13.1	8.1
Middle-sized city	7.1	3.2
Wealthy rural areas	4.1	1.9
Poor rural areas	2.3	0.7

TABLE 13.4: Prevalence of overweight and obesity in Chinese children aged 7–17 years old in 2002
(Source: Wang et al 2005)

To fully understand the global epidemic of obesity, especially in developing countries, we need to move beyond individual physiology and personal characteristics to examine collective social, economic and political structures, and cultural changes (Sobal 2001). These include factors such as urbanisation, technological shifts, economic forces and cultural factors (Kawachi & Wamala 2007b). Table 13.5 examines the range of factors contributing to the global epidemic of obesity. Among the cultural factors, which have changed people's food choices and dietary patterns in many developing countries, we will examine two aspects, large shifts in food imports and modern advertising.

	FACTORS	CONTRIBUTION (%)
Cultural factors	Modern advertising Other elements affecting food choice and dietary patterns	25%
Economic forces	Food and price changes	30%
Technological shifts	Energy expenditure decreases at work, travel, home production and leisure	30%
Urbanisation	Urbanisation and others	15%

TABLE 13.5: Factors contributing to global epidemic of obesity
(Source: Kawachi & Wamala 2007b)

Large changes in food imports are evident, for example between 1989 and 1998, sales by US-owned food-processing affiliates in South America grew from US$5 billion to US$15 billion, and sales in Asia increased from US$5 billion to US$20 billion (Bolling & Somwaru 2001). In China in 2004, there were more than 1,000 Kentucky Fried Chicken (KFC) restaurants, and they were increasing at a rate of 200 each year. A new KFC restaurant opens every second day in China (China Daily 2004). Having arrived in China in the early 1990s, McDonald's has more than 600 restaurants in nearly 100 cities and in 2004 was growing at a rate of 100 restaurants per year (China Daily 2004). The most obvious expressions for this phenomenon are the 'burgerisation' or 'coca-colonisation' or 'McDonaldisation' of food culture (Lang 1998, Zimmet 2000).

The marketing of brands and shifts in cultural norms can actually influence people's tastes (Chopra et al 2002). This particularly applies to young people and populations longing for a 'Western' lifestyle. Marketing and product branding have the ability to transform food culture in surprisingly short periods of time (Lang 1998). This has enormous implications both for state budgets and for health inequalities. How can a government with a limited budget hope to influence a population with a health education message, when a transnational company can spend almost unlimited amounts of money on advertising to promote brand recognition and consumption (Lang 1998)?

A transformation in food cultures, including an increase in meat consumption, also has a negative effect on our living environment. Worldwide, agriculture, particularly livestock production, makes up approximately 20% of total greenhouse-gas emissions, thus contributing to global climate change (McMichael et al 2007). Worldwide, the current average meat consumption is about 100 g per person per day, with about a tenfold difference between high- and low-consuming populations. To prevent increased greenhouse-gas emissions from this production sector, '90 g per day is proposed as a working global target, shared more evenly, with no more than 50 g per day being red meat from ruminants (i.e. cattle, sheep and goats)' (McMichael et al 2007 p 1253). Reducing the consumption of meat will not only benefit population health, but also the natural environment of our world.

ACTIVITY

- As a health professional, what would you do to promote a healthy diet among school students in a developing country where fast food restaurants are emerging as a major source of dietary intake?
- Who would you work with? Are there other professionals you would consider important to collaborate with?
- How might you use the school curriculum to help you?

REFLECTION

Did you think about the role a country's food policy plays in promoting a healthy diet or, conversely, how might it make it more difficult to adopt a healthy lifestyle? Did you consider the food industry's contribution to choices and opportunities? Did you consider using health education and school health promotion activities to support healthy dietary messages? One of the negative aspects of the 'Western' lifestyle is the risk of children and older young people in particular, adopting unhealthy dietary habits because of their desire to adopt a particular lifestyle that they think is better than their own.

Globalisation is a two-way street. While 'Western' food cultures are imported into developing countries, 'Eastern' food cultures are also exported from developing countries, but mainly as raw and unprocessed foods. For example, exports of poultry to Japan from China almost quadrupled during the period 1988–1993 (McMichael 2000). This rapid increase has the financial and technical support of the multinational food company Charoen Pokphand of Thailand, which now has 80 establishments across China. They develop feed mills, breeder farms, broiler chicken farms, processing factories and chicken fast-food stores (McMichael 2000). The quality of food exports is of potential national public health concern. For example, in 2007 low levels of banned antibiotics were identified in one-third of the samples of prawns, fish, crabs and eels imported from Thailand, Indonesia, China and Vietnam into Australia (Mitchell & Wilson 2007). This discovery of prohibited antibiotics in imported seafood was a major concern for the Australian public because Australia imported $1.03 billion worth of edible fish and seafood in 2005–06, which is about 70% of Australia's annual seafood consumption (Mitchell & Wilson 2007).

Globalisation has a considerable impact on the spread of communicable diseases, such as SARS. Furthermore, it plays an important role in the development of non-communicable diseases, such as those resulting from tobacco use and unhealthy diets. Accordingly, because of globalisation's role in the health of the world's population, it is a pragmatic focus for modern public health practice.

The global burden of disease

The 'global burden of disease' is a statistical concept that is useful for tracking changes in patterns of health, for policy development and analysing the effectiveness of public health programs. It provides a significant tool in facilitating cross-national comparison during the process of globalisation. The global burden of disease (GBD) is a comprehensive regional and global assessment of mortality and disability from 107 diseases and injuries and 10 risk factors. It is assessed using WHO's GBD study and is an example of an evidence-based input to public health policy debate. The aim of the study was to provide information and projections about the global burden of disease.

In 1996 WHO conducted a GBD project, which was updated in 2006 (Mathers & Loncar 2006b). The work produced estimates of the rates of deaths and DALYs for 2005, 2015 and 2030. These estimates can be downloaded from the WHO website by causes of death, age and sex, for several different regional groupings of countries. The full details of the methodology and data sources were published by Mathers and Loncar (2006a).

A summary of those results and the methodology used are presented here as an example of the impact of income and other factors on health. In its report, the GBD estimates included a limited number of socioeconomic variables: (1) average income per capita, measured as gross domestic product (GDP) per capita; (2) the average number of years of schooling in adults, referred to as 'human capital'; and (3) time, a proxy measure for the impact of technological change on health status. Time is an important variable as it captures the effects of accumulating knowledge and technological development. It allows the implementation of more cost-effective health interventions (both preventive and curative) at constant levels of income and human capital. And variable (4), tobacco use, was included in the projections for cancers, cardiovascular diseases and chronic respiratory diseases (Mathers & Loncar 2006b).

Using historical death registration data for 107 countries between 1950 and 2002, death rates from all major causes (excluding HIV/AIDS and tuberculosis) were related to the four variables outlined above (Mathers & Loncar 2006b). The study conclusively demonstrated the importance of income, human capital and tobacco use in determining global public health. The report predicts a shift in the distribution of deaths from 2002 to 2030: from younger ages to older ages; and from communicable diseases, and maternal, peri-natal and nutritional causes to non-communicable disease causes. Other important projected results regarding the change between 2002 and 2030 include:

- the risk of death for children aged under five will probably fall by nearly 50%
- the proportion of deaths due to non-communicable disease will likely rise from 59% to 69%
- global HIV/AIDS deaths will probably rise from 2.8 million to 6.5 million per annum.

Projected changes in HIV/AIDS status assumes that coverage of patients with anti-retroviral (ARV) drugs reaches 80% by 2012. Assuming increased prevention activity in HIV/AIDS (under the optimistic scenario), deaths would drop to 3.7 million in 2030 (Mathers & Loncar 2006b).

There are some shifts in the ranking of the world's top 15 leading causes of death between 2002 and 2030 (see Table 13.6), reflecting the change from communicable to non-communicable diseases (except HIV/AIDS) (Mathers & Loncar 2006a). For example, diarrhoeal diseases and tuberculosis, which were ranked seventh and eighth respectively in 2002, are not expected to feature in the top 15 by the year 2030. Although ischaemic heart disease is expected to be the leading cause of death in low-income countries in 2030, lower respiratory disease is still going to be the fifth highest cause of death, contributing about 5.1% of total deaths in this group of countries (see Table 13.7). Perinatal conditions, road traffic accidents, diarrhoeal diseases and malaria are

DISEASE OR INJURY	2002 RANK	2030 RANK
Ischaemic heart disease	1	1
Cerebrovascular disease	2	2
Lower respiratory infections	3	5
HIV/AIDS	4	3
COPD	5	4
Perinatal conditions	6	9
Diarrhoeal diseases	7	16
Tuberculosis	8	23
Trachea, bronchus, lung cancers	9	6
Road traffic accidents	10	8
Diabetes mellitus	11	7
Malaria	12	22
Hypertensive heart disease	13	11
Self-inflicted injuries	14	12
Stomach cancer	15	10
Nephritis and nephrosis	17	13
Colon and rectum cancers	18	15
Liver cancers	19	14

TABLE 13.6: The world's top 18 leading causes of death in 2002 and 2030

(Adapted from Mathers & Loncar 2006a)

still expected to be in the top 10 causes of death in low-income countries, contributing to about 12% of total deaths. This study indicates that there will be a 'double burden' of disease in developing countries over the next couple of decades, which is an important consideration in policy development. (For more information on policy development, see Chapter 3.) Comprehensive health policies need to target this 'double burden' to ensure improvements in population health in developing countries.

RANK	DISEASES OR INJURY	PERCENTAGE OF TOTAL DEATHS
1	Ischaemic heart disease	13.4
2	HIV/AIDS	13.2
3	Cerebrovascular diseases	8.2
4	COPD	5.5
5	Lower respiratory infections	5.1
6	Perinatal conditions	3.9
7	Road traffic accidents	3.7
8	Diarrhoeal disease	2.3
9	Diabetes mellitus	2.1
10	Malaria	1.8

TABLE 13.7: Top 10 leading causes of death in low-income countries in 2030 (projected)
(Adapted from Mathers & Loncar 2006a)

Fatal health outcomes can be clearly related to mortality and causes of death. On the other hand, non-fatal health outcomes are also important when considering the burden of disease. DALYs is a variable that measures premature mortality and non-fatal conditions (Murray & Acharya 1997). It is not the purpose of this chapter to cover the last decade's debate about DALYs, although we do acknowledge that using DALYs as a measure is not without limitations (Arnesen & Kapiriri 2004, Barker & Green 1996, Mont 2007, Üstün et al 1999).

Measured by DALYs, the top four contributors to the global burden of disease in 2030 are projected to be HIV/AIDS, unipolar depressive disorders, ischaemic heart disease and road traffic accidents (see Table 13.8), which together will be responsible for almost one-third of the total DALYs (Mathers & Loncar 2006b).

HIV/AIDS ranks number one and contributes to 12% of the total DALYs, while number two, unipolar depressive disorders, contributes to almost 6% of the total. After ischaemic heart disease, road traffic accidents rank number four in the world and contribute to about 4% of the total DALYs. It is important to note that lower respiratory infections, diarrhoeal diseases, malaria and cataracts are expected to remain in the top 10 causes of burden of diseases in low-income countries by 2030. Prevention, diagnosis and treatment of these diseases is well developed, and explains why these diseases are not projected to be included in the top 10 contributors to the burden of disease in the world as a whole (Mathers & Loncar 2006a).

Finally, it is important to be aware that the projections of causes of death and burden of disease were developed under an explicit set of assumptions. If, for example, additional efforts are made to address the United Nations' (UN's) *Millennium Development Goals* (MDG), or some major scientific breakthroughs are made, then the world may achieve faster progress than that projected. Conversely, if economic growth in low-income

	RANK	DISEASE OR INJURY	PERCENT OF TOTAL DALYS
World	1	HIV/AIDS	12.1
	2	Unipolar depressive disorders	5.7
	3	Ischaemic heart disease	4.7
	4	Road traffic accidents	4.2
	5	Perinatal conditions	4.0
	6	Cerebrovascular disease	3.9
	7	COPD	3.1
	8	Lower respiratory infections	3.0
	9	Hearing loss, adult onset	2.5
	10	Cataracts	2.5
Low-income countries	1	HIV/AIDS	14.6
	2	Perinatal conditions	5.8
	3	Unipolar depressive disorders	4.7
	4	Road traffic accidents	4.6
	5	Ischaemic heart disease	4.5
	6	Lower respiratory infections	4.4
	7	Diarrhoeal diseases	2.8
	8	Cerebrovascular disease	2.8
	9	Cataracts	2.8
	10	Malaria	2.5

TABLE 13.8: Ten leading causes of disability adjusted life years in 2030 (projected)

(Adapted from Mathers & Loncar 2006a)

countries is lower than the forecasts used (due to war or natural disasters, for example), then the world may achieve slower progress and an increase in the health inequalities between developed and developing countries (Mathers & Loncar 2006a). Nevertheless, WHO's 2006 report on the global burden of disease provides a foundation for the global public health community to work towards to the UN's MDG.

ACTIVITY

In 2030 the number one leading cause of death globally will be ischaemic heart disease. It will contribute to approximately 13%, 14%, and 16% of total deaths in low-, middle-, and high- income countries respectively.

● Why do you think the burden of heart disease is expected to be fairly equally distributed between income levels in the future?

Consider the contribution of HIV/AIDS to global morbidity by 2030: It is projected to be listed as the number one cause of death in low-income countries (nearly 15%), the number one cause of death in middle-income countries (almost 10%), but not listed in the top 10 in high-income countries, yet listed as number one in the world (12%).

● Can you think of three explanations for this pattern of morbidity projected to 2030?

- Why do you think the death rates from HIV/AIDS are low in affluent countries?
- Might there be some social and medical explanations for these differences?

Unipolar depressive disorders have been projected to be the number one cause of morbidity in high-income countries (almost 10%), the number two cause of morbidity in middle-income countries (almost 7%), and the number three cause in low-income countries (nearly 5%).

- What does this data tell us? Does it mean that 'the richer you are the more unhappy you are?'
- What are some of factors that may be contributing to these trends?

REFLECTION

For each of these questions you need to have an understanding of the disease process you are considering, and the risk factors and determinants that influence the development of the disease. For the first question did you consider the 'double burden' of diseases in developing countries? Did you think about some of the social, economic and medical factors for the HIV/AIDS question? Did you take into account the possibility of under-diagnosis and poor management of unipolar depression in low-income countries? For further discussion regarding the physical, environmental, social and emotional determinants of health, refer to Chapters 5 and 6.

This leads us into a discussion about the structure and achievements of the global public health community.

The global public health community

The global public health community has a 150-year history of working together to deal with international health problems. In this section, we will briefly describe the current international health organisations, their programs and their contributions to global public health.

The first international meeting of the public health community was held in 1851 in Paris. In the mid 20th century the collaboration was formalised through the UN and its various agents including WHO (Walt 1998). During that meeting it was agreed that resources for health development would be channelled through multilateral (global system) and bilateral (government-to-government) organisations, and non-government organisations (NGOs). In addition to WHO, the World Bank has been an increasingly significant contributor to the global public health community, through providing financial and technical support. Private sector organisations, such as non-government foundations (e.g. the Rockefeller Foundation and the Bill and Melinda Gates Foundation) and for-profit organisations (e.g. pharmaceutical and insurance companies), have been very active as well. Some of the main international players in the global public health community are introduced below.

The United Nations (UN) is a multilateral organisation that was officially established on 24 October 1945 in San Francisco with 50 member countries (UN 2008b). The five purposes of the UN articulated at that time were:

1 'to maintain international peace and security;
2 to develop friendly relations among nations;
3 to cooperate in solving international economic, social, cultural and humanitarian problems;
4 to cooperate in promoting respect for human rights and fundamental freedoms; and
5 to be a centre for harmonizing the actions of nations in attaining these ends' (UN 2008b).

As history shows, the UN has been an active and effective player in numerous aspects of international politics and health through its agencies. In September 2000, at the *Millennium Summit,* member states of the UN (e.g. Australia) reaffirmed their commitment to eliminate global poverty and hunger, to improve health, gender equality, education, environmental sustainability, and to create a global partnership for development (UN 2008b). One of the outcomes of this historic assembly was the announcement of eight MDG (introduced in Chapter 1), which are listed in Table 13.9 (Wamala et al 2007, UN website).

	GOAL	TARGETS
1	Eradicate extreme poverty and hunger	Between 1990 and 2015, halve the proportion of people whose income is less than $1 a day and who suffer from hunger
2	Achieve universal primary education	By 2015, every child (boy or girl) complete a full course of primary schooling
3	Promote gender equality and empower women	Eliminate gender disparity in all levels of education by 2015
4	Reduce child mortality	Between 1990 and 2015, reduce mortality by two-thirds in children under five years of age
5	Improve maternal health	Between 1990 and 2015, reduce maternal mortality by 75%
6	Combat HIV/AIDS, malaria, and other diseases	By 2015, have halved and begun to reverse the spread of HIV/AIDS By 2015 have halved and begun to reverse the incidence of malaria and other diseases
7	Ensure environmental sustainability	For example: integrate the principles of sustainable development into country policies and programs and reverse the loss of environment resources
8	Develop a global partnership for development	For example: develop further an open, rule-based, predictable, non-discriminatory trading and financial system, including a commitment to good governance, development, and poverty reduction – both nationally and internationally.

TABLE 13.9: The UN Millennium Development Goals

(Source: United Nations website, Wamala et al 2007)

Despite the daunting task ahead, the UN has taken a number of steps in collaboration with member states to achieve the eight goals listed in Table 13.9. Consider climate change as one example to demonstrate the commitment of the UN's member states. One hundred and eighty seven countries were present at the *United Nations Climate Change Conference* in Bali, Indonesia, held in December 2007. The purpose of the conference was to try to reach a consensus on parameters for the negotiation of a new international climate change agreement. Such a consensus could then begin to make a significant contribution to achieving the MDG goal of 'ensuring environmental sustainability'. This new agreement, with a new global emissions reduction objective, will go some way towards achieving targets. However, it will require the major carbon emitters like the United States to make a commitment.

Within the UN system, there is a wide range of agencies that undertake work directly or indirectly to support international health. These include WHO, the World Bank, UNICEF, the UN Development Program, the UN Educational, Scientific and Cultural Organization (UNESCO), the Food and Agriculture Organization, UN High Commission for Refugees, International Labour Organization, UN Environment Program, UN Fund for Drug Abuse Control and the WTO. Some of the activities in these agencies are directly related to public health. For example, the World Bank has become the largest single international financier of health services in low- and middle-income countries, the world's largest external funder of education, and one of the world's largest external funders in the fight against HIV/AIDS (World Bank 2008). It is not difficult to imagine that not all commentators agree with the World Bank's focus on improving population health.

Other UN programs have indirect links to health. For example, UNESCO works to promote pride and engagement in cultural activities and to preserve cultural heritage. One important outcome is that this improves the wellbeing of both the individual and the population.

National governments are essential players in this global public health community. Under the initiative on global health and foreign policy, launched in New York in September 2006, the foreign affairs ministers of Brazil, France, Indonesia, Norway, Senegal, South Africa and Thailand issued an official statement in Oslo on 20 March 2007 (Ministers of Foreign Affairs 2007). These ministers agreed to work towards greater links and the recognition of the importance of foreign policy deliberations on health. Box 13.2 describes the major areas of commonality identified by the group.

The *Oslo Statement of Ministers of Foreign Affairs* clearly articulates a need to broaden the scope of foreign policy to include health, and the impact of policy decisions on the health of the population, saying:

> In today's era of globalisation and interdependence there is an urgent need
> to broaden the scope of foreign policy …We believe that health is one of the

---

Box 13.2: Major areas of commonality identified in the Oslo Statement

'Increase awareness of our common vulnerability in the face of health threats by bringing health issues more strongly into the arenas of foreign policy discussions and decisions, in order to strengthen our commitment to concerted action at the global level.'

'Build bilateral, regional and multilateral cooperation for global health security by strengthening the case for collaboration and brokering broad agreement, accountability, and action.'

'Reinforce health as a key element in strategies for development and for fighting poverty, in order to reach the Millennium Development Goals; ensure that a higher priority is given to health in dealing with trade issues and in conforming to the Doha principles, affirming the right of each country to make full use of TRIPS (Trade-Related Aspects of Intellectual Property Rights) flexibilities in order to ensure universal access to medicines.'

'Strengthen the place of health measures in conflict and crisis management and in reconstruction efforts' (Ministers of Foreign Affairs 2007 p 1373).

---

most important, yet still broadly neglected, long-term foreign policy issues of our time … We believe that health as a foreign policy issue needs a stronger strategic focus on the international agenda. We have therefore agreed to make impact on health a point of departure and a defining lens that each of our countries will use to examine key elements of foreign policy and development strategies, and to engage in a dialogue on how to deal with policy options from this perspective.

(Ministers of Foreign Affairs 2007 p 1373).

Another example of foreign policy deliberations that have an impact on health is Australia's foreign aid programs. The Australian Agency for International Development (AusAid) was established in 1974 (AusAid 2008). It is the main agency responsible for managing Australia's overseas aid program, and has representatives in 25 Australian diplomatic missions overseas. AusAid programs and projects cover more than 35 countries in our region. Its objectives are to assist developing countries to reduce poverty and achieve sustainable development, in line with Australia's national interest (AusAid 2008).

As mentioned in Chapter 7, Australia's 2007-08 budget for the *Overseas Aid Program* was $3.155 billion (about 0.30% of GDP and 1% of federal government expenditure). This aid supports a range of initiatives in health, education, infrastructure, governance and the environment. The budget is expected to increase to $4.3 billion in 2010–11, which could provide a significant opportunity to make further progress towards achieving the UN's MDG in the region (AusAid 2008). Every Australian contributes to Australia's aid programs. On average, every week, each person puts in around $2.40 to pay for the aid program, which is less than the cost of a loaf of bread.

ACTIVITY

- Would you like to work in a developing country to improve the population's health status? Even if this meant earning less income than a person working in a developed country?
- Make a list of the reasons for and against working in a developing country to improve the health of the population.
- Add all the lists together and then discuss with the whole class.

REFLECTION

What factors would motivate you to work in a health-related position in a developing country? One of the obvious reasons would be the satisfaction gained from trying to make a difference, no matter how small, to the lives of people, rather than the money you would be earning.

Why do Australians give aid? This is not a simple question – whether or not people give aid is influenced by their beliefs, knowledge, experiences and motivations, as well as their perceptions about their financial status. Many individuals believe that giving aid is the right thing to do because it makes a real difference to other people's lives, especially those who are less fortunate. Conversely, the Australian Government gives aid because it improves security in the region. Furthermore, it helps partner governments to improve law and order, and prevent and recover from conflict; it assists in managing a range of transnational threats, such as people-trafficking, illicit drugs and HIV/AIDS; and it improves Australia's own economic and security interests by helping to build stronger communities and more stable governments in the region (AusAid 2008).

Philanthropic organisations also play significant roles in the global public health community. Consider the Bill and Melinda Gates Foundation (Gates Foundation) as an example. The foundation was established in 2000, and focuses on two main areas: improving access to existing vaccines, drugs and other tools to fight diseases common in developing countries; and research to develop health solutions that are effective, affordable and practical (Gates Foundation 2008). For the year ending September 2007, the Gates Foundation had contributed US$14.45 billion in grants and US$8.5 billion of that was on global health. In the latter half of 2007, the Gates Foundation had distributed substantial financial support to the international public health community for the prevention, management and treatment of the global HIV/AIDS epidemic, including:

- *United Nations Programme on HIV/AIDS* – $547,400 over six months to provide an analysis of the past responses, present actions, and possible futures of the HIV/AIDS epidemic in a consortium of partners from multiple disciplines including economics, epidemiology, and the biomedical, social and political sciences
- *University of Maryland* – $15,000,000 over five years to develop a vaccine in both developing and developed nations that prevents the transmission of HIV
- *AIDS Vaccine Advocacy Coalition* – $14,050,295 over five years to create a favourable social environment for accelerated ethical research and global delivery of HIV/AIDS vaccines
- *Global HIV Vaccine Enterprise Secretariat* – $20,000,000 over four years to provide an operational support grant to the Global HIV Vaccine Enterprise (Gates Foundation website).

In addition to non-government organisations such as philanthropic agencies, government international aid organisations such as AusAid, and multilateral organisations such as the UN, WHO and the World Bank, there are also professional organisations working together to address specific health issues. One of these is the International Society for Prevention of Child Abuse and Neglect (ISPCAN 2008), which was established in 1977.

ACTIVITY

Go to ISPCAN's website (www.ispcan.org) and answer the following questions:
- How many members are there, and how many countries are represented?
- What professional activities are undertaken?
- How is the society supported financially?

REFLECTION

It is not difficult to find the answers for the above questions when you explore the website. Consider the effort required for health professionals to form a global organisation like ISPCAN, especially the effort required to organise funding and develop professional activities. Then you should be able to appreciate the achievements of this organisation and its potential impact in improving the health status of children.

While there are examples of immense achievements, there are still challenges ahead, and some clear shortcomings in activity and focus. It has been suggested that some essential functions had been neglected by international public health agencies, such as the creation of comprehensive information systems to promote cooperation in health policy development, at both the national and international levels, and the sharing of experiences in health reforms between countries (Frenk et al 1997).

Others have suggested that WHO needs to move from traditional disease governance approaches to new public health governance approaches, which would include WHO's global leadership in public health education and interventions.

It has been suggested that WHO should use data from a range of resources, including treaties, regulations, recommendations and travel advisories, to provide for global public health security (Aginam 2006). However, WHO faces many challenges to implement the above ideas, one of these being finances.

When established in 1948, WHO's funding relied largely on a budget made up of member states' contributions (US$6 million in 1950) (Merson et al 2006). Then some high-income member states started to give additional funds to WHO for particular programs, which is called extra-budgetary funding. This accounted for 25% of WHO's total budget in 1971, and increased to 66% by 2004 (Merson et al 2006). Therefore, a few donor countries seem increasingly to dominate WHO's activities while WHO is expected to be a universalist, keeping its reputation for being neutral in dealing with its member states (Merson et al 2006).

Investigations have shown 'that national autonomy over health policy is not preserved under' the WTO's *General Agreement on Trade in Service* (GATS), 'and that accordingly, there is a role for international standards that protect public services from the adverse effect of trade and market forces' (Pollock & Price 2003 p 1072). Sustainability, an issue for any international aid program, needs to be appropriately addressed. To provide support for sustainability, Edwards and Roelofs (2006) recommend the 'development of strong and transparent partnerships'; the management of 'planned transition points'; and the use of 'local champions who led integration efforts' (Edwards & Roelofs 2006 pp 47–48).

Looking to the future of the global public health community, it has been predicted that global cooperation will be:

- likely to focus on global public health governance and regulations, such as environmental issues and cross-national trade of health products and services
- likely to have a public–private partnership as an increasing characteristic
- unlikely to be dominated by the UN or its agencies such as WHO, but will be represented by a more diverse set of actors including private sectors, NGOs, consumer and professional groups, environmental groups, and civil society organisations (Merson et al 2006 p 675).

It is with confidence that the global public health community will continue to work closely together to overcome challenges and improve global population health.

A final word

This chapter is an introduction to the concept of globalisation and its impacts on population health, particularly on communicable and non-communicable diseases. We discussed the distribution of the global burden of diseases in high-, middle- and low-income countries and introduced the role of the global public health community by describing some of their achievements and current challenges. If you are interested in further exploring globalisation and health, there have been numerous textbooks published recently (Kawachi & Wamala 2007a, Merson et al 2006), and there are also formal university courses on international health.

REVIEW QUESTIONS

1 What is globalisation?
2 How does globalisation impact on population health, for example, with reference to infectious diseases, tobacco use and unhealthy diet?
3 There are differences between high- and low-income countries in the leading causes of death. What are the main factors contributing to this pattern?

4   What are the major challenges for the global public health community in responding to globalisation?

REFERENCES

Aginam O 2006 Globalization of health insecurity: the World Health Organization and the new International Health Regulations. Med Law 25(4):663–672

Allen I 2007 Pipe Dreams: The Next Big Thing 2008. Available: http://www.abc.net.au/http/pipe/nextbig.htm 22 Jan 2008

Arnesen T, Kapiriri L 2004 Can the value choices in DALYs influence global priority-setting? Health Policy 70:137–149

AusAid 2008 Australia's Aid Program 2008 Available: http://www.ausaid.gov.au 21 Jan 2008

Australian Bureau of Statistics 2007 3101.0 – Australian Demographic Statistics, Jun 2007. Available: http://www.abs.gov.au/ausstats/abs@.nsf/mf/3101.0/ 7 Mar 2007

Australian-Transport 2007 Aviation Statistics 2008. Available: http://www.infrastructure.gov.au/aviation/index.aspx 24 Jan 2008

Bakan J 2004 The Corporation: The Pathological Pursuit of Profit and Power. Simon & Schuster, New York

Barker C, Green A 1996 Opening The Debate On DALYs. Health Policy and Planning 11(2):179–183

Bolling C, Somwaru A 2001 US food companies access foreign markets through investment. ERS Food Rev 24(3):23–28

Centers for Disease Control and Prevention 2008 Severe Acute Respiratory Syndrome (SARS). Available: http://www.cdc.gov/ncidod/sars/ 10 Jan 2008

Chanda N 2002 What is Globalization? Available: http://yaleglobal.yale.edu/about/essay.jsp 8 Jan 2008

Cherniavsky B, Dachis B 2007 Excess Baggage: Measuring Air Transportation's Fiscal Burden. C D Howe Institute, Toronto

Cherry J D 2004 The chronology of the 2002–2003 SARS mini pandemic. Paediatric Respiratory Reviews 5:262–269

China Daily 2004 KFC and McDonald's – a model of blended culture. China Daily Beijing 1st June 2004. Available: http://www.chinadaily.com.cn/english 8 Jan 2008

Chopra M, Galbraith S et al 2002 A Global Response to a Global Problem: the epidemic of overnutrition. Bulletin of the World Health Organization 80:952–958

Edwards N C, Roelofs S M 2006 Sustainability: The Elusive Dimension of International Health Projects. Canadian Journal of Public Health 97(1):45

Ezzati M, Lopez A D 2003 Estimates of global mortality attributable to smoking in 2000. The Lancet 362(9387):847–852

Fischer S 2003 Globalization and Its Challenges. American Economic Review, American Economic Association, 93(2):1–30

Formiguera X, Canton A 2004 Obesity: epidemiology and clinical aspects. Best Practice & Research Clinical Gastroenterology 18(6):1125–1146

Frenk J, Sepúlveda J, GómezDantés O et al 1997 The future of world health: The new world order and international health. BMJ 314:1404–1407

Gates Foundation 2008 Global Health Program. Bill & Melinda Gates Foundation. Available: http://www.gatesfoundation.org 15 Jan 2008

Hui L, Bell A C 2003 Overweight and obesity in children from Shenzhen Peoples Republic of China. Health & Place 9(4):371–376

International Society for Prevention of Child Abuse and Neglect 2008 ISPCAN Celebrates 30 Years. Available: http://www.ispcan.org/16 Jan 2008

James P T 2004 Obesity: The worldwide epidemic. Clinics in Dermatology 22(4):276–280

Jones K E, Patel N G, Levy M A et al 2008 Global trends in emerging infectious diseases. Nature 451:990–994

Kawachi I, Wamala S 2007a Globalization and Health. Oxford University Press, New York

Kawachi I, Wamala S 2007b Globalization and Health: Challenges and Prospects. In: Kawachi I, Wamala S (eds) Globalization and Health. Oxford University Press, New York, pp 3–15

Kickbusch I 2003 SARS: Wake-Up Call for a Strong Global Health Policy. Available: http://www.yaleglobal.yale.edu 7 Jan 2008

Knai C, Suhrcke M, Lobstein T 2007 Obesity in Eastern Europe: An overview of its health and economic implications. Economics & Human Biology 5(3):392–408

Lang T 1998 The new globalisation food and health: is public health receiving its due emphasis? Journal of Epidemiology and Community Health 52(9):538–539

Lee K 1999 Globalisation and the need for a strong public health response. European Journal of Public Health 9(4):249–250

Liu J-M et al 2007 Prevalence of Overweight/Obesity in Chinese Children. Archives of Medical Research 38(8):882–886

Liu Y et al 2006 Cigarette smoking and poverty in China. Social Science & Medicine 63(11):2784–2790

Masson P 2001 Globalization: Facts and Figures IMF Policy Discussion Paper: 1–18

Mathers C, Loncar D 2006a Projections of global mortality and burden of disease from 2002 to 2030. PLoS Med 3(11):e442

Mathers C, Loncar D 2006b Updated projections of global mortality and burden of disease 2002–2030: data sources methods and results. Evidence and Information for Policy Working Paper. WHO, Geneva, pp 1–12

McMichael A J, Powles J W, Butler C D et al 2007 Food livestock production energy climate change and health. The Lancet 370(9594):1253–1263

McMichael P 2000 A Global Interpretation of the Rise of the East Asian Food Import Complex. World Development 28(3):409–424

Merson M 2003 SARS Proved Health is Global Public Good. Available: http:www.yaleglobal.yale.edu 23 Jan 2008

Merson M H, Black R E, Mills A 2006 International Public Health: Diseases, Programs, Systems and Policies. Jones and Bartlett Publishers, Boston

Ministers of Foreign Affairs 2007 Oslo Ministerial Declaration – global health: a pressing foreign policy issue of our time. The Lancet 369(9570):1373–1378

Miniwatts Marketing Group 2007 Internet Usage Statistics: The Internet Big Picture - World Internet Users and Population Stats. Available: http://www.internetworldstats.com/stats.htm 21 Jan 2008

Mitchell S L Wilson 2007 Fish bans raise poison risk. The Australian, 4th August 2007. Available: http://www.theaustralian.news.com.au 23 Jan 2008

Mont D 2007 Measuring health and disability. The Lancet 369:1658–1663

Murray C J L, Lopez A D 1996 The global burden of disease: a comprehensive assessment of mortality and disability from diseases, injuries and risk factors in 1990 and projected to 2020. Global Burden of Diseases and Injury Series. Harvard University Press, Cambridge, Vol 1

Murray C J L, Acharya A K 1997 Understanding DALYs. Journal of Health Economics 16(6):703–730

Pollock A, Price D 2003 The public health implications of world trade negotiations on the general agreement on trade in services and public services. Lancet 362(9389):1072–1075

Sachs J 2005 The End of Poverty. The Penguin Press, New York

Smith R D 2006 Trade and public health: facing the challenges of globalisation. Journal of Epidemiology and Community Health 60(8):650–651

Sobal J 2001 Commentary: Globalization and the epidemiology of obesity. International Journal of Epidemiology 30(5):1136–1137

Sturm R, Wells K B 2001 Does obesity contribute as much to morbidity as poverty or smoking? Public Health 115(3):229–235

United Nations 2008a Globalization Must Benefit 'Bottom Billion' Of Poor. Available: http://www.un.org/news 9 Mar 2008

United Nations 2008b About the UN: Introduction to the structure & work of UN. Available: http://www.un.org 11 Jan 2008

Üstün T B, Saxena S, Bedirhan Ü T et al 1999 Are disability weights universal? The Lancet 354:1306

Walt G 1998 Globalisation of international health. The Lancet 351(9100):434–437

Wamala S, Kawachi I, Mpepo B P 2007 Poverty Reduction Strategy Papers: Bold New Approach to Poverty Eradication or Old Wine in New Bottles? In: Wamala S, Kawachi I (eds) Globalization and Health. Oxford University Press, New York, pp 234–249

Wang H, Sindelar J L, Busch S H 2006 The impact of tobacco expenditure on household consumption patterns in rural China. Social Science & Medicine 62(6):1414–1426

Wang L et al 2005 Preventing chronic diseases in China. The Lancet 366(9499):1821–1824

World Bank 2008 The World Bank Projects and Operations. Available: http://www.worldbank.org 14 Jan 2008

World Health Organization 2006 World Health Report – working together for health. Geneva World Health Organization, Geneva. Available: http://www.who.int/whr/2006/en/index.html 15 Jan 2008

World Health Organization 2008 Programs and Projects. Available: http://www.who.int 25 Jan 2008

WorldPublicOpinion.org, University of Maryland 2007 World Public Favors Globalization and Trade but Wants to Protect Environment and Jobs A publication of the Program on International Policy Attitudes at the University of Maryland. Available: http://worldpublicopinion.org/pipa/articles/btglobalizationtradera/349.php?lb=btgl&pnt=349&nid=&id= 9 Jan 2008

Yale 2003 SARS – Special Reports on YaleGlobal. Available: http://yaleglobal.yale.edu/display.article?id=2503 24 Jan 2008

Yin P et al 2007 Passive smoking exposure and risk of COPD among adults in China: the Guangzhou Biobank Cohort Study. The Lancet 370(9589):751–757

Zhong N-S, Wong G W K 2004 Epidemiology of severe acute respiratory syndrome (SARS): adults and children. Paediatric Respiratory Reviews 5:270–274

Zimmet P 2000 Globalization, coca-colonization and the chronic disease epidemic: can the doomsday scenario be averted? J Intern Med 247:301–310

The author would like to thank Professor Michael Dunne and Associate Professor Mary Louise Fleming of the School of Public Health, QUT.

CHAPTER 14

The new epidemics

Gerry FitzGerald

Learning objectives

After reading this chapter you should be able to:

- outline the nature and threat of current and emerging epidemics
- identify the risks and impact of epidemics on the health of the community
- describe the population health strategies required to reduce the risk and mitigate the impact of epidemics
- outline your role as a health professional in reducing the likelihood and/or impact of an epidemic
- describe the key elements of health disaster management.

Introduction

This chapter aims to outline the impact that infectious diseases have on population health, to identify the risks of major outbreaks of infectious diseases, to discuss the factors influencing those risks and to identify the strategies required to reduce the risk and to manage any outbreak.

Infectious diseases are those diseases caused by microorganisms such as helminths (parasitic worms), protozoa, viruses, bacteria, fungi and prions (Irving et al 2005) (see Ch 11). These microorganisms have the capacity to spread from individual to individual and, therefore, to cause an outbreak of disease in the community, which is known as an epidemic. An epidemic has been defined as an excess of cases in the community from that normally expected; or the appearance of a new infectious disease (Webber 2005). The term pandemic is used when epidemics occur in multiple communities. These terms are meant to distinguish outbreaks of disease from those diseases that continue to occur at constant or relatively low levels within any community. Such diseases are said to be endemic within the community.

In developed countries we once thought that the scourge of infectious diseases was tamed. Vaccination prevented many illnesses, and antibiotics were able to control infection in individual patients. The community had great faith in the capacity of science to confound the most cunning organism. However, in the new millennium we are confronting a host of new and resurgent challenges to community health arising from infectious diseases. These challenges have the capacity to cause major outbreaks (or epidemics) of disease, and therefore, may have a significant impact on community health and wellbeing.

The old epidemics

Throughout human history, infectious diseases have had a major impact on community mortality and morbidity. This impact has been both from endemic disease and from major disease outbreaks.

In developed countries such as Australia, infectious diseases once had a much greater impact on health than they now have. Table 14.1 reflects the change in causes of death in Australia between 1907 and 2000 (AIHW 2006). In 1907, infectious diseases accounted for four of the top 10 causes of death. In 2000, there were no infectious diseases among the top 10 causes of death in Australia.

1907		2000	
DISEASES	**% OF DEATHS**	**DISEASES**	**% OF DEATHS**
Organic heart disease	8.3	Ischaemic heart disease	21.0
Tuberculosis (TB)	8.2	Cerebrovascular	7.4
Diarrhoea	7.1	Lung cancer	6.9
Senility	6.6	Other heart disease	4.9
Congenital conditions	6.1	Chronic obstructive pulmonary disease (COPD)	4.7
Bronchitis	4.8	Prostate cancer	4.0
Pneumonia	4.3	Colon cancer	3.8
Nephritis	4.1	Suicide	2.8
Cerebrovascular disease	3.8	Diabetes	2.4
Unspecified or ill-defined	3.1	Transport accidents	2.0
Top 10	**56.4**	**Top 10**	**59.9**

TABLE 14.1: Cause of death of males in Australia 1907, 2000

(Source: AIHW 2006)

However, infectious diseases continue to be a major cause of death and disability in underdeveloped countries. In South-East Asia infectious diseases account for 40% of deaths and 28% of morbidity (WHO 2005a). Such countries lack the economic capacity to provide the community with public health and health management infrastructure required to prevent or manage infectious diseases. Infectious diseases still account for five of the top 10 causes of death in low-income countries (see Table 14.2).

Because of the large populations in developing countries, infectious diseases still cause one in five deaths throughout the world. Table 14.3 identifies the challenge not only from well-known and predictable diseases such as HIV/AIDS (human immunodeficiency virus/ acquired immune deficiency syndrome), tuberculosis and malaria, but also a host of diseases that are more easily preventable, through simple vaccination, nutrition and other public health measures. Globally, over one million children died in 2002 from childhood diseases, most of which are readily preventable by well-known public health measures (WHO 2004).

	HIGH INCOME	MIDDLE INCOME	LOW INCOME
1	Coronary artery disease	Stroke and other cerebrovascular disease	Coronary artery disease
2	Stroke and other cerebrovascular disease	Coronary artery disease	Lower respiratory infection
3	Trachea, bronchus and lung cancer	COPD	HIV/AIDS
4	Lower respiratory infection	Lower respiratory infection	Perinatal conditions
5	COPD	HIV/AIDS	Stroke and other cerebrovascular disease
6	Colon and rectum cancer	Perinatal conditions	Diarrhoeal diseases
7	Alzheimer and other dementia	Stomach cancer	Malaria
8	Diabetes mellitus	Trachea, bronchus and lung cancer	TB
9	Breast cancer	Road traffic accidents	COPD
10	Stomach cancer	Hypertensive heart disease	Road traffic accidents

TABLE 14.2: The top 10 causes of death in high-, middle- and low-income countries

(Source: WHO 2007)

DISEASE CATEGORY	DEATHS PER ANNUM
HIV/AIDS	2,777,175
Diarrhoeal diseases	1,797,972
TB	1,566,003
Malaria	1,272,393
Childhood diseases	1,124,365
STDs excluding HIV	179,673
Meningitis	173,031
Japanese encephalitis	134,957
Tropical diseases	129,167
Hepatitis B	102,819
Hepatitis C	53,762
Dengue	18,561
Intestinal nematodes	11,771
Leprosy	6,167
Trachoma	154
Subtotal	9,226,970
Maternal peri natal and nutritional diseases	7,420,280
Non-communicable diseases	3,353,583
Injuries	5,168,315
TOTAL	47,931,868

TABLE 14.3: Deaths from infectious diseases (2002)

(Source: WHO 2004)

Malaria

Malaria is one of the principal causes of the burden of infectious disease. Malaria is caused by the *Plasmodium* genus and is transmitted from individual to individual by mosquitoes. Over three billion people are exposed to malarial risk, which is estimated to cause between one and three million deaths each year with massive social and economic costs. It has been difficult to eliminate, although some countries including Australia have eliminated native malaria (Guinovart et al 2006).

In addition to these endemic diseases, pandemics of infectious diseases have from time to time caused massive adverse health effects and, consequently, have had a fundamental impact on society – including the destruction of civilisations.

The Plague

The term 'plague' is often used to describe any endemic or pandemic illness. However, the disease known as 'The Plague' or the 'Black Death' is caused by the organism *Pasteurella pestis* (or *Yersinia pestis*). The organism is spread by fleas, which transmit the disease directly from human to human or via an intermediate host, typically rats. The organisms may lodge in the lungs causing a 'pneumonic plague', or spread to regional lymph nodes where they cause lymphadenitis (buboes) and hence the 'bubonic' form of The Plague. From there, the disease spreads via the lymphatic drainage system to the principal organs of the body including the liver, spleen, lungs and kidney resulting in septicaemia.

The Black Death has been known for centuries and is reputed to have caused the downfall of the Greek civilisation 500 years BC, and to have contributed to the collapse of the Roman Empire 1000 years later. The Plague spread throughout Europe during the Middle Ages, where it is thought to have caused the death of one-third of Europe's population. The Plague continues to cause small outbreaks around the world, mostly in sub-equatorial Africa.

The Spanish flu

At the end of the First World War, a highly virulent form of influenza broke out, firstly in military camps in Europe, but the disease subsequently spread to every continent and all countries. The disease was a highly virulent form of influenza caused by the modification of a human influenza virus (H1N1), and was estimated to have caused the deaths of up to 50 million people in a world whose total population was approximately 1.7 billion. The epidemic caused more deaths than the First World War, and had long-term economic consequences, contributing indirectly to the economic collapse of the 1930s and, subsequently, the Second World War.

Smallpox

Smallpox is a human disease that has been identified as a cause of epidemics in ancient Egypt, and continued to cause widespread disease until officially declared eradicated by the World Health Organization (WHO) in 1980. Smallpox was reputed to have killed one in every five children at the height of its impact, and as recently as 1967 caused 10–15 million cases, and two million deaths, worldwide per year (Tucker 2001). The eradication of smallpox is not only significant because of its impact on human health, but also because it demonstrates that it is possible to eliminate a disease. Conquering smallpox was ultimately achieved through widespread vaccination programs.

ACTIVITY

● Write a paragraph about the possible effects of a new 'Spanish flu' outbreak today; that is, what are the differences between the current social and structural conditions and those of 1918 that would alter the impact of the flu on the health and wellbeing of the community?

REFLECTION

Since 1918, the world has changed considerably in regard to the standards of health of the community and our capacity to treat people. However, at the same time we have become a more integrated world characterised by rapid transport, global trade and instantaneous communications. The net effect of these differences makes it difficult to assess the impact of a modern pandemic.

The nature of epidemics

Epidemics occur when an infective agent becomes established within a vulnerable community. Epidemics may result either from a common source, or by person-to-person spread (Webber 2005).

A common source of infection occurs with a contaminated food or water source. The exposure may be a single event as may occur with a contaminated meal served in a restaurant or repeated exposure to a source of infection, such as contaminated water. A propagated source of infection occurs when the disease is spread from infected patients to non-infected individuals, either directly or indirectly via intermediate vectors or hosts.

Epidemics may occur unexpectedly due to the emergence of a new disease or the movement of a disease into a community where it was previously non-existent or occurred only at low levels (Webber 2005). For example, in 2004 SARS (severe acute respiratory syndrome) was a novel virus that was previously unknown and caused an outbreak that spread to several countries, having a significant economic and social impact. Epidemics may also occur regularly as a result of seasonal or other factors, for example, influenza epidemics in the winter.

The pattern of the disease is related to the nature of its infectious agent. Organisms must grow to sufficient numbers in the host before they cause disease. There also must be sufficient numbers of organisms in the infected person before they become infective to others. Infectivity persists while enough organisms are still circulating in the host to risk transmission. The period between infection and the presence of symptoms is called the 'incubation period'. The period during which the host is infectious to others is known as the 'infective period'. This often commences before the onset of symptoms and may last until symptoms begin to resolve.

In population terms the incubation period corresponds to the latent period of the epidemic, during which the disease begins to cause infections and the number of cases starts to increase. The length of this period is determined by the agent, population and environmental characteristics. Public health and other community interventions may also affect the pattern of the disease by slowing the transmission of the agent.

The pattern of the epidemic varies according to the nature of the exposure, the nature of the disease and the particular demographic and environmental characteristics of the community (Webber 2005).

A single-point exposure will produce a single peak of cases. The size of the peak will be affected by the size of the population at risk and the infectivity of the agent. The delay between exposure and the cases is determined by the nature of the exposure and the latent (pre-symptomatic) period of the disease.

Repeated exposure will produce a prolonged pattern of cases. The nature of the exposure and the size and density of the population at risk will determine the pattern of cases.

With propagated exposure, cases may occur in waves. The first wave results from the first appearance of the agent in a vulnerable population. Rapid response and the growth of immunity among recovered patients will limit the immediate spread and thus reduce the frequency of new cases. However, a second wave may then occur as restraints are lessened and people tire of the restrictions imposed in an attempt to address the original outbreak. The third wave is associated with the appearance of new vulnerable people, as life returns to normal and people begin travelling, then new vulnerable populations are brought into contact with the agent. The number of waves, and the size and time lag, are affected by the latent period of the organism, the infectivity of the agent, the population at risk and the effectiveness of population health controls.

ACTIVITY

- An outbreak of a mysterious illness occurs in an Indonesian village. Over three days, more than 30 people become ill and 10 of those die. What are some possible causes, and how would you investigate the incident?

REFLECTION

The pattern of cases is often a significant clue to the cause of the illness. In this instance, the sudden onset of a single wave of cases suggests a single point of contact for the illness. More detailed examination may link the outbreak to a particular food or water source, and help identify the cause, and therefore, prevent the continuance or repetition of the incident.

WHO phases of pandemics

WHO describes pandemics in three periods, which are divided into six phases (WHO 2005b). This description was designed specifically for the *WHO Pandemic Preparedness Plan* but may be applied generically to any disease epidemic or pandemic. Different diseases may be present in different phases at any particular time.

The *inter-pandemic period* describes the time when there is no active epidemic of the particular disease in humans. In Phase 1, the disease may be present in animals but there is no evidence of spread to humans. In Phase 2, there is evidence of a circulating animal disease, which has the potential to cause disease in humans but there is no evidence currently of disease (WHO 2005b).

The *pandemic alert period* describes the situation where there is evidence of human disease but there is no major outbreak of the disease in humans. In Phase 3 there may be a small number of human cases but no person-to-person spread, except in rare circumstances of very close contact. In Phase 4 there is evidence of person-to-person spread in very small clusters involving common exposure or intimate contact. In Phase 5 there are large clusters of cases arising from person-to-person contact, but the disease remains localised (WHO 2005b).

The *pandemic period* describes the time when there is evidence of person-to-person spread of the disease. In Phase 6 there is increased and sustained person-to-person spread with widespread distribution of the disease (WHO 2005b).

At present it may be said that avian influenza is at Phase 3, although there have been two small clusters in Indonesia that could result in a Phase 4 classification.

Factors influencing the risk of new epidemics

The impact of infectious diseases has been progressively reduced throughout the 20th century, through the combined effects of improved public health, enhanced personal protection, including immunisation, and the developments in treating infected patients.

The key influences include providing clean drinking water; immunisations; reductions in overcrowding; improved nutrition; safe sewage and waste disposal; control of vectors such as rats and mosquitoes; and changes in personal habits, such as hand washing, clothes laundering and banning public spitting. In addition, the development of effective antibiotic agents, particularly penicillin in the 1940s, provided a means of managing patients with infectious diseases, to further limit the spread and personal impact of those organisms.

The proliferation of new epidemics depends on the combination of population, agent and environmental factors. The interaction of these factors determines the extent and impact of the epidemic.

Population factors

The size, density, health status and socioeconomic characteristics of the population will have an impact on the size and impact of epidemics. Larger more densely populated communities increase the number of 'at-risk' people and their risk of exposure to the infective agent. Epidemics will spread in poorer communities that do not have high standards of social infrastructure. The health status of the community, and in particular their immune status, will influence the disease spread and impact. The presence of comorbidities, such as TB or AIDS, will increase the vulnerability of the population.

Thus, at a population level, increased population growth and density, and migration (particularly into congested urban areas) are increasing the risks and impact of epidemics. These risks are augmented by the health problems associated with poverty and overcrowding. People living closer together often lack the social distancing that characterises rural life or wealthier communities. Rapid growth in many cities is often associated with a failure of community infrastructure such as sewerage and water supplies, and leads to a lack of adequate social support, including medical services. Often people in these circumstances are unable to access health services, including immunisation, thus creating a fertile environment with low 'herd immunity' that leads to disease outbreaks. In addition, large human populations are developing in locations where diseases have previously been rife, but affected few people. This vulnerability is intensified by the presence of vector breeding grounds near large human populations.

Poverty also increases the individual risk of infectious disease by lowering nutrition levels and, therefore, the body's capacity to produce an immune response and to resist disease. Changes in societal norms are increasing the exposure of communities. Children accumulate in childcare centres and schools, which are potent sources of infection. People indulge in leisure activities, which may involve mass gatherings. Changes in food management, including massive increases in international trade, are increasing the risks of transmission of contaminated foodstuffs between communities.

Advances in health care technology are increasing the exposure of vulnerable people to disease. Chemotherapeutic agents reduce immunological capacity. Large groups of people close together in health care institutions, such as hospitals, create an environment in which (antimicrobial) resistant organisms can flourish. Antimicrobial chemotherapy is used commonly, resulting in an increase in resistant organisms. Patients often fail to complete their courses of medication, resulting in the ability of organisms to evolve resistant forms. Invasive medical procedures, such as transplantation, are compromising human resistance, thus increasing the risks of infection.

Increased population mobility and the rapidity of travel are resulting in an increased exposure of people to diseases, which previously would have had little opportunity to spread beyond the immediate vicinity. For example, an infected patient walking through Singapore airport may transmit that virus to individuals in every continent of the world within 24 hours, and certainly within the incubation period of most viruses. Thus traditional methods of control based on quarantine will prove less effective in a rapidly mobile world.

Major conflicts and natural disasters produce sudden and unpredictable movements of large numbers of people, who are often then forced to live in refugee camps where infrastructure is inadequate, and where safe waste disposal, safe food and clean water are difficult to provide. International awareness, cooperation and collaboration have often sought to minimise the potential impact on human health from such circumstances.

Environmental factors

Increased population density also intensifies the exposure of humans to disease vectors and animals, as both struggle for room in congested living environments and humans rely on the animals for meagre food supplies. Thus people are increasingly exposed to animal diseases, and their shared environment offers opportunities for microorganisms to evolve and new or resistant organisms to develop.

Global warming poses significant risks to human health from a variety of factors (McMichael et al 2006). Population displacement from low-lying areas will lead to further congestion and population density. Global warming will permit microbial variations and alter the patterns of animal and disease distribution; associated climatic change will expose large populations to severe weather events such as heatwaves, tropical storms or flooding, and the public health challenges those events bring. Changes in weather will lead to changing patterns of vectors and disease exposure to new, more vulnerable and unprepared populations. New food production technologies are leading to increased farming intensity. Mass animal congregations for food production provide a fertile ground for genetic adaptation of microorganisms, which may in turn pose a risk to human health.

Disease factors

While the developed world perceives that it has controlled infectious diseases, the majority of people in the world are at risk of contracting existing and new infectious diseases. The risks of epidemics relates to the ongoing challenge of old diseases, new challenges from old diseases and new emerging diseases.

The ongoing challenge of old diseases

Common infections continue to impact, particularly in societies in which social, economic or other factors – including military conflict – prevent the application of known effective public health strategies. TB causes more than 1.5 million deaths per year, principally in poorly nourished, poor and overcrowded societies. Malaria causes 1.3 million deaths per year in societies in which the public health strategies of vector control, personal protection and prophylactic agents are unavailable because of poverty or social disruption. Common viruses can have a disproportionate impact on poorly nourished people and common vaccine-preventable diseases exist because of the failure of vaccination programs.

The most significant risk of a new epidemic is human influenza. Influenza causes annual epidemics in most countries and the variability of the influenza virus results in ineffective natural or artificial immunity. The virus continues to mutate which means that immunity to previous strains does not prevent infection from new variations of the virus. Influenza is a highly infectious disease that causes significant mortality among the very young, the elderly or immuno-suppressed people. However, previous experience with influenza epidemics has demonstrated that highly lethal varieties are often associated with an immunological over-reaction, which leads to the rapid onset of respiratory distress; most commonly among the young and healthy. Mutation of common human influenza viruses into a highly lethal form is the highest risk of a major epidemic. However, there is also a risk that animal influenza viruses such as avian influenza could mutate into a human-to-human transmissible form; or could exchange genetic material with a human influenza virus and thus produce a new virus with the lethality of the avian influenza virus and the infectivity of the human influenza virus.

New challenges of old diseases

New challenges are emerging with many of the old infectious diseases. Public complacency is permitting the re-emergence of diseases that have previously been better controlled. The decreasing levels of herd immunity in some communities increase the probability of outbreaks. Some people are suspicious of vaccines, and some see them as a conspiracy, sometimes with political overtones. As a result of the low level of disease and the resultant low level of natural immunity, populations without good public health services have become a fertile ground for further outbreaks.

The emergence of resistant organisms is challenging our capacity to prevent or treat infection at either the individual or community level. Multiple drug-resistant TB is continuing to spread and is common among infected people in Papua New Guinea and the Torres Strait Islands (Gilpin 2007). Vancomycin and methicillin-resistant *Staphylococcus aureus* is a significant concern to hospitals around the world, as it exposes people to infection with an agent that is largely untreatable. Resistant *Staphylococcus* strains are a particular concern in health facilities because of the presence of immuno-compromised vulnerable people, often with surgical implants or undergoing surgical procedures.

The presence of many people in the community with poor immune status, often resulting from infection with HIV/AIDS and/or by poverty-related malnourishment, is leading to the emergence of low-pathogenic organisms as a cause of disease, and combinations of disease, for example TB and AIDS.

Finally, advances in medical science continue to enhance the capacity to intervene in a range of complex medical conditions. The new technology creates vulnerable people who can form the locus of infectious diseases. For example, antiviral agents are increasing the life expectancy of people living with AIDS. However, the effect is that there are more people living with AIDS in the community who are vulnerable to AIDS-related diseases that require close monitoring.

Emerging infectious diseases

'Emerging infectious diseases are diseases of infectious origin whose incidence in humans has increased within the recent past or threatens to increase in the near future' (WHO 2005a p 10). New diseases such as HIV/AIDS, Ebola, hepatitis C and E, H5N1, Japanese encephalitis and Nipah virus are now recognised but there is no effective response at either the individual or community level with many of these diseases.

These novel viruses are emerging as a significant threat to population health either because of close contact with other animals, or because population mobility, treatment effectiveness and rapidity of transportation allows some highly virulent, fatal diseases to spread quickly. The following examples demonstrate the impact that new viruses can have on the community.

SARS

SARS was caused by an animal (coronavirus) virus that made the transition to humans and caused a highly contagious and highly fatal disease. This disease originated in Guangdong province in China, but came to international awareness when a doctor from Guangzhou travelled to Hong Kong and became ill. The disease spread from the emergency department of the hospital where he was treated to five continents, and caused over 800 deaths. The outbreak had immeasurable economic and social impact. The disease was ultimately brought under control through public health controls, and led to enhanced international awareness of the risks of epidemics and thus considerably enhanced precautions and preparedness (Wong & Yuen 2005).

HIV

HIV, which causes AIDS, was first identified in 1983 and is now the most common cause of death by infectious diseases. It causes 2.7 million deaths per year, with infection rates in some communities of almost 50% (WHO 2007). There is no effective prevention strategy – vaccines remain ineffective. Personal protective strategies, such as safe sexual practices, are the only effective preventative measures. Public health strategies aimed at health promotion and disease prevention are of mixed effectiveness.

AVIAN INFLUENZA

Avian influenza is an example of an animal disease that has the capacity to cause human disease. This current avian influenza virus (H5N1) has been shown to be highly lethal to chickens but causes low-pathogenic or non-pathogenic disease in other migratory birds. Hence the disease has spread around the world. Humans with close contact with the infected birds can catch the disease and there is the capacity for human-to-human spread, but only from very close contact with infected people. The principal risk of this disease is that it could modify or mutate into a human transmissible disease and cause a widespread pandemic.

Bioterrorism and biological warfare

Biological agents have been part of military tactics, either intentionally or inadvertently, for centuries. In 1519, Cortes led an army of 500 men into Mexico (Tucker 2001). After suffering heavy losses he retreated to the coast, but was not completely conquered because of a subsequent outbreak of smallpox among the Aztecs; consequently, he was able to defeat the Aztec army. In 1763, an alliance of Shawnee, Mingo and Delaware tribes began a siege of Fort Pitt (now Pittsburgh). When a small party from this force visited the fort to advise the inhabitants to surrender, officers gave them two blankets and a handkerchief from the smallpox hospital. The subsequent epidemic led to the raising of the siege (Tucker 2001). Soon after the attacks on New York City in September 2001, letters containing anthrax spores were received at several news agencies in the US. More than 22 people developed anthrax disease and five died.

A vast array of biological agents has been identified as potential agents of biological warfare. The US Centers for Disease Control and Prevention (COC) identify Category A agents as those that:

- 'can be easily disseminated or transmitted from person to person;
- result in high mortality rates and have the potential for major public health impact;
- might cause public panic and social disruption; and
- require special action for public health preparedness' (CDC Emergency Preparedness & Response website).

These agents include smallpox, plague, botulism, anthrax, tularaemia, Ebola, Lassa fever and Marburg haemorrhagic fever (CDC Emergency Preparedness & Response website).

There are concerns that rogue nations or terrorist organisations could obtain or manufacture smallpox viruses. Smallpox demonstrates the risks confronting the community from an affective biological agent. Smallpox would be very dangerous because it is highly infectious, highly lethal, there is no (or little) residual immunity left in the community and there are limited vaccines to restore the herd immunity. In addition, the vaccine is a relatively dangerous live virus vaccine, so massive preventive vaccination programs without a credible threat would not be tolerated by the community. Smallpox was manufactured in weapons-grade standards by several countries. President Nixon banned further experimentation by the US in 1969, but evidence exists that the former USSR continued to maintain weapons grade virus until the early 1990s (Tucker 2001).

Unlike most terrorist or military attacks, a biological attack is less likely to be publicly heralded. Terrorists would not warn people, as their intent would be to cause chaos and maximum injury. Diagnosis would be difficult because of the lack of specific diagnostic clues, and the likelihood that health service personnel who respond to such an attack will be infected, which will result in significant weakening of the health system's capacity to manage those affected. The key defences to biological attack, therefore, remain effective public health systems based on risk reduction and mitigation, planning and preparedness, surveillance and laboratory capacity, vaccination of key personnel where possible, standard infection control and biosecurity of facilities and viruses.

The impact of new pandemics

New and emerging pandemics will have not only a significant effect on the health of communities, but also significant economic, social and environmental effects. The outbreak of SARS was estimated by the Asian Development Bank to have cost between $10 billion and $30 billion (Fan 2003). Many tourist and transport ventures failed due to the sudden reduction in travel, with long-term consequences on those who owned or worked for those organisations. The CDC estimated the health care costs alone of a significant pandemic in the US would be between $71.3 billion and $166.5 billion, with unmeasurable additional costs in terms of economic consequences, failed ventures, lost productivity and support for the bereaved (Meltzer et al 1999).

Widespread pandemics would have significant social impacts. People would cease travel and be reluctant to move from the safety of their own homes. People would avoid public locations, including workplaces, leading to further economic impacts both individually and to the community. Rivalry for scarce resources would likely lead to interpersonal conflict. Loss of family and friends would have long-term personal impacts on communities and their future productive capacity.

These impacts are particularly significant to health services. In contradistinction to most other disasters, health staff may be reluctant to expose themselves to the risks associated with caring for epidemic victims. In a 'normal' disaster volunteers are common, because the staff are not generally at further risk. However, during an epidemic the collection of highly infective patients in hospitals and other health facilities could reduce the willingness of staff to come to work.

Epidemics, particularly those derived from animal illnesses, may result in significant changes to the environment; certain animal species may be at risk, either from the virus, or from attempts to control spread by culling animal sources or carriers.

The extent and nature of the health impact of any epidemic will depend on the characteristics of the agent, the characteristics of the community and the effectiveness of control strategies. The interplay of these factors will directly affect the rapidity of the onset of the epidemic, the number of people infected, and the morbidity and mortality of the affected population.

Agent-related factors

The nature of the organism determines the nature of the disease, its pathological impact and its capacity to efficiently spread. Upper respiratory infections are highly contagious as they are often associated with symptoms such as sneezing or coughing, which are efficient dispersers of virus-laden water droplets. The virus is protected by the water droplet, until another person inhales the droplet or it comes into contact with their hands and they then transfer the virus to their mouth. On the other hand, diseases associated with blood-borne infections (e.g. HIV/AIDS) are less efficiently spread to others. They rely on exchange of bodily fluids, which is a more complicated transmission process.

The infectivity of the agent is dependent on the number of organisms required to produce infection in an individual person. The nature of the organism will determine its capacity to cause disease in humans. This may vary between organisms of the same species or within the same species over time. The infectivity of a particular organism and its ability to cause disease may change over time as it adapts to new environments through changes in its genetic structure.

Population factors

The spread of an epidemic will depend on the characteristics of the population and the community environment. The rapidity of spread will depend on the density of the population, the nutritional status of the community, the presence of other diseases and the immunological status of the community. The spread of the epidemic will also depend on the extent and effectiveness of routine infection control procedures and public health preparedness within the community.

The success of interventions

The spread of the epidemic will depend on the effectiveness of public health and community intervention strategies. Early recognition of the disease, which is dependent on effective surveillance, will enable a rapid response and thus limit the disease's impact. The extent of possible containment, and the presence of effective treatment or prevention measures such as vaccines will also determine the extent and impact of the epidemic.

As introduced in Chapter 10, the average number of people who any given infected patient may infect is defined as the 'R factor' of the epidemic. If the R factor exceeds one then the epidemic will continue to expand. If the R factor is less than one then the epidemic will decline. The pathogenicity of the agent paradoxically limits its ability to spread rapidly. A disease that kills rapidly is more likely to limit the mobility of infected people, and thus their ability to make contact with vulnerable individuals or populations. Thus the current pandemic of avian influenza is contributed to by the ability of the virus to cause asymptomatic or low-grade disease in migratory birds, which can then spread the virus to other communities where it causes the highly lethal, pathogenic form in chickens.

ACTIVITY
- The world is better prepared for the outbreak of disease than ever before, yet the risk remains and is amplified by the density and rapid growth of the world's population.
- What are the microbiological issues that increase the risk of epidemics?

REFLECTION

Worldwide, people are at significant risk from drug-resistant organisms, novel viruses that humans have not previously been exposed to and the transmission of animal organisms that cause diseases in humans. We need to remain vigilant.

Managing epidemics

There is a community and professional expectation that health services and population health services will do everything possible to minimise the likelihood and impact of any current or potential epidemic. The key challenge for these services is to ensure an organised and comprehensive approach to prevention and management.

Management of the current epidemics requires strategies that are directed to the system failures that led to the ongoing problem. While multiple strategies are generally appropriate, emphasis should be placed on strategies directed at the principal system failure. Table 14.4 identifies the existing pandemics and broadly explains the population-wide strategies required to deal with existing pandemics.

	DISEASE GROUP	PRINCIPAL STRATEGIES
1	Childhood diseases, e.g. measles, mumps, chicken pox, tetanus	Vaccination programs
2	Vector diseases, e.g. malaria, dengue	Vector control and personal protection
3	Sexually transmitted infections and lifestyle diseases, e.g. AIDS	Behavioural modification
4	Diseases of poverty, e.g. diarrhoeal diseases, meningitis	Improved public health and living conditions
5	Diseases of failed diagnosis, e.g. TB, pneumonia, nematode diseases	Improved health care

TABLE 14.4: The current epidemics

The principal community-wide strategies should be tailored to the particular disease group and to the systematic failure that is most relevant to that group. In effect each of these disease groups occurs in epidemic levels because of fundamental failures in community infrastructure or public health strategies and the remedy should be directed at the fundamental failure.

In Australia, initial management of any epidemic would be based on the population health management strategies in place for routine disease surveillance and management. However, if the epidemic reached major proportions, then it would be managed in accordance with the national disaster management arrangements with health services providing a lead agency role. A major pandemic will be a 'disaster' and will be managed in accordance with national and international disaster response arrangements. Pandemics not only impact on health, but also on society as a whole. Health services would play a leading role, particularly providing advice on system strategy and patient management. A major outbreak would have a massive impact outside of the health environment and, therefore, national and jurisdictional disaster management arrangements would be involved in preparing and managing the response.

Management of new epidemics is based on the principles of disaster management. In Australia, these principles are determined by Emergency Management Australia, and include:

- an all hazards approach whereby preparation, planning and response are based on standard approaches regardless of the incident
- ensuring that all agencies are engaged cooperatively in the response – epidemics have a widespread community impact and while health services may lead the response, involvement of all response agencies will be essential in effective management

- a comprehensive approach involving a consistent approach through prevention, preparedness, response and recovery
- leveraging off existing infrastructure and procedures to provide the necessary response.

There is growing international concern in regard to the risk of pandemics driven by the SARS experience and the risks identified with avian influenza. WHO has developed a suite of international standards that complement the latest update of the *International Health Regulations* (WHO 2005c). The International Health Regulations are a legally binding agreement by member states to work cooperatively on the management of new outbreaks at their source, and not just at national borders. WHO has also produced the *Global Influenza Preparedness Plan* (WHO 2005b) as a model for nations and other standards documents relating to infection control. Most countries have now developed pandemic preparedness plans based on the WHO model.

Epidemics do not respect international borders. International cooperation is essential in order to manage the consequences and limit the impact. Poorer countries are most susceptible to disease outbreaks, and have fewer resources and less capacity to sustain the economic and social impact (Cash & Narasimhan 2000). International cooperation must be directed towards protecting the interests of reporting countries, in order that they may have an incentive to report new epidemics.

Management strategies

As we saw in Chapter 10, protecting the community against potential epidemics relies on both individual and population strategies. At the individual level, strategies aim to prevent infection and to break the chain of transmission. This is achieved by ensuring maximum personal protection through immunisation; the use of physical protective devices, for example, mosquito nets or condoms; and the use of prophylaxis, for example, anti-malarial drugs. Second, by practising universal personal infection control procedures, such as hand washing after using the toilet and before handling food, personal hygiene measures relating to sneezing and avoidance of spitting, cleaning of the personal environment and avoidance of risks. Finally, appropriately managing individual infection should occur through early recognition, isolation and treatment.

At the population level, strategies that aim to reduce the spread of disease include monitoring, surveillance, early recognition and early intervention. Monitoring the presence of risk factors including vectors and the incidence of infections through reporting of disease will support early recognition and intervention. Maintaining laboratory capacity will ensure accuracy of diagnosis to aid both recognition and management. Rapid case investigation and response will ensure the potential for individual cases to become epidemics is minimised. All countries have a responsibility under the *International Health Regulations* to maintain a system of disease surveillance, monitoring and reporting including reporting to international authorities regarding the outbreak of infectious diseases.

Managing risks is an essential component of preparedness. Communities must identify, evaluate and manage the risks to human health. We should reduce human exposure to potential animal sources of disease through biosecurity initiatives, for example, controlling entry to animal breeding areas and monitoring animal diseases.

Epidemics, however, will occur and the capacity of the community to respond will rely on the cycle of planning, preparation, response and recovery. There are several key strategies necessary to maximise the degree of preparation of the society. Outlined below, these strategies are planning, preparedness, response management and recovery.

Planning

The process of planning is an important and valuable element of preparation in that it engages key stakeholders to consider community needs and establishes personal and official links, which will facilitate management of any major incident. Planning also helps to identify the resource requirements, and strategies to increase resources, in the event of a major outbreak. This is particularly important in regard to health resources.

Preparedness

Preparation for major incidents, including pandemics, depends largely on the maintenance of general public health infrastructure and processes. Furthermore, eliminating common risk sources by strategies that ensure clean food, water, air and the safe disposal of waste reduce the risk of major outbreaks. In addition, appropriate infection control procedures should be maintained in health facilities, including both universal and special precautions. Universal precautions are those that should be implemented at 'all times', based on the assumption that all patients are potentially 'infectious'.

Some countries have the capacity to stockpile stores and equipment that may be in sudden demand during an epidemic. These stockpiles include drugs (e.g. antiviral agents), masks, vaccines and equipment. They include 'physical stockpiles' such as those stored in warehouses or 'embedded stockpiles', which refers to the items that at any time are in the manufacture, distribution and supply and storage pathways. In the event of an outbreak it may be important to identify the latter and secure this stockpile for priority usage.

Educating key personnel so they can assist with response management is an essential element of disaster preparation. A comprehensive multidisciplinary approach to disaster education is a critical component of preparation and should include exercises that test the state of preparedness.

Response management

In the event of an outbreak, the key strategies are those of major incident or disaster management. The key elements of health response management are command and control, communication, coordination, capacity of both human and physical resources, containment of the event and clinical care of those affected.

In the event of significant outbreak, effective management will depend on strategies that seek to localise the disease and to protect the vulnerable. Personnel required to help manage the patients will be further reduced by illness among health staff as well as a lack of preparedness of staff to place themselves and their families at risk. Priority may need to be given to protecting those required for ongoing management particularly health and other essential workers. Strategies need to be in place to manage the required expansion in health facilities to cope with the rapidly increasing demand. Rapidly creating capacity will involve reducing alternative services, closing non-essential services, for example, cancelling non-urgent surgery, and strategies to rapidly expand health facility capacity including, for example, using hotels and field hospitals.

Recovery

Following any major event, the health consequences continue. For the individual they must contend with the personal health consequences and the ongoing medical care required. They must also contend with the personal loss and grief that may accompany the death of family and friends. Health systems must recuperate as well. Learning from any event is an important part of system development. Reporting the outcomes, identifying issues to be incorporated into future planning and preparedness helps the system recover. Facilities, personnel and other resources must be restored. In particular those involved in the care of others should be cared for in turn and helped to recover from the threats, challenges and injuries that may be the consequence of any major incident including epidemics.

ACTIVITY

● As a health professional, what should your particular role be in preparing for epidemics?

REFLECTION

Public health professionals including clinicians will be the key to minimising the impact of any epidemic. We need to remain vigilant; maintaining the system of surveillance, which will detect any outbreak early. We should be involved in planning and preparation, becoming knowledgeable and participating in education and raising people's awareness. In the event of an epidemic we will be responsible for investigation, containment and treatment. This has great significance to professionals and their families and you should think through how you would react in such a situation.

The role of public health in disaster management

Public health officials will be involved in the full cycle of disaster preparedness, planning, response and recovery. In particular public health has a leading role to play in certain aspects of disaster response including:

- events in which public health will take a leadership role such as pandemic or bioterrorism
- managing the health consequences of disasters relating to injuries
- preventing secondary public health outbreaks by managing the public health requirements following a disaster, such as safe waste disposal, clean food, water supplies
- surveillance and early detection and intervention of any possible outbreaks that may follow major incidents.

A final word

Experience with SARS, avian influenza and the biological attack in the US following the events of '9/11' have reawakened awareness of the potential impact of epidemics. The world is overdue for a major outbreak although the modern endemic infections such as HIV, TB and malaria continue to cause significant mortality and morbidity.

In the developed world, these infectious diseases are less prevalent, but they remind us of the potential impact of a new infectious epidemic on the structure and functioning of our community. As health professionals, it is important that you comprehend the risks that epidemics pose to the community, and the factors that influence those risks. It is also essential that you understand the strategies that are necessary to minimise those risks, and in the event of an epidemic, to help manage the outbreak and minimise the impact on the community.

This chapter aimed to outline these factors and to provide you with an understanding of how those factors may influence the new epidemics; why the maintenance of public health measures is critical to the task of preventing epidemics; and why it is so important to provide the infrastructure necessary to manage an epidemic should one arise.

REVIEW QUESTIONS

1 Define the following terms: 'epidemic', 'pandemic' and 'endemic'.
2 Identify infectious diseases that continue to cause significant effects on the public's health.
3 What are the factors that may influence the risk and impact of any epidemic?
4 What strategies should a community adopt to ensure that it is prepared for any potential epidemic?
5 As a health professional how can you help reduce the likelihood or impact of an epidemic, before the outbreak and during the outbreak?
6 What are the key elements of health disaster management?

USEFUL WEBSITES

Australian Department of Health and Ageing, communicable disease section: http://www.health.gov.au/internet/main/publishing.nsf/Content/Communicable+Disease+Control-4

Australian Department of Health and Ageing, emergency health section: http://www.health.gov.au/internet/wcms/publishing.nsf/Content/phd-health-emergency.htm

State and territory government sites are generally at www.health.<state abbreviation>.gov.au (e.g. New South Wales: www.health.nsw.gov.au)

US Centers for Disease Control and Prevention: www.cdc.gov

World Association for Emergency and Disaster Medicine: http://wadem.medicine.wisc.edu

World Health Organization: www.who.int/infectious-disease-news

REFERENCES

Australian Institute of Health and Welfare 2006 Mortality over the 20th century in Australia. AIHW

Cash R, Narasimhan V 2000 Impediments to global surveillance of infectious diseases: Consequences of open reporting in a global economy. Bulletin of the World Health Organization 78(11):1358–1368

Fan E X 2003 ERD Policy Brief SARS: Economic impacts and implications. Asian Development Bank 2003. Available: http://www.adb.org/economics 30 Jan 2008

Gilpin C 2007 Migration and Tuberculosis: Evaluation of current tuberculosis control strategies among migrants and emerging issues for Queensland. Unpublished Masters Thesis. Queensland University of Technology, Brisbane

Guinovart C, Navia N M, Tanner M et al 2006 Malaria: burden of disease. Curr. Mol Med 6(2):137–140

Irving W, Boswell T, Alaalden D 2005 Medical Microbiology. Taylor and Francis Group, New York

McMichael A J, Woodruff R E, Hales S 2006 Climate change and human health: present and future risks. Lancet 367:859–869

Meltzer M, Cox N, Fufuda K 1999 The economic impact of pandemic influenza in the United States: Priorities for intervention. Emergency Infectious Diseases 5(5):659–671. Available: http://www.cdc.gov/ncidod/EID/vol5no5/meltzer.htm 30 Jan 2008

Tucker J B 2001 Scourge: The Once and Future Threat of Smallpox. Grove Press, New York

US Centers for Disease Control n.d. Categories of Bioterrorist agents. Available: http://emergency.cdc.gov/agent/agentlist-category.asp#catdef 28 Jan 2008

Webber R 2005 Communicable disease epidemiology and control: a global perspective. CABI Pub, Cambridge

Wong S, Yuen K Y 2005 The severe acute respiratory syndrome (SARS). Journal of Neurovirology 11:455–465

World Health Organization 2004 World Health Report 2004. WHO, Geneva

World Health Organization 2005a Combating Emerging Infectious Diseases. WHO SouthEast Asia. WHO. Available: http://www.who.int/csr/resources/publications/influenza/WHO_CDS_CSR_GIP_2005_5/en/ 28 Nov 2007

World Health Organization 2005b Global influenza preparedness plan. Available: http://www.who.int/csr/resources/publications/influenza/WHO_CDS_CSR_GIP_2005_5/en/ 28 Jan 2008

World Health Organization 2005c International Health Regulations. Available: http://www.who.int/csr/ihr/en/ 23 Jan 2008

World Health Organization 2007 The top 10 causes of death. Available: http://www.who.int/mediacentre/factsheets/fs310/en/ 10 Oct 2007

CHAPTER 15

The future for public health

Mary Louise Fleming

Learning objectives

After reading this chapter you should be able to:

- identify and describe the major challenges facing public health in the 21st century
- analyse the importance of ecological sustainability to the survival of the planet and its impact on public health activity in the future
- discuss the varying roles of the public health worker in the future in light of emerging infectious diseases and the development of a range of chronic illnesses
- consider the important place of politics in decision making about public health resources, infrastructure and strategies, and learn to advocate effectively at various levels of government for public health
- critique the issues that have influenced the globalisation of health and the impact of this development on public health in Australia
- utilise your research skills to engage in research that addresses the underlying causes of mortality and morbidity.

Introduction

What is the future for public health in the 21st century? Can we glean an idea about the future of public health from its past? As Winston Churchill once said, 'The further backward you look, the further forward you can see'. What then can we see in the history of public health that gives us an idea of where public health might be headed in the future?

In the 20th century there was substantial progress in public health in Australia. These improvements were brought about through a number of factors. In part, improvements were due to increasing knowledge about the natural history of disease and its treatment. Added to this knowledge was a shifting focus from legislative measures to protect health, to the emergence of improved promotion and prevention strategies and a general improvement in social and economic conditions for people living in countries like Australia. The same could not, however, be said for poorer countries, many of whom have the most fundamental of sanitary and health protection issues still to deal with. For example, in Sub-Saharan Africa and Russia, the decline in life expectancy may be an aberration or it may be related to a range of interconnected factors. In Russia, factors such as alcoholism, violence, suicide, accidents and cardiovascular disease could be contributing to the falling life expectancy (McMichael & Butler 2007). In Sub-Saharan Africa, a range of issues such as HIV/AIDS, poverty, malaria, tuberculosis, undernutrition, totally inadequate infrastructure, gender inequality, conflict and violence, political taboos and a complete lack of political will, have all contributed to a dramatic drop in life expectancy (McMichael & Butler 2007).

Within Australia, subpopulations still suffer adverse health effects. For Indigenous Australians, mortality rates are higher for almost all causes of death. The major risk factors for poor health in Indigenous populations include low birth weight, obesity, poor nutrition, high levels of alcohol and other drug use, poor housing and living conditions, and inadequate access to health care. Some of the leading causes of death for Indigenous Australians are diabetes, kidney disease and suicide (AIHW 2006). These issues have been canvassed extensively in Section 2 of the book.

The multidisciplinary nature of contemporary public health has become evident in the range of developments that have advanced public health during the 20th century. Biomedical scientists have identified many of the disease-causing organisms and have developed control methods to manage them. Epidemiologists have identified the determinants that underpin many chronic diseases, enabling this information to be used to reduce people's risk of illness. Efforts to improve the environment through clean air and water have resulted in cleaner environments than was the case 50 years ago (Schneider 2006).

Improvements such as these have advanced the health of Australians and meant that life expectancy has also increased substantially; a large part of these improvements have been attributed to public health interventions. The 10 great American public health achievements in the 20th century are listed in Box 15.1. It is interesting to note that none of these achievements had a focus on the ecosystem or ecological sustainability. However, these issues are now firmly on the world stage, and on the public health agenda, for action in the 21st century.

Box 15.1: Ten great public health achievements – United States, 1900–1999

1 Vaccination
2 Motor-vehicle safety
3 Safer workplaces
4 Control of infectious diseases
5 Decline in deaths from coronary heart disease and stroke
6 Safer and healthier foods
7 Healthier mothers and babies
8 Family planning
9 Fluoridation of drinking water
10 Recognition of tobacco use as a health hazard

(Source: CDC MMWR Weekly 1999)

We can clearly see the re-emergence of infectious diseases as a major challenge for public health in the 21st century. The challenge of HIV/AIDS has been with the community for more than 20 years, but new diseases such as SARS and avian influenza have also emerged as major diseases that may affect the public's health into the future, and this underscores the importance of surveillance and monitoring strategies to control such outbreaks.

In the late 1990s the National Public Health Partnership (NPHP 1998) produced an overview of the public health system and its activities. In that document, a section outlined recent key achievements for public health. Many of these achievements are similar to the United States list presented in Box 15.1. Countries like Australia and the United States have a similar set of public health successes, in which they have demonstrated improvements in mortality and morbidity over the past century. Others on the Australian list have a more contemporary flavour, as shown in Box 15.2.

Box 15.2: Key achievements within the public health sector

Recent achievements in the Australian public health sector include:

- increasing community awareness and behaviour change in relation to risk factors for tobacco-related cancer and skin cancers
- reducing the transmission of communicable diseases specifically HIV/AIDS
- early detection of breast and cervical cancers
- reducing the rates of mortality of motor vehicle crashes
- providing communities with access to public health information, including the development of innovative techniques in social marketing of public health policy
- focussing on evidence-based practice (e.g. Cochrane Collaborating Centres) developing communicable disease control (vaccine preventable diseases and food-borne diseases)
- antivenom research
- improved approaches to using data by applying epidemiological principles to statistical analysis (e.g. injury surveillance)
- medical entomology.

New health challenges require a changing set of strategies for public health action into the future. This is an ambitious agenda of growing urgency, with daunting challenges. Tang et al (2005) provided the context, noting that since the 1986 *Ottawa Charter for Health Promotion* (WHO 1986) new patterns of consumption and communication, urbanisation, environmental changes and public health emergencies – along with accelerating social and demographic changes to work, learning, family and community life – have become critical factors influencing health. Similarly, Baum (2008) argues for public health strategies in the future that have developing supportive societies and communities as their central plank (Baum 2008). She goes on to state:

> Social support, high self-esteem and a sense of personal control are important determinants of health, best achieved in societies and communities that are relatively equal and that have reasonable levels of social solidarity.

> (Baum 2008 p 576)

Public health challenges in the 21st century: balancing re-emerging issues and new developments

As we begin the 21st century, public health faces new challenges, yet it also needs to remember its roots. While we have discussed some of these issues in Sections 2, 4 and parts of Section 5 of the book, the challenges into the future are more complex and bring together the importance of fundamental public health with the emergence of global issues like climate change. In some countries, basic sanitation is still a major challenge for public health. There are renewed threats from infectious diseases, such as HIV/AIDS, food-borne pathogens and ecological issues that threaten the planet, such as climate change. An ageing population brings its own issues, including the associated increased costs of health care. While there has been a decline in cigarette smoking, this decline has slowed; and among adolescents, rates of alcohol abuse and illicit drug use have remained largely unchanged for the past decade (Schneider 2006). More recently, the emergence of the problems associated with physical inactivity and unhealthy diets have contributed to increasing levels of overweight and obesity among the Australian population.

In the 21st century, one of the major challenges for health systems and governments around the world will be the increasing cost of health and medical care. Advances in the medical model and a focus on curing health problems, rather than preventing them, have meant that more resources have been expended on medical care and treatment. However, as that type of care has become more and more sophisticated the costs have also increased.

The importance of public health was noted by the 1988 Institute of Medicine (IOM) report, *The Future of Public Health* in the United States. The report prompted public health agencies, policymakers and academic institutions to initiate a national discussion on the importance of and role of public health in advancing population health (IOM 1988). In 2003, a further report was produced by the IOM titled *The Future of the Public's Health in the 21st Century*. Like the 1988 report, the 2003 report noted that the United States was not meeting its potential in the area of population health. It highlighted three important issues: (1) the focus on medical care rather than prevention; (2) the attention to biomedical research rather than prevention research; and (3) the ongoing disparity in health between different population groups by issues such as race and ethnicity, gender and socioeconomic status (IOM 2003). A health system for the future needs to shifts its attention from funding high-tech infrastructure that supports a small percentage of the population to a continuum of care that enhances health promotion and comprehensive primary care strategies.

In developed countries there has been a general call for better education and training of the public health workforce to meet the diverse needs of population health in the 21st century (Baum 2008, Schneider 2006, Watterson 2003).

Solutions to public health issues

A future orientation for public health is one of the strategies that Lin et al (2007) argue for in their book on public health. Table 15.1 summarises some of the issues presented by a range of authors (Beaglehole & Bonita 2004, Hancock 2007, Lin et al 2007, McMichael

FUTURE ISSUES	IMPLICATIONS FOR PUBLIC HEALTH
Influence of globalisation (markets, technology and communications)	Epidemics, terrorism and environmental concerns have expanded to international as well as domestic implications for population health
Global issues – poverty, urbanisation, globalisation, and social and economic inequalities	Obstacles to sustainability, impact on the level and equity of population health
Global environmental changes	Depletion and degradation of natural capital is not sustainable; need to focus on dependence on maintaining Earth's life support system; population wellbeing and health are the real bottom line of sustainability

➡

FUTURE ISSUES	IMPLICATIONS FOR PUBLIC HEALTH
Risk management – necessary to predict, influence and minimise risks in major systems on which society depends	Protect and improve population health through mitigation and management of risk
Social factors – values, demography, education, housing, mobility, migration, social inequality, literacy, health status	Social determinants influence patterns of health, access to health, understanding of health issues and health care
Technological factors – developments in information technology and telecommunications, and medical technology	Information technology developments enhance knowledge and analysis of health patterns to enable health management and care; costs, however, mean that society will not be able to support the increasing technological sophistication
Economic factors – employment, income, inflation, consumer spending on health resources, demand and supply issues	Socioeconomic gradients and health, unemployment and associated health consequences, social isolation, increasing costs for consumer and sophistication of health care
Resource factors – use of resources, particularly energy, and impact	Maintaining viable ecosystem for sustainable development, renewable energy sources, implication of current systems on long-term sustainability
Political factors – government stability, ideological climate, policy priorities	Level of investment in public health, and the focus of that investment, priority issues, state–federal collaboration and divisions
Re-emergence of infectious diseases	Need for public health researchers and practitioners to transmit to the public information about the risks inherent in current modes of social and economic development and the resultant large-scale environmental changes, and to find ecologically attuned ways of managing social change to minimise health risk. Surveillance and monitoring of new diseases and ways of preventing widespread mortality will need to be an important part of public health activity in the future.
Decline in life expectancy in several regions	After some gains, declines in life expectancy in poor countries as a result of the re-emergence of infectious diseases, new infectious diseases, poor basic health services, poverty, malnutrition, lack of affordable drug therapies, lack of political support and will

TABLE 15.1: Future issues impacting on public health activity in the 21st century

(Source: Beaglehole & Bonita 2004, Lin et al 2007, McMichael 2006, McMichael & Butler 2007, Hancock 2007)

2006, McMichael & Butler 2007) that articulate future developments that will impact on public health. It is amazing how similar the lists are for many different authors. The focus is clearly on the big social, environmental and economic issues that have a direct and indirect affect on the health of the population. Consider the range of issues presented and the implications for public health, and complete the reflection activity after the table.

ACTIVITY

- Consider the issues raised in Table 15.1. What do you think are the three major challenges for public health in the 21st century?
- How prepared do you think the public health workforce needs to be, and what skills would you identify as important for a public health worker in this century?
- Can you, as a health professional in Australia, have an impact on global issues? What impact do you think you can have?

REFLECTION

You might like to consider the impact of globalisation on health; the issues of social and economic inequalities and their impact on health; or the advances in science and technology that might lead health systems further down the pathway of specialised technologies that are enormously expensive with limited population health returns.

We have discussed the public health workforce and its development in Section 1 of the book as well as in this chapter. Reflect back on what you have read and think about the skills that a public health worker might need to meet the challenges of the 21st century.

Public health workers will probably need to specialise more as public health practice becomes more complex. What other health professionals have moved in this direction? The catch cry of 'think global act local' is already in our vocabulary, but what does that really mean for health workers? Does it mean that no matter how small your actions you can have an impact if others in the profession are working in similar ways to you?

Challenges of predicting future public health activity

The challenge of predicting trends in health, and strategies to address these issues, are often predicated on decisions about service types and locations, and resourcing matters. Eager et al (2001) provide a useful list of the nature and types of decisions that are often made to determine service type and resourcing:

- incidence or prevalence of conditions
- behavioural and environmental determinants of health
- factors that influence consumers to seek medical care, such as income, household structure, socio-cultural factors and other variables
- technological advancement and clinical patterns of care
- consumer selection of provider and preferences referral patterns
- health expenditure and government outlay of funds.

Globalisation and health

Issues such as free trade, modern economic theory (that asserts 'that increased per capita income will offset the non-costed losses'), mobility of capital and the deregulation of labour conditions all contribute to social and economic inequalities and environmental risk (McMichael & Butler 2007 pp 21–22). As McMichael and Butler state:

> Tackling these more systemic health issues requires multisectoral policy coordination at community, national and international levels. Via an expanded repertoire of bottom-up, top-down and 'middle-out' approaches … The central task is to promote sustainable environmental and social conditions that confer enduring and equitable gains in population health.
>
> (McMichael & Butler 2007 pp 22–23)

Public health will have to be global to be effective and take on a strong advocacy role in order to deal with global inequalities, and inequities within countries.

Sustainable ecological public health

Accomplishing sustainable social, economic and environmental conditions underpins achieving population health. However, environmental changes, including climate change, loss of biodiversity, productivity downturns in land and oceans and freshwater depletion have all contributed to the potential of serious health risks to current and future human societies (Baum 2008, Beaglehole & Bonita 2004, McMichael & Butler 2007).

Reflecting on 20 years since the *Ottawa Charter* (WHO 1986), Hancock (2007) commented that he would strengthen four major areas for debate and discussion if he was to present now on the role of public health and health promotion into the future. These areas are:

1 an explicit link between human health and ecosystem health: 'Global environmental change, including climate and atmospheric change, resource depletion, ecotoxicity, habitat destruction and species extinction, is the ultimate threat to health…' (Hancock 2007 p 7)
2 more emphasis on the built environment, and how we design, build and operate our built environments is of major importance to our health and it also has a profound impact on the natural environment
3 a broadening of the focus on social capital to include 'formal' social capital, such as the system of social programs and institutions, as well as 'invisible' social capital that includes the legal, political and constitutional infrastructure that underpins our societies and communities
4 a focus on a new economics based on human wellbeing. As Hancock states: '…real capitalists in the 21st century will be those who simultaneously build all four forms of capital – natural, social and human as well as economic capital' (Hancock 2007 p 8).

Further, McMichael (2006) says that health researchers have been slow to engage with the issue of 'ecological sustainability' and its impact on health. He suggests that the reason for this is the reluctance of scientists to look beyond defined professional boundaries and paradigms, and the enormity of a task that asks researchers to examine how changes in whole natural systems can affect health (McMichael 2006 p 580). Nevertheless, these are issues that must be addressed if we are to be able to sustain a way of life that is based on recognition of the centrality of maintaining viable ecosystems for a sustainable world future.

Emerging and re-emerging infections

Infectious diseases have re-emerged in recent years, associated with mobility, shifts in the ecology of human living, technologies and economic activity. This has required public health researchers to undertake study and surveillance of infectious disease transmission patterns (McMichael 2006 p 580). A recent upturn in the range, burden and risk of infectious diseases has been produced by a variety of factors, including increased population density, persistent poverty, the vulnerability of younger population groups, as well as many environmental, political and social factors. These causes are compounded by gender, economic and structural inequalities, by political denial, vaccine obstacles and the mismatch between health resource distribution and major causes of illness (McMichael & Butler 2007 p 17).

Effectively managing infectious diseases in society is reliant on a range of complementary strategies, which together aim to prevent, monitor or treat disease. These strategies include those targeted at disease prevention, those involved with surveillance and early detection, and strategies aimed at managing disease when it occurs. This approach is equivalent to primary, secondary and tertiary prevention. Accordingly, the three key aspects of managing infectious diseases are: (1) disease prevention; (2) surveillance, early recognition and early intervention; and (3) managing a disease outbreak.

Genetics, biotechnology and information technology

Molecular and genetic approaches to controlling disease are well underway. Supporters of such approaches argue that money will be well spent because of the potential that understanding genes and molecular structures have for promoting health and improving life expectancy (Baum 2008). Baum (2008) argues that public health practitioners will have to take a critical and sceptical view of genetic technology, questioning its potential for impact on population health status and the impact its availability would have on equity.

Using biotechnology holds great promise in advancing medical care and treatment but these activities will also contribute to the spiralling costs of health care (Schneider 2006). Technology has a number of other possibilities that raise both ethical and legal issues and will need to be resolved through public debate and difficult policy choices. Included in this list are genetic engineering, cloning, stem cell research and slowing the ageing process. The bottom line with respect to biotechnology is not that these advances might occur, but the ultimate challenge to public health in the 21st century is the cost of these innovations and the limited resources available to pay for them (Schneider 2006).

Advances in information technology have led to improvements in public health surveillance capabilities. However, as technology has improved, ethical and legal questions have arisen about the need to be able to keep information private as well as ensuring that information that should be made public is available in the public domain. The rise of the internet as a source of information and commerce also poses many challenges for consumers with regard to how to evaluate the information, and for governments and policymakers, about on how to protect consumers from inappropriate advice and information (Schneider 2006).

The public health workforce: skills for a complex future

The public health workforce is an important consideration in advancing public health activity into the 21st century. In Australia, a wide range of universities offer Master of Public Health degrees with a range of specialisations, such as environmental health, epidemiology, health promotion, health management and occupational health and safety. Regardless of the institutional base for public health training, the nature and orientation of that training are fundamental to advancing public health in this century. A key focus for public health education is the link between the processes of education and the practice of public health. There is a gap between academic and practical public health, which does not well serve either the public health workforce or the public health academic community. Clearly, what we need is strong institutional support and leadership for public health education and training, to ensure that students understand and adopt the fundamental values of public health.

Beaglehole and Bonita (2004) argue strongly for links between public health practice and the delivery of medical care, in order to support the implementation of preventive programs. They suggest that this is particularly important in poor countries (2004 p 260).

Public health workers not only need an understanding of the core competencies of practice, they also need a clear appreciation of the complexity of the task and the multiple drivers of population health patterns. The development of competencies for public health and health promotion have been well researched in Australia, including the work of Rotem et al (1995); more recently there has been research from Western Australia (Shilton et al 2006) to update the Australian health promotion competencies. The study by Shilton et al (2006) is a collaboration between the Australian Health Promotion Association (AHPA), the Public Health Association of Australia Health Promotion Special Interest Group (PHAA HPSIG), and the International Union for Health Promotion and Education (IUHPE) SW Pacific Regional Committee. This work further reinforces the importance of a public health worker who understands the complexity of the task.

Public health workers need to have a focus on equity and equality, and values that acknowledge the right to self-determination of the Indigenous population. However, they also need to understand that public health now has a global perspective to consider and, importantly, must acknowledge and act on the issues that impact on ecological sustainability.

Strategic planning for public health: political will and action

The need for planning and coordination of public health activities is, as ever, the underlying priority for advancing a national public health agenda in Australia. Federation in 1901 marked the development of State and Commonwealth divisions of responsibility and the establishment of a Commonwealth Department of Health. State health departments technically take responsibility in Australia for delivering population health services to the public, while the federal government determines the national agenda and the strategic direction, in consultation with states and territories. This consultation process is often fraught with difficulty, particularly if at the federal level there is, for example, a Labor federal government and Liberal state governments.

As we saw in Chapter 2, the various levels of government in Australia are responsible for different levels of public health activity, at times with some overlap. We also discussed the role of the non-government sector and private industry in the complex web of activity that makes up the public health agenda in Australia. In Chapter 3 we also discussed the policy process and the levels of activity and influence that local, state and federal governments have in that process.

However, public health is as much about democracy, empowerment, accountability, transparency and communication as it is about professional skill sets. In many of the developed countries the focus for government is still on treating disease rather than promoting public health. In addition, where public health has taken a somewhat front seat in debate and discussion, it has often been focussed on lifestyle approaches to health rather than life circumstance approaches (Watterson 2003 p 11).

Following on for this perspective, Baum (2008) argues that a strong state should see its role as balancing social, environmental and economic concerns in order to support the goals of public health, which focus on equity, sustainability and achieving health for the majority of the population.

Return on investment to improve health

Health is determined by health behaviours and genetics, and by social, physical, environmental and economic factors that impact on how people go about their daily lives. However, the majority of resources, both human and material, are expended on medical care. As Schneider (2006 p 548) indicates, 'it is becoming increasingly apparent that advances in high technology medical care have become economically unsustainable'. The challenge for public health is to continue to work towards educating the public and policymakers that the role of public health is to protect and promote the health of the population, a far more economically and socially responsible position.

Leadership and public health: establishing a research agenda

Internationally, both the World Bank and WHO have already identified the major public health research challenges; these are presented in Box 15.3.

Box 15.3: Major public health research challenges

These have been identified as:

- continuing epidemics of preventable childhood infectious diseases, which are aggravated by poverty and undernutrition
- economic, social and environmental changes, which lead to emerging and re-emerging infectious diseases
- growing epidemics of non-communicable diseases and injuries
- assessing the effectiveness and efficiency of public health programs.

(Source: Beaglehole & Bonita 2004 p 261)

McMichael (2006) quite rightly points out that in addition to the current research activity in public health we need research that focuses on the health risks posed by global environmental changes. He proposes three types of research; first, empirical studies that are designed to describe how variations in environmental and ecological systems affect health risks; second, evidence about whether global environmental changes already affect health; and third, the need to make 'credible estimates of future changes in the health risks due to plausible scenarios of ongoing changes in large-scale environmental systems' (McMichael 2006 p 580).

Beaglehole and Bonita (2004) very succinctly sum up the focus for public health research when they state:

> Public health research is a multidisciplinary activity … All too often, however, it is limited to epidemiology and health systems research. The real research challenge is the exploration of the interaction between social, economic and environmental factors and disease.

> (Beaglehole & Bonita 2004 p 260)

Population ageing

Older Australians are people aged 65 years or over (AIHW 2006), and this group makes up 13% of the population (2,604,900 people in 2004) (AIHW 2006). During the past several decades, the number and proportion of the population aged 65 years or over have increased rapidly in Australia. The increase in the population aged 85 years or over was even more marked (AIHW 2006).

Maintaining good health among older Australians helps to moderate the demand for health and aged care services, which is important as Australia's population ages over the coming decades. In response to population ageing, Australia has made improving older people's health a national research priority (AIHW 2006). One area of special interest is adopting a healthy lifestyle at older ages because its benefits include preventing disease and functional decline, extending longevity and enhancing quality of life (WHO 2002).

At age 65, Australia's males now expect to live for a further 17.8 years and females for another 21.1 years, which is about six years more than their counterparts at the beginning of the 20th century (AIHW 2006). Males and females aged 85 years can expect to live for a further 5.7 and 6.9 years respectively, which is about two years more than for the early 1900s. Most of these gains in life expectancy among older Australians occurred during the latter three decades of the last century, when mortality from cardiovascular diseases (notably heart disease and stroke) fell rapidly.

Maintaining good health for older people in Australia is essential not only for their own wellbeing, but also because the costs of curative and long-term care for an ever-increasing subpopulation will not be sustainable into the future. As we mentioned earlier in this chapter the public health workforce needs to work towards maintaining the health of our ageing population through fundamental promotion strategies such as good nutrition, moderate physical activity and enhanced mental health and wellbeing.

Dietary imbalance and physical inactivity

In the past two decades there has been a striking increase in the prevalence of obesity observed in many countries. Decreasing levels of physical activity and a high intake of kilojoules have both made significant contributions to the epidemics of overweight and obesity. It is interesting to note that public health workers in wealthy countries are concerned about the health effects of over-nutrition, but from a global perspective hunger is a much more important problem (Beaglehole & Bonita 2004). Participation in physical activity is an important protective factor for health, furthermore, physical inactivity, according to Keleher and Murphy (2004), is second only to tobacco smoking in terms of its contribution to the burden of disease.

One of the major concerns for public health workers in countries like Australia is that the contribution of both the lack of physical activity and the over consumption of food has a strong association with cardiovascular risk factors, obesity and diabetes. It also compounds the risks when associated with smoking, alcohol consumption and poor nutrition (AIHW 2006, Keleher & Murphy 2004).

Many of the factors that contribute to overweight and obesity in wealthy countries are social and economic factors, including longer working hours, limited leisure time and appropriate facilities, and a range of labour-saving devices that have reduced our opportunities to engage in adequate physical activity. The challenge for public health is not only about reorienting the health system but working in concert with other sectors to promote a balance between work and leisure. In addition, it is important to ensure that people have the opportunities to achieve such a balance, and an understanding of the health implications of long working hours or limited opportunities for physical activity. It means health professionals working in collaboration with governments, architects and builders to reorganise living spaces to facilitate physical activity. True multisector collaboration for enhancing health is likely to be a central strategy for public health into the future.

REFLECTION

The progress that has been made in public health over the 20th century has been remarkable in many respects, particularly in wealthy countries. However, progress in the health of subpopulations within these countries, such as Indigenous health in Australia, and within developing countries, where basic sanitation and food supply are still inadequate, remains a major challenge of public health.

On a positive note, in Australia infectious diseases have been reduced, risk factors for chronic diseases such as diabetes have become well understood, environmental issues have to some degree been improved and we have a lot of knowledge about the contribution of health behaviours to illness and disease. Life expectancy has increased for both men and women over the decade and this has brought potentially new challenges as the population ages, and more and more people are living with chronic disease. Health information is far more comprehensive and readily available and we understand more clearly the impact of a range of social, economic and physical determinants of health on patterns of mortality and morbidity.

What challenges will public health face in the 21st century? Some of those challenges were already emerging late in the 20th century, such as the development of new infectious diseases and the fundamental question of ecological sustainability.

Schneider (2006) believes that the most important challenge facing public health in the 21st century will be to 'encourage a society-wide debate on how public resources should be allocated to most effectively improve the health of the population as a whole' (Schneider 2006 p 550). McMichael (2006), on the other hand, clearly sees our future as one of a focus on sustainability, about ensuring positive (and equitable) human experience – of which health is fundamental. He says, 'If our way of living and of managing the natural environment do not underwrite current and future population health, then that trajectory represents non-sustainability' (McMichael 2006 p 581).

The public health war on disease and death is moving in and out of the shadows of issues such as the War on Terrorism, but all too often it remains in darkness, especially when the politics of disease treatment means secondary and tertiary care continues to consume the vast amount of global health resources (Watterson 2003 p 14).

Public health also faces many challenges. As we have seen in this chapter, issues such as ecological sustainability, inequitable resource distribution and political conditions impact on health, and there seems to be limited political will to restructure resources and infrastructure to ensure the equitable distribution of health in our society. In addition, we face issues of social isolation, an ageing population and problems of overweight and obesity, particularly among young Australians.

However, the future of public health is an exciting one. Health professionals of the future working to improve the public's health will need to be multi-skilled, flexible and adaptable to meet the challenges they will face. Challenges in public health are there to be met and we are all well placed to make a difference to the health of the population.

REVIEW QUESTIONS

1 Draw up a chart that displays developments that have advanced the health of the Australian population in the 20th century, and then the beginnings of this century.
2 What are the major challenges? For example, is over-consumption a problem across the world?
3 How do these challenges differ for wealthy countries compared with poor countries?
4 What part has globalisation played in the emerging patterns of mortality and morbidity?
5 How important is ecological sustainability and, if it is important, for what reasons is it important?
6 What skills and expertise do the health workforce of the 21st century need that may not have been as important in the previous century?

REFERENCES

Australian Institute of Health and Welfare 2006 Australia's Health 2006. AGPS, Canberra

Baum F 2008 The new public health. Oxford University Press, Melbourne

Beaglehole R, Bonita R 2004 Public Health at the Crossroads: Achievements and prospects, 2nd edn. Cambridge University Press, Cambridge

CDC MMWR Weekly 1999 Ten Great Public Health Achievements – United States, 1900–1999, 48(12):241–243

Eager K, Garrett P, Lin V 2001 Health Planning: An Australian Perspective. Allen and Unwin, Sydney

Hancock T 2007 Creating environments for health – 20 years on. IUHPE – Promotion and Education Supplement 2:7–8

Institute of Medicine 1988 The Future of Public Health. National Academy Press, Washington DC

Institute of Medicine (IOM) 2003 The Future of Public's Health in the 21st Century. National Academy Press, Washington DC

Keleher H, Murphy B 2004 Understanding health: a determinants approach. Oxford University Press, South Melbourne

Lin V, Smith J, Fawkes S 2007 Public Health Practice in Australia. The organised effort. Allen and Unwin, Sydney

Martens P, Huynen M 2003 A future without health? Health dimension in global scenario studies. Bulletin of the World Health Organization 81(12):896–901

McMichael A J 2006 population health as the 'bottom line' of sustainability: a contemporary challenge for public health researchers. European Journal of Public Health 16(6):579–582

McMichael A J, Butler C D 2007 Emerging health issues: the widening challenge for population health promotion. Health Promotion International 21(S1):15–24

National Public Health Partnership (NPHP) 1998 Public Health in Australia: The Public Health Landscape: person, society, environment. National Public Health Partnership, Melbourne

Rotem A, Walters J, Dewdney J 1995, 'The public health workforce education and training study', Australian Journal of Public Health, vol. 19, no. 5, pp. 437–438

Schneider M J 2006 Introduction to Public Health, 2nd edn. Jones and Bartlett, Sudbury

Shilton T, Howat P, James R et al 2006 Revision of Health Promotion Competencies for Australia 2005. Western Australia, Western Australian Centre for Health Promotion Research and The National Heart Foundation of Australia (WA Division)

Tang K C, Beaglehole R, O'Byrne D 2005 Policy and partnership for health promotion – addressing the determinants of health. Bulletin of the World Health Organization 83: 884–885

Watterson A (ed) 2003 Public Health in Practice. Palgrave Macmillan, UK

World Health Organization 1986 Ottawa Charter. WHO, Geneva

World Health Organization 2002 Active ageing: a policy framework. WHO/NMH/NPH/02.8. WHO, Geneva

Reflection

Public health achievements and challenges in the 21st century

Introduction

Public health is essentially about 'the science and the art of advancing health through organised efforts that promote, protect and restore the health of the population' (Last 2001 p 145). As we have discussed in this book, public health is both an art and a science, it is about organised efforts and it works on multiple fronts to advance the health of the population or subsections of the population. Public health practitioners will need to be advocates for public health, and for groups within society without a voice, and there will continue to be a need for strong professional associations to advocate at government level. Practitioners need to advocate for the communities they serve and to stress the importance of community participation (Baum 2008).

Public health is also a global enterprise. The major challenge for us is to sustain and increase the health gains made over the past half century despite some worrying trends that suggest that this may be difficult to achieve. As Beaglehole and Bonita (2004) point out there are several interrelated global developments that continue to have a profound effect on public health. These include 'the unequal relationship between wealthy and poor countries; the prevailing ideology that stresses the role of the "free market" and "individualism"; and the threats to the environment' (Beaglehole & Bonita 2004 p 266).

Globalisation and health

A global agenda for public health is a major challenge for practitioners, public health advocacy groups and governments. Throughout this book we have discussed the emerging issues associated with the globalisation of health and we have noted the implications. There are a number of international organisations that have played, and continue to play, a significant role in advocating for global health advances. However, these roles are sometimes overlapping and there is a serious lack of coordination between agencies and their activities. For example, the World Health Organization (WHO) is the lead technical agency for public health (Lee et al 1996); however, the World Bank is, financially, the most important agency in world health (Lancet 1996). Other agencies also play a role including the UN Children's Fund (UNICEF); UN Population Fund (UNFPA); and the UN Development Programme (UNDP).

Beaglehole and Bonita (2004) suggest that more recently the World Bank has acknowledged that inequalities are a substantial barrier to prosperity and growth and that there is a need for strong government leadership, an active trade union movement and greater equality in poor countries. However, these messages are not always consistent. Similarly, the influence of WHO has been less evident recently with times of solid achievement followed by less success, some successful programs that have seen real achievement internationally or programs that have not been at all successful, such as *Roll Back Malaria* (RBM). Pressures from vested interests, such as the tobacco industry and more recently the food industry in the United States, have always been a part of the nature of WHO and its activities (Ashraf 2003). Balancing the important global public health challenges against the needs of member countries, and pressure from vested interest groups, will always be a struggle for WHO. Strong and consistent leadership will be required for WHO in the 21st century. The issue of public–private partnerships will also continue to be a challenge for WHO. A recent international health promotion conference had the notion of public–private partnerships as its theme, and while in theory these partnerships have many potentially positive aspects, the reality requires much more stringent rules of engagement. Most recently the *Millennium Development Goals* (MDGs), established by the UN member states in 2000, mark a watershed for the alleviation of world poverty. Three of the eight goals refers to health. However, all of the goals are important for health as, for example, achieving the education goal is also essential to achieving improvements in health (Beaglehole 2003).

Before we conclude this book we need to gaze into the future for what we think might be the agenda for public health.

Future challenges

Public health practitioners need an opportunity to think about public health futures, the trends and challenges, and the possible ways forward. Can public health practitioners anticipate and react to potential future scenarios or can they, in fact, act to shape futures? What are the implications of global warming and ecological sustainability on public health and the health of the population? What do we currently know about likely futures and how can we take this information into account in making decisions that range from the local to the global level, to pursue preferred futures (Lin et al 2007 p 389)?

Martens and Huynen (2003 p 899) propose three possible futures for public health (see Box R.1). Each of these stages is affected by economic, political, social and environmental events, which means that some countries may stagnate or reverse their position, depending on the influence of the factors listed above.

More recently, Lin et al (2007) predicted three new issues that will challenge public health to find a solution or a set of solutions for their resolution. These are described in Table R.1 with brief reference to some of the issues that the authors identify within each of the areas of challenge. Many of the implications are based on changing technologies, infrastructure and systems, although changes in consumer behaviour are also discussed as is the impact of globalisation on health.

Public health will, by necessity, meet many of the challenges put before it, as it has in the 20th century. However, a word of caution for public health in the 21st century: practitioners will need to meet the needs of their communities and local constituencies, as well as being aware of the impact of global issues on local agendas. The principles of public health that have stood the test of time, such as equity, equality, advocacy and social, economic and environmental responsibility, will need to continue to be placed at the

Box R.1: Possible public health futures

AGE OF EMERGING INFECTIOUS DISEASES OR THE RE-EMERGENCE OF 'OLD' DISEASES

Unfavourable changes in population health will be brought about by changes in global social, political and economic factors that will influence trade, travel, microbiological resistance, human behaviour, health systems and the environment. Responses to increasing disease threats will be limited by antibiotic resistance, insecticides and inadequate public health infrastructure. These problems will lead to an increase in infectious diseases and reduced life expectancy. The economic consequences of ill health will lead to increased environmental degradation, reduced income and poor health. Control of infectious diseases will be hampered by an inability to manage existing technologies, and political and financial barriers.

THE AGE OF MEDICAL TERMINOLOGY

Increased economic growth and technological improvements will offer new opportunities for health gain even though lifestyle and environmental issues may pose a threat to health. If sustainable economic development is not realised then increased environmental pressure and social imbalances might propel societies into the age of emerging infectious diseases. If a balance can be achieved between all of these factors then sustained health might be achieved.

THE AGE OF SUSTAINED HEALTH

Reduction in lifestyle diseases and eradication of most environmentally related infectious diseases will occur if investments in social services can occur. Resources needed for future generations will not be depleted and even though infections might emerge, effective and timely handling of these outbreaks will occur because of improved worldwide surveillance and monitoring systems. Health systems will meet the needs of an ageing population and inequalities in health between countries will disappear.

(Source: Martens and Huynen 2003 p 899)

forefront, not just for public health practitioners but for politicians and the community at large. As Beaglehole and Bonita succinctly state:

> … there is a need for a collective, international responsibility that addresses the requirements of future generations through coordinated multisectoral action at local, community, national, regional and international levels. If public health practitioners are successful in framing these debates and in communicating their importance, public support for public health activities will increase and, collectively, we will be able to reduce the threats to the health of all populations.

(Beaglehole & Bonita 2004 p 278)

Conclusion

This introductory text to the principles and practices of public health has been designed to help you understand the fundamental issues that have shaped public health, and will continue to do so into the future. We hope that, as a result of reading this book, you have

CHALLENGE	IMPLICATIONS
New forms of health care	Innovation in communication and diagnostic technologies that lead to, for example, home monitoring, track personal health histories, take charge of health care decisions.
	Better informed and more demanding health care consumers, greater choice around service delivery and nature of care.
	Technology to create human life, cloning, genetically altered babies.
	Emergence of social and technological innovations such as molecular nanotechnology, cognitive sciences, biotechnology, information technology. Some of these opportunities may in fact increase inequalities in health among population subgroups.
Globalisation and security	The positive and negative impact of cultural globalisation, globalisation of trade and globalisation in relation to health, for example, products and lifestyle, places in which we live and work.
	Implications of capitalism on public health, global population movement through travel, and the accelerated pace of change as examples.
	The impact of 'mega-cities', the needs of local communities and the impact of globalisation on local issues all present challenges.
Science, technology, environment	The impact of global risks factors such as natural disasters, terrorism and new diseases on public health.
	Ethical, social, legal and religious questions associated with gene therapy and genetic engineering.

TABLE R.1: New issues that will challenge public health in the future

(Source: Lin et al 2007)

a fundamental understanding of the nature and scope of public health, the factors that provide the evidence that underpins public health activity, the range and scope of public health interventions and the emerging issues that will challenge public health into the 21st century and beyond.

REFERENCES

Ashraf H 2003 WHO's diet report prompts food industry backlash. Lancet 361:1142

Baum F 2008 The New Public Health, 3rd edn. Oxford University Press, Melbourne

Beaglehole R (ed) 2003 Global Public Health: A New Era. Oxford University Press, Oxford

Beaglehole R, Bonita R 2004 Public Health at the Crossroads: Achievements and Prospects, 2nd edn. Cambridge University Press, Cambridge

Editorial 1996 The World Bank. Listening and Learning. Lancet 347:411

Last J M 2001 A dictionary of epidemiology, 4th edn. Oxford University Press, New York

Lee K, Collinson S, Walt G et al 1996 Who should be doing what in international health: a confusion of mandates in the United Nations? British Medical Journal 312:302–307

Lin V, Smith J, Fawkes S 2007 Public Health Practice in Australia: The organised effort. Allen and Unwin, Sydney

Martens P, Huynen M 2003 A future without health? Health dimensions in global scenario studies. Bulletin of the World Health Organization 81(12):895–901

Schneider M J 2006 Introduction to Public Health, 2nd edn. Jones and Bartlett Publishers, Boston

Glossary

Acquired immunity – Immunity specific to a single organism or group of organisms that is acquired through either active or passive mechanisms.

Active immunity – Immunity that is produced by a person's own immune system.

Additional precautions – Additional infection control practices taken for patients known or suspected to be infected or colonised with disease agents that may not be contained by standard precautions alone.

Advocacy for health – 'A combination of individual and social actions designed to gain political commitment, policy support, social acceptance and systems support for a particular health goal or programme' (WHO 1998 Glossary).

Biodiversity – The variability among living organisms from all sources including terrestrial, marine and other aquatic ecosystems and the ecological complexes of which they are part. This includes diversity within species, between species and of ecosystems.

BMI – Body Mass Index (kg/m^2): Underweight less than 18.5; normal weight over 18.5 and less than 25; overweight (but not obese) 25 and above, but less than 30; obese 30 and above (AIHW Chronic Disease website).

Commensal relationship – In communicable terms is one in which the microorganism and the human co-exist for mutual benefit.

Communicable (or contagious) disease – A disease that can spread from one individual to another.

Community empowerment – 'An empowered community is one in which individuals and organizations apply their skills and resources in collective efforts to address health priorities and meet their respective health needs' (WHO 1998 Glossary).

Critical appraisal – The process of determining how useful the evidence is.

Determinants of health – 'The range of personal, social, economic and environmental factors which determine the health status of individuals or populations' (WHO 1998 Glossary).

Disability-adjusted life years (DALYs) – 'A health gap measure that extends the concept of potential years of life lost due to premature death (PYLL) to include equivalent years of "healthy" life lost in states of less than full health, broadly termed disability. One DALY represents the loss of one year of equivalent full health' (WHO website).

Disease – An abnormal condition of an organism that impairs bodily functions, and that is associated with specific symptoms and signs.

Dose–response assessment – A step in the risk assessment process in which information on the toxicity of the hazardous agent is considered to determine the relationship between various exposure levels and their effects.

Ecological footprint – A measure of sustainability that is based on the concept of 'appropriate carrying capacity' and is defined as 'the land area which is needed exclusively to produce the natural resources that population consumes and to assimilate the waste that it generates indefinitely' (Wackernagel et al 1993).

Ecology – The branch of biology that deals with the inter-relationships between organisms and their environment.

Ecosystem – A dynamic complex of plant, animal and microorganism communities and the non-living environment interacting as a functional unit. Humans are an integral part of ecosystems, with ecosystems varying enormously in size, for example from a temporary pond in a tree hollow to an entire ocean basin.

Ecosystem services – All ecological systems perform essential functions for humans, and these 'ecosystem services' are essential for sustaining human life. In addition to providing goods (e.g. food and medicine), ecosystems provide 'services' such as purification of air and water, accumulation of toxins, decomposition of wastes, mitigation of floods, stabilisation of landscapes and regulation of climate.

Empowerment for health – 'In health promotion, empowerment is a process through which people gain greater control over decisions and actions affecting their health' (WHO 1998 Glossary).

Endemic – A disease that occurs at low or consistent levels within a community.

Environmental determinant of health – Any external physical, chemical and microbiological exposures and processes that impact on the health of individuals and the community at large, and that are beyond their immediate control (i.e. they are involuntary).

Environmental health – Those aspects of human health, including quality of life, that are determined by physical, chemical, biological and social factors in the environment (enHealth Council 1999)

Environmental health practice – The assessment, correction, control and prevention of environmental factors that can adversely affect health, as well as the enhancement of those aspects of the environment that can improve human health (enHealth Council 1999).

Epidemic – An excess of cases in the community from that normally expected; or the appearance of a new infectious disease (Webber 2005).

Evaluation – 'The process by which we decide the worth or value of something' (Suchman 1967).

Evidence-based medicine – The conscientious, explicit and judicious use of current best evidence in making decisions about the care of individual patients.

Evidence-based practice (EBP) – Uses various methods (e.g. summarising research, educating professionals in how to understand and apply research findings) to encourage, and in some instances to force, professionals and other decision makers to pay more attention to evidence that can inform their decision making.

Exposure assessment – A step in the risk assessment process that involves determining the magnitude, frequency, extent, character and duration of exposures in the past, at present and in the future. It also includes identifying the exposed populations and potential exposure pathways (e.g. exposure through the air, food, water or soil).

Global climate change – A change of climate that is attributed directly or indirectly to human activity, alters the composition of the global atmosphere, and which is in addition to natural climate variability observed over comparable time periods (United Nations 1992).

Goal – What you ultimately want to achieve by implementing your program plan.

Hazard assessment – A key stage in the risk assessment process that consists of two parts: hazard identification and dose–response assessment.

Hazard identification – A step in the risk assessment process that involves determining what types of adverse health effects might be caused by the implicated agent, and how quickly the adverse health effects might be experienced.

Health education – The provision of learning experiences that encourage voluntary modifications of behaviour that are conducive to health.

Health impact assessment – A process that systematically identifies and examines, in a balanced way, both the potential positive and negative health impacts of an activity (e.g. policy, program, project or development) (enHealth Council 2001).

Health promotion – The process of encouraging and enabling individuals and communities to increase their control over the determinants of health and thereby improve their health (WHO 1986).

Human wellbeing – There are a range of components that interact to produce human wellbeing and these include the basic material for a good life, freedom and choice, health, good social relations, and security. Wellbeing is considered to be at the opposite end of a continuum from poverty, which has been defined as a 'pronounced deprivation in wellbeing' (World Bank 2000, p 15).

Infectious diseases – Diseases caused by pathogenic microorganisms, such as bacteria, viruses, parasites or fungi.

Innate or non-specific immunity – Immunity present from birth and includes the physical barriers (e.g. intact skin and mucous membranes), chemical barriers (e.g. gastric acid, digestive enzymes and bacteriostatic fatty acids of the skin), phagocytic cells and the complement system.

Intergovernmental Panel on Climate Change – An international body that was established by the World Meteorological Organization (WMO) and the *United Nations Environment Program* (UNEP) to assess scientific, technical and socioeconomic information relevant for the understanding of climate change, its potential impacts and options for adaptation and mitigation.

Interpandemic period – Describes the time when the particular disease is not affecting humans although there may be a risk.

Intersectoral collaboration – 'A recognised relationship between part or parts of different sectors of society which has been formed to take action on an issue to achieve *health outcomes* or *intermediate health outcomes* in a way which is more effective, efficient or sustainable than might be achieved by the *health sector* acting alone' (WHO 1998 Glossary).

Lay beliefs about health and illness – Commonsense understandings and personal experience, imbued with professional rationalisation (Blaxter 2007).

Medical microbiology – The study of microbes that cause diseases in humans (Irving et al 2005).

Meta-analyses – Identify relevant primary research studies and aggregate the results and come up with a quantitative estimate of the overall effect (Naidoo & Wills 2005).

Meta-ethnography – The systematic synthesis of qualitative research studies.

Mode of transmission – The way in which a communicable disease may be spread from one source to another.

Modern environmental health hazards – Any hazards that are related to any rapid development that lacks health and environment safeguards, and also to the unsustainable consumption of natural resources.

Morbidity – State of illness, or the occurrence of illness in a population.

Mortality – Death, or death rates, in a population.

Neutral relationship – In communicable terms is one in which the organisms and the humans live in harmony without any adverse or mutual beneficial effects.

Nipah virus – A member of the family *Paramyxoviridae*, Nipah virus is a newly recognised zoonotic virus. The virus was 'discovered' in 1999. It has caused disease in animals and in humans.

Objectives – Specific statements about the changes you want to see as a result of the program (adapted from Hawe et al 1990 p 42). For example, the proportion of students who eat a healthy lunch at school.

Organisation for Economic Co-operation and Development (OECD) – A Paris-based intergovernmental organisation of 30 wealthy nations whose purpose is to provide a forum for governments to compare experiences to achieve the highest sustainable economic growth and employment and improving living standards in member and non-member states.

Outbreak – The sudden occurrence of a disease in a community.

Pandemic – The occurrence of an epidemic in multiple communities.

Pandemic alert period – The time when the disease may be causing isolated human disease or small clusters of patients without rapid spread or significant outbreak.

Pandemic period – The situation when there is a pandemic with human-to-human spread and significant number of affected persons.

Passive immunity – The protection that is provided by the transfer of antibodies derived from immune people.

Pathogen – A disease-producing microorganism.

Pathogenic relationship – In communicable terms is one in which the microorganism causes disease in the larger organism.

Plan – Overall structure of intended set of activities to get you to what you want to achieve.

Policy – The process by which governments translate their political vision into programs and actions to delivery 'outcomes' – desired changes in the 'real world' (Cabinet Office 1999 in Naidoo & Wills 2005). For example, the national policy on diabetes.

Population health – The study of health and disease in defined populations.

Precautionary approach/principle – When credible scientific evidence or concern is raised regarding activities or agents that may harm human health or the environment, this principle states that precautionary measures should be taken even when there is uncertainty and where the cause and effect relationships have not yet been fully established.

Prion – An infectious agent.

Program – A grouping of resources including people, funds, equipment and supplies performing activities that enable the scope of the program and its activities to be measured, fulfilling a definable set of goals and objectives (adapted from Health and Welfare, Canada 1977). Sometimes called an intervention.

Program Logic Model – A graphic depiction of relationships between all planned program components and the desired results.

Propagated exposure – Occurs when affected people pass on the disease to other affected people.

Propagated source – Spread from person to person rather than from a single common source.

Repeated exposure – Occurs when the community is repeatedly exposed to the cause of an outbreak as may occur when people continue to drink from an infected water source.

Risk assessment – The process of estimating the potential impact of chemical, physical, microbiological or psychosocial hazards on a specified human population or ecological system under a specific set of conditions and for a certain timeframe (enHealth Council 2004).

Risk characterisation – Final step in the risk assessment process that seeks to integrate the information from the hazard assessment and exposure assessment steps and describe the risks to individuals and populations in terms of the nature, extent and severity of potential adverse health effects.

Risk communication – An interactive process involving the exchange among individuals, groups and institutions of information and expert opinion about the nature, severity and acceptability of risks and the decisions taken to combat them (enHealth Council 2004).

Risk management – The process of evaluating alternative actions, selecting options and implementing them in response to risk assessments. The decision-making process will incorporate scientific, technological, social, economic and political information. The process requires value judgement, such as on the tolerability and reasonableness of costs (enHealth Council 2004).

Risk transition – Used to describe the reduction in 'traditional environmental health risks' and increase in 'modern environmental health risks' that takes place with advances in economic development.

Settings for health – 'The place or social context in which people engage in daily activities in which environmental, organizational and personal factors interact to affect health and wellbeing' (WHO 1998 Glossary).

Single-point exposure – Occurs when the source of an outbreak can be traced to a single event or focus as may occur with an episode of food poisoning.

Social capital – Social resources developed through networks, relationships, reciprocity, exchange and connectedness.

Social cohesion – The connections and relations between societal units, such as individual, groups and associations, or the 'glue' that holds communities together (AIHW 2005a).

Stakeholders – Everyone who has an interest in the program, particularly decision makers and the community for whom the program is planned.

Standard precautions – Involves a series of systems and structures that should always be used in patient management so as to minimise the risks associated with infection.

Strategies – The methods employed to assist you to reach your objectives, for example, providing healthy foods in a tuckshop. This is about what your plan is going to provide and/ or deliver, for example, education programs, brochures, media campaigns, action by parents to change the tuckshop menu and advocacy to ban 'junk' food advertisements during children's television programs.

Sustainability – A balance that integrates protection of the ecological processes and natural systems at local, regional, state and national levels; economic development; and maintenance of the cultural, economic, physical and social wellbeing of people and communities (Queensland Integrated Planning Act 1997).

Sustainable development – Defined by the 'Brundtland Commission' as development that meets the needs of the present without compromising the ability of future generations to meet their own needs.

Target group – The group of people the program is aiming to reach, for example, teenage students in Years 9 and 10.

Traditional environmental health hazards – Hazards that are often associated with poverty and a lack of development and include a lack of access to safe drinking water and inadequate basic sanitation in the household and the community.

Urban sprawl – A land use/urban planning term to describe haphazard growth or extension outward, especially that resulting from real estate development on the outskirts of a city.

Vector – A carrier, especially one that transmits disease.

Zoonotic diseases – Infectious diseases of animals that can cause disease when transmitted to humans.

REFERENCES

Australian Institute of Health and Welfare 2008 Chronic diseases and associated risk factors. Available: http://www.aihw.gov.au/cdarf/

Australian Institute of Health and Welfare 2005 Australia's welfare 2005. AIHW cat. no. AUS65. AIHW, Canberra

Blaxter M 2007 How is health experienced? In: Douglas J, Earle S, Handsley S et al (eds) A reader in promoting public health. Sage Publications, London

enHealth Council 1999 National environmental health strategy. enHealth Council, Canberra

enHealth Council 2001 Health impact assessment guidelines, Commonwealth Department of Health and Aged Care, Canberra

enHealth Council 2004 Environmental health risk assessment: Guidelines for assessing human health risks from environmental hazards. Commonwealth Department of Health and Ageing, Canberra

Hawe P, Degeling D, Hall J 1990 Evaluating health promotion. MacLennan & Petty, Sydney

Health and Welfare Canada 1977 Evaluation guidelines. Ontario

Irving W L, Ala'Aldeen D, Boswell T 2005 Medical microbiology. Taylor & Francis, New York

Naidoo J, Wills J 2005 Public health and health promotion: developing practice. Baillière Tindall, Edinburgh

Queensland Government 1997 Integrated Planning Act 1997. GoPrint, Brisbane

Suchman E A 1967 Evaluative research. Russell Sage Foundation, New York

United Nations 1992 United Nations Framework Convention on Climate Change. United Nations, New York

Wackernagel M, McIntosh J, Rees W E et al 1993 How big is our ecological footprint? A handbook for estimating a community's appropriated carrying capacity. Task Force on Planning Healthy and Sustainable Communities, Vancouver

Webber, R 2005 Communicable disease epidemiology and control: a global perspective, 2nd edn. CABI Publishing, Oxfordshire, p 22

World Bank 2001 World Development Report 2000–2001: Attacking poverty. Oxford University Press, New York

World Commission on Environment and Development 1987 Our common future. Oxford University Press, Oxford

World Health Organization 1986 The Ottawa Charter for Health Promotion First International Conference on Health Promotion, Ottawa, 21 November 1986. Available: http://www.who.int/healthpromotion/conferences/previous/ottawa/en/ 6 Nov 2007

World Health Organization 1998 Health promotion glossary. Available: http://www.who.int/healthpromotion/about/HPR%20Glossary%201998.pdf

World Health Organization 2008 Disability adjusted life years (DALY). Available: http://www.who.int/healthinfo/boddaly/en/

Index

(*b* denotes box, *cs* denotes case study, *f* denotes figure, *t* denotes table)